Crossroads:
A Reader for
Psychosocial Occupational Therapy

Edited by
Anne K. Briggs, M.S., OTR and Alice R. Agrin, Ed.M., OTR

ISBN 0-910317-04-6

Crossroads:
A Reader for Psychosocial Occupational Therapy

Introduction

The paths of practice are converging. Practitioners and educators are discussing, defining, and debating the central juncture, the common theoretical basis, of practice. *Crossroads,* the reader, begins at this point. In Section One: *Juncture at the Crossroads,* King, Fidler, and others examine core concepts of occupational therapy practice. Concepts such as adaptation, purposeful activity, mastery, life space, and life tasks are described.

Frames of reference, or the paths of practice, are explored more closely in Section Two. These frames of reference guide the occupational therapist in selecting a course of action. Although these directions may vary, they begin and end at the same place . . . at the crossroad of the core concepts.

The client also stands at a crossroad. He or she must choose a future direction (determine goals) and develop the means (necessary skills) to attain the goals. To assist the client in this process, the occupational therapist joins the client in a therapeutic relationship and uses specific evaluation and treatment techniques to enhance the client's functioning and to promote growth.

What is a therapeutic relationship? What are the qualities of a "helpful" person, and how much of these qualities can be learned and maintained? These questions are addressed in Section Three: *The Helpful Guide.*

Section Four: *Daily Life Analysis and Programming* presents the application of theory to occupational therapy practice. Analysis involves evaluation. Harry Stack Sullivan posed the primary question of evaluation: "Who is this person and how has he come to be here?" The "who" part of the question focuses on the individual personality, the "how" part on the sequence of events that led the person to seek help. Occupational therapists would add to Sullivan's question the following: And what has she or he been doing? This concern with the quality and the activity of daily life, a characteristic of occupational therapy since its inception, has also distinguished occupational therapy from more primarily intrapsychic approaches. The question, what has the person been doing, is addressed in Section Four. Some articles provide the means for assessing specifics such as time management, role acquisition and performance, and daily living skills. Other articles describe programs to implement change in these areas.

The articles in the four sections comprise a blend of the classic and the contemporary. The content reflects the uniqueness and breadth of occupational therapy, but it does not cover any one topic in depth; that is a goal of a text, not of a reader. *Crossroads* is meant to supplement texts, not to replace them. It provides a reference for students, practitioners, and that growing number of "others" interested in the field of occupational therapy.

To keep this reader of publishable size, the editors recognized and exercised some constraints. It is not possible to include everyone's "favorites," not even our own. With a 50-year-plus history, the field of occupational therapy is rich with articles of merit. Omission of any article is therefore not a statement on its value. Inclusion of an article does reflect the editors' belief in its current usefulness. In selecting these articles, the editors have tried to incorporate the suggestions of students, faculty, and clinicians. The editors tried to avoid duplication of material already covered in depth in psychosocial occupational therapy texts.

The editors believe that psychosocial occupational therapy is a component of the practice of occupational therapy, regardless of the specialty area or the population receiving the services. Function, the orientation of the field, is an integrative concept with psychological aspects. Numerous articles from all aspects of practice could have been included in this reader. Our most taxing constraint was to limit the reader to articles that primarily address an adult population with a primary functional problem of a psychosocial nature.

Occupational therapists also assume many roles: clinician, administrator, educator, consultant, supervisor, among others. The reader is oriented toward the direct service role: working with clients. The other roles the editors leave to other texts.

Now that we have recognized some of the constraints, we do want to reiterate the merit of the reader, which lies in the value of the individual articles. Credit, of course, goes to the authors who developed the included works. Their inspiration was probably followed by long hours of sometimes tedious work. Fortunately, they persisted, and we reap the benefits. The articles are informative, thought-provoking, creative, and, occasionally, even humorous. They offer a perspective on the past, the present, and the future of the field. Undoubtedly the future direction of occupational therapy, the future paths of practice, will be influenced by their work.

Contents

v

Section Four
The Journey: Daily Life Analysis and Programming

Environmental Occupational Therapy

Helen Dunning, M.A., O.T.R.

It is important that occupational therapists in all disciplines visualize the patient in his total environmental context. Toward this end, the present study, exploratory in nature, proposes a classification system that permits examination of the environment by analyzing its parts—space, people, and task. The conceptual basis of this system is derived from an emerging field of study called environmental psychology. The variables of space, people, and task are operationalized through the use of a questionnaire designed to measure the interaction between the psychiatric outpatient and his home environment.

Introduction

There is reason to believe that occupational therapists, in the role of environmental managers, can profit from continued surveillance of research emerging from environmental studies. Findings in this field not only add support to the practice of occupational therapy but provide a conceptual basis for assessing the treatment environment through the variables of space, people, and task.

These aspects of the environment have been basic to our practice for over fifty years. Space is designed to promote stimulation. People are arranged to encourage social interaction. Tasks are used to develop skills. Yet, while occupational therapists concentrate on the doing aspect of work, they overlook the need for a theoretical orientation that encompasses all the environmental factors used in treatment.

Depending on the specialty practiced, therapists tend to focus on one aspect of the environment to the exclusion of others. In physical disabilities, attention is directed toward the patient's ability to function in space, or what is termed the physical environment. In psychosocial disorders, treatment focuses on psychological and social processes and frequently overlooks the physical environment from which the patient came and to which he must return. It is important that therapists in all disciplines visualize the patient in his total environmental context. The present work, exploratory in nature, is, directed toward this end.

Environmental Psychology

The theoretical foundation that permits the environment to be analyzed through the examination of its parts is the work being done in environmental studies and drawn together by Proshansky, Ittelson and Rivlin in a discipline called "environmental

Helen Dunning was formerly staff therapist at the Los Angeles Day Treatment Center.

The American Journal of Occupational Therapy
1972, Vol. 26, No. 6, 292—298

psychology."[1] The aim of this science is to study the interactional patterns between human behavior and man-made modifications in the physical environment. This is a complex task, multidisciplinary in nature. As such, it encompasses a variety of concepts, methods, theoretical approaches, and empirical research findings. Areas of study are: (1) the function and meaning of space, (2) the satisfaction of needs through spatial organization, (3) the effect of the environment on social interaction and role performance, (4) environmental influences as these shape psychological processes of learning, perception, cognition, and emotion, and (5) the importance of environmental design and urban planning on human behavior and the quality of life.

Systematic investigations of man and his transactions with the environment are relatively recent. In the past, social scientists concentrated on the influence of the social environment on the individual while psychologists were absorbed with rat behavior and isolated stimuli. Little research was done outside the laboratory in physical settings where man lived and worked.

In the cities, problems of overcrowding, urban blight, and pollution mounted. In the natural environment, symptoms of ecological imbalances surfaced. What man had taken for granted—air, earth, and water—was seriously endangered. Clearly a reordering of research priorities was necessary with environmental studies high on the list. As a result, sociologists, psychologists, anthropologists, architects, urban planners, and others have joined forces to find possible solutions to complex problems.

In an effort to synthesize research being done in these fields, Proshansky, Ittelson, and Rivlin propose a basic framework. Drawn from this foundation are a number of orienting statements that serve as a guide to the study of environment and behavior.

1. There is no dichotomy between the person and the environment. There is only the total environment of which man is simply one kind of component in relationship with other components.

2. For the purpose of analysis and research, it is possible to extract from the total environment a social, physical, or even a personal or psychological environment. Yet, these are not separate environments but different ways of analyzing the same situation.

3. While the environment is a total process, components can be extracted for the purpose of analysis and investigation. However, no component is in itself an entity. Whatever component is extracted, it is clearly evident that it not only acts upon other components and thereby changes them, but in so doing it changes the environment and thereby induces changes in itself. Environmental process is one of reciprocal or circular feedback.

4. The study of man in relation to the environment should be made at a social psychological level. With this approach the emphasis is not placed primarily at the individual level of psychological analysis but on behavior as it is expressed at all levels of social organization.

5. While human goals are many and varied, their sum and substance depends on where and how particular groups of individuals are socialized. For any given role the person not only learns to behave in certain ways and to expect certain behavior from others, but he also has expectations about the nature and conditions of the physical setting in which he is to play a role.

6. Human psychological functioning is not necessarily a reflection of the inherent nature of the organism but is more frequently an indication of the demands made upon the organism by the environment. Therefore, if one wants to know how the normal human being functions, studies must be conducted in environments that are representative of those in which actual behavior occurs.

7. The individual's response to his physical environment is never determined solely by the properties of structures and the events that define it. Spaces, their properties, the people in them, and the activities that involve these people represent significant systems for the individual participant and thereby influence his responses to the physical setting.

Statements one and two permit an analysis of the environment by examination of its parts. Statement three is consistent with the learning theory of White who stresses the interplay between individual and environmental forces that lead to the development of competence.[2] Statements four and five provide a social psychological context that describes role behavior as it develops in the process of socialization, a concept congruent with Reilly's occupational behavior theory.[3] Statement six gives cause for assessing the patient's home environment, and statement seven provides the subcategories of the environment to be investigated, however, with one modification. While the properties of space are considered to be the physical environment, and the people in the space comprise the social environment, the environment of activity will henceforth be

designated the task environment. This substitution of the concept of task in preference to activity is based on the work of Breer and Locke and reflects the specific concern of occupational therapists with the quality of daily life performance.[4]

An examination of the literature on environment and behavior, within the parameters set forth in environmental psychology, reveals a number of ways in which space, people and task are studied. Selected from this large multidisciplinary body of knowledge are: (1) some concepts empirically tested that serve as a basis for measuring man's relationship to the environment, and (2) several theories that are untested but serve the process of heuristics by raising questions as to how this relationship should be studied. Both concepts and theories contribute to a classification system of the environment called "the environmental grid" (Table 1). The construction of this grid is discussed in the sections that follow.

Space

The study of the relationship between space usage and behavior is known as environmental design. It seeks to answer the question: Can environments be designed to accomplish specific objectives in terms of human response? Systematic efforts in this direction have just begun and recent research is reported in the journal *Environment and Behavior*.[5]

Architects claim their most effective work comes about when the goals of the institution are clearly stated. Only then is there a close relationship between physical design, behavior, and purpose. Osmond's work is a case in point.[6] He was able to define the social needs of psychiatric patients and design the environment accordingly. Working closely with architect Izumi, he planned a "sociopetal" building where the physical layout fostered sociability. Sommer, a psychologist working with Osmond, later measured the before and after effect of a sociopetal arrangement of furniture on a geriatric ward.[7] He found there was an increase in social interaction. This suggests that the grouping of objects in space provides cues as to their use. How these cues are perceived and interpreted depends in part upon the individual's subjective needs and expectations.

While the measure of individual response to physical modifications in space is studied through environmental design, there are other ways of examining this relationship. One of these is through the framework of territoriality which is defined as a biological need to possess and defend space, a concept based on animal behavioral studies.

Writing on the subject are ethnologists who draw parallels from animal to human behavior[8,9] and social scientists who accept this linkage as part of their theoretical construct.[10,11] Altman takes exception to analogies made between animal and human territoriality because they tend to ignore obvious differences between the species. These are man's thinking and feeling nature, his need to occupy a greater variety of geographic areas, his subtlety in

TABLE 1
The Environmental Grid

Givens	Possibility for Change	Preference
	SPACE	
Physical properties of home, neighborhood and larger community as perceived by the individual.	Givens amenable to change through individual initiative.	Attitudes about present living arrangement.
	Givens changed by altered modes of behavior.	The expressed desire to organize objects and arrange space.
	Givens amenable to change by one way action of subject upon the environment.	The need to personalize space.
	Givens that can be organized for more efficient use.	The expressed wish to make greater use of resources outside the home.
	PEOPLE	
Social role relationships of marriage, nuclear family, extended family, friends, peers and neighbors.	Narrowing of distance between the individual and those with whom he wishes to communicate.	Attitudes toward others.
		Expressed satisfaction or dissatisfaction with present relationships.
Patterns of propinquity and distance the individual establishes between himself and others.	Selection of environments that increase the possibility for social stimulation and interaction.	The wish to increase social contacts and develop closer relationships.
	TASK	
Task expectancies in the environment.	Developing competence with objects at hand.	Skill areas the individual desires to improve.
Sources of task stimulation.	Developing activities of daily living skills.	The expressed need for improved competence in activities of daily living skills.
Availability of objects.	Enriching the environment with new stimulus material.	
Spatial behavior as related to task performance.	Modifying space for task performance.	The expressed need for greater task responsibility
Satisfaction derived from accomplishment.	Using community resources for task stimulation.	

behavior which is part of territorial defense, his personalization of space, and his unique object possessiveness.[12]

Directly related to human territoriality are concepts of privacy and crowding. The need for privacy is seen by Proshansky, Ittelson and Rivlin as a need to maximize freedom of choice. A study of bedroom size and social interactional patterns on a psychiatric ward showed that the proportion of activity devoted to isolated passive behavior rose with an increase in the number of beds per room. They concluded that the concept of privacy was not strictly "being alone" but having the widest range of personal choice. This the small bedroom provides.[13]

As for crowding, the authors believe it should be seen as psychological as well as an objectively viewed social phenomenon. How space is organized, for what purpose it is designed and the kinds of activities that are involved, are factors that contribute to the phenomenology of crowding. Crowding may be pleasurable as well as painful depending on the individual's past experiences. In this, culture and subculture play an important part. Therefore, crowding as a psychological phenomenon is only indirectly related to the density of people and directly related to privacy and territoriality.

As a step toward measuring territoriality and human needs, Hall proposes a system for organizing spatial information in three ways: fixed-feature, semifixed-feature, and informal.[10] Fixed-feature space describes the material objects and internal design of rooms and buildings that govern human behavior. Semifixed-feature space is more flexible and can be modified and rearranged to meet the behavioral needs of its occupants. Informal space is a category of spatial experience which is significant for the individual because it includes the distances encountered in human transactions within space.

In summary, space and its properties are studied as part of environmental design. Physical factors of bounded space (territoriality), the quantity and quality of space (privacy and crowding), the interior design, furniture arrangement and objects in the environment, are considered in light of their effect on life style, human satisfaction, and behavior.

Because there are few quantitative measures of the properties of space as they affect human behavior, the environmental grid can only suggest a descriptive method for estimating the individual's interaction with his physical space. This is done by identifying architectural and object givens as they are perceived by the individual in accordance with Hall's classification of fixed-feature and semifixed-feature space.

People

The concept of territoriality is linked to fixed geographic areas. Different from this is territory that is portable, has the body as its locus and moves with the individual. Through body positions and body cues

the individual establishes distances from others in an attempt to satisfy psychological and interpersonal needs. These distances Sommer[11] calls "personal space" and Hall[10] "the study of proxemics." Bodily movements in space are also referred to as spatial behavior.

Sommer has observed a number of ways in which people satisfy their needs through manipulation of personal space—seating arrangements for conversation in a cafeteria;[14] seating patterns for casual, cooperative and competitive small groups;[15] preferred positions vis-a-vis a leader;[16] and the use of library chairs to establish privacy.[17]

Hall measures personal space through the study of proxemics. Space is conceived as invisible concentric circles that he classifies according to the distance established between people. Descriptive measures of space are: intimate, personal, social-consultive, and public. Within these "space bubbles" men communicate not only with language but with visual, kinesthetic, thermal, olfactory, and aural body cues. The extent to which these senses are brought into play is culturally determined.

The concept of personal space is called into question by Liebman who claims it is a catchall term for a number of variables with different conceptual and operational definitions.[18] The model she proposes centers on intrinsic factors of personality as these are expressed and shaped by the environment. Liebman's model includes: *the psychological variable* which is the set of expectations held by the individual that his own and others' behavior related to distance and position in space will satisfy interpersonal goals in the most appropriate way; *the task performance* which involves physical distance and configurations specific to the task as well as spacing related to the desired level of psychological distance; *the antecedent conditions* in which the individual's desire for closeness or separation is worked out spatially; *the interpersonal goals* which are defined by the nature of the antecedent conditions—task, mood, presence of others; *the physical space* such as room size, number of chairs, and other factors that permit psychological distance to be translated into physical terms; and *the use of body cues or symbolic distance* to convey individual attitudes when the choice of physical distance is unavailable.

Briefly then, man is studied in relation to his social environment through concepts of spatial behavior, personal space, and proxemics. Drawing from this work, criteria are established in the environmental grid to identify the individual's interaction with his social environment. Social role relationships are investigated as are patterns of propinquity and distance the individual establishes between himself and others.

Task

Liebman is the single researcher who speaks to task in a manner useful to the present work. Her focus is on task as it relates to mutually satisfying goals between individuals in the environment. The present discussion of task includes this interpersonal aspect but in addition adds White's concept of competence as it develops in the interactional process between the individual and objects in the environment. Therefore, task is seen as it relates to personal satisfaction derived from accomplishment and interpersonal satisfaction obtained from role performance.

Personal space variables set forth by Liebman are useful in assessing the relationship between humans, objects and space in any given situation. Thus, we are able to evaluate the individual's daily life performance within the context of his roles, the task expectancies of others who share his living arrangement, the physical characteristics of space, and the availability of objects and materials.

Criteria developed in the environmental grid for assessment of the task environment are based on the potential use of objects and space according to: (1) presence, (2) availability, (3) desirability, and (4) feasibility. By identifying available space and kinds of objects the givens of the environment are determined or what may be termed the *presence* of objects and space. By determining social restrictions placed upon the use of space and objects, a measure of *availability* is provided. By estimating if the individual wishes to act upon the objects or space, a baseline is established for *desirability*. By considering personal constraints such as skill level, physical/social psychological dysfunction, age, and other factors as these influence goal success, a measure of *feasibility* is obtained.

Objects in the environment can be classified according to Matsutsuyu's interest categories of manual skills, physical sports, social recreation, activities of daily living, and cultural/educational.[19] For example, objects for manual activity could be a sewing machine or car tools, and objects for social recreation activity could be cards, a record player, and television set.

In summary, givens of the task environment are classified: task expectancies in the environment; sources of task stimulation; availability of objects; spatial behavior as related to task performance; and satisfaction derived from accomplishment.

The Environmental Grid

Thus far criteria established for the variables of space, people, and task serve as a guide for determining givens in the patient's home environment. Another dimension of the grid that helps to identify the possibility for interaction with these givens, is based on the concepts of preference and planned change.

Phillips states that preference is a measure of the individual's attitudes based on modes of behavior and levels of aspiration. "Each individual strives to establish that type of environment and those relationships with it that provide an optimum balance between security and fulfillment of his goals, values, and aspirations."[20] The measure of preference is used

in this study to make a gross estimate of the individual's expressed desire to improve his level of functioning in terms of his physical, social, and task space. However, it should be noted that the possibility for effecting change will depend upon the ability of the patient to meet the conditions of planned change set forth by Lippitt, Watson, and Westley.[21]

These authors state that planned change is change that derives from a purposeful decision to effect improvement in a personality or social system which is achieved with professional help. In their vernacular, the personality or social system is the "client system" and the professional person who assists is the "change agent." The key to planned change is the participation of the client system in the change process.

Change agents who work with changing the relationship between the client system and its environment have several orientations. One orientation emphasizes the skills and strategies needed by the client system to solve problems presented by the external environment.

It is here proposed: (1) that the occupational therapist is a change agent and the patient is a client system, (2) that the patient must be a participant in decisions for change as well as in the process of change itself (in this case the occupational therapy process), and (3) the solving of problems related to change must be amenable to the skills and strategies that can be provided by the occupational therapy process.

The Questionnaire

The instrument chosen to operationalize the environmental grid is a questionnaire designed to be used as an interview guide.[22] The degree of the investigator's control over questioning and the depth of potential responses desired, fits Berelson and Steiner's category of the semistructured interview.[23]

The interview is preferred over a self-administered questionnaire because it has greater flexibility, the interviewer can observe what the respondent says and how he says it, and follow-up questions can be asked to elicit further information. The quality of the data obtained will depend on the interviewer's skill and experience.

The validity of the individual's self-report can be brought into question. While direct observation of the individual in his home setting would further validate his responses, this is not always feasible. Therefore, the self-report will be accepted in accordance with the rules of history-taking.[24]

It is recognized that further refinement of the instrument is necessary to meet standards of validity and reliability. These conditions are difficult to meet at the exploratory level.

A pretest of the questionnaire was made with five male and five female psychiatric outpatients attending the Los Angeles Day Treatment Center. Ages ranged from 16 to 66. The respondents were patients who volunteered to answer the questionnaire. Data from the instrument should be viewed in light of the limitations inherent in size and selection of the sample. Generalizations to a larger population should not be made.

Organization of the Data

Suggestive trends in the data were used to develop a series of propositional statements about the physical, social, and task environment of the psychiatric outpatient. At the clinical level these propositions provide information for treatment planning. In terms of research, they help to narrow the focus for future investigation.

Proposition 1. Psychiatric outpatients residing in the community tend to live in protected environments.

The term protected environment is used to suggest a dependency relationship based on the individual's inability in all cases to provide his own source of income, and in many cases to manage an independent living arrangement. Half of the population sampled lived in board and care homes.

Proposition 2. Disability factors as well as economic constraints limit the individual's ability to select his own residence.

Living arrangements of psychiatric outpatients tend to be made by professional workers or families of patients.

Proposition 3. The possibility of change in the environment is affected by extrinsic environmental factors as well as intrinsic factors of personality.

Extrinsic factors are personal ownership of space, the amount of space, and the attitudes of others who share the space and will be affected by the change. Intrinsic factors of personality are the individual's level of anxiety about change, and the individual's ability to perceive the range of possibilities for change in the environment.

Proposition 4. Objects and personal possessions in the individual's environment help to identify past and present interests.

For those people living in board and care homes, there were few expressions of these interests. In these homes, objects related to social recreational activity are most prevalent, the television set being of major importance.

Proposition 5. The availability and proximity of social stimulation space, and the number of people in the space, appear to affect the degree of sociability of the resident.

Individuals living in board and care homes report that they enjoy conversing with others in dining rooms, patios, and lounge areas. The probability of finding people with whom the individual feels compatible is greater in the larger board and care homes which ranged in size from 72 to 120 residents.

Proposition 6. Families of psychiatric outpatients are not a resource for affiliative social activities.

While most of the respondents were in touch with some member of their family through telephone,

letters, and limited personal contact, activity with family members was negligible except for two respondents who lived with their families.

Proposition 7. Conflict in the social environment is apt to arise between the individual and others in social areas that must be regulated.

This area in the board and care home is generally bedroom space that is shared by one to three people. Differences over sleeping habits, neatness in organizing personal belongings, and television viewing habits are potential sources of conflict.

Proposition 8. Conflict in the task environment is promoted when space is shared and differences in task expectancies arise.

This conflict was most obvious with respondents who lived with their families and were having difficulty working out their role relationships.

Proposition 9. Psychiatric outpatients tend to live with the situation that exists and do not project alternative solutions.

While psychiatric outpatients express the desire to improve their social life and have closer relations with others, they evince few ideas of how this can be done. In a similar fashion, preferences expressed about the desire to move and find paid work, are not set forth as part of a plan.

Proposition 11. Economic constraints are perceived by the individual as limiting his ability to use community resources.

One of the economic constraints is personal transportation. While most of the respondents use public busses, it was those individuals who had cars or access to family owned cars who made greater use of parks and recreational facilities. Although the respondents mention economic constraints as limiting their ability to buy tickets, eat out, go shopping, there appears to be a general lack of awareness of the range of possibilities that exist in the community.

Summary and Recommendations

As a step toward assessing the patient in his total environmental context, this study developed a classification system based on the work of Proshansky, Ittelson, and Rivlin in environmental psychology. This system, designated the Environmental Grid, combined the variables of space, people, and task with givens, possibility for change, and preference. A questionnaire was used to test the proposed relationships. While the data from the questionnaire provided a gross measure of the individual's current life space and life style, a closer assessment requires that it be used in conjunction with other instruments, such as those measuring task,[25] time,[26] and interests.[19]

Drawing upon the work being done in environmental studies, the ability to determine the relationship between environment and behavior will increase. This should add to occupational therapists' skill as managers of space, people, and task toward the end of improved patient care.

REFERENCES

1. Proshansky HM, Ittelson WH, Rivlin LG (eds): Environmental Psychology: Man and His Physical Setting, New York, Holt Rinehart and Winston Inc, 1970
2. White RW: Motivation reconsidered: the concept of competence. Psychol Rev 66: 297-333, 1959
3. Reilly M: The educational process. Am J Occup Ther 23: 299-307, 1969
4. Breer PE, Locke EA: Task Experience as a Source of Attitudes, Homewood, Illinois, The Dorsey Press, 1965
5. Environment and Behavior, Beverly Hills, California, Sage Publications
6. Osmond H: Some psychiatric aspects of design, in Who Designs America?, Holland LB (ed) Garden City, New York, Anchor Books, Doubleday and Co, 1966
7. Sommer R: Small group ecology in institutions for the elderly, in Spatial Behavior of Older People, Pastalan LA, Carson DH (eds) Ann Arbor, Michigan, University of Michigan, 1970
8. Ardrey R: The Territorial Imperative, New York, Atheneum, 1966
9. Morris D: The Naked Ape, New York, McGraw-Hill Book Co, 1967
10. Hall ET: The Hidden Dimension, Garden City, New York, Anchor Books, Doubleday and Co, Inc, 1969
11. Sommer R: Personal Space, Englewood Cliffs, New Jersey, Prentice-Hall Inc, 1969
12. Altman I: Territorial behavior in humans, in Spatial Behavior of Older People, Pastalan LA, Carson DH (eds) Ann Arbor, Michigan, University of Michigan, 1970
13. Ittelson WH, Proshansky HM, Rivlin LG: The environmental psychology of the psychiatric ward, in Environmental Psychology: Man and His Psysical Setting, Proshansky HM, Ittelson WH, Rivlin LG (eds), New York, Holt, Rinehart and Winston Inc, 1970
14. Sommer R: Studies in personal space. Sociometry 22: 247-260, 1959
15. Sommer R: Further studies of small group ecology. Sociometry 28: 337-348, 1965
16. Sommer R: Leadership and group geography. Sociometry 24: 99-110, 1961
17. Sommer R: The ecology of privacy. Library Q 36: 234-248, 1966
18. Liebman M: The effects of sex and race norms on personal space. Environ Behav 2: 208-246, 1970.
19. Matsutsuyu JS: The interest check list. Am J Occup Ther 23: 323-328, 1969
20. Phillips L: Human Adaptation and its Failures, New York, Academic Press, 1968, p 7-8
21. Lippitt R, Watson J, Westley B: Planned Change, New York, Harcourt, Brace and Co Inc, 1958
22. Dunning H: Environmental Occupational Therapy. Master's thesis. Occupational Therapy Department, University of Southern California, 1972
23. Berelson B, Steiner GA: Human Behavior: An Inventory of Scientific Findings, New York, Harcourt, Brace, 1964
24. Barzun J, Graff HF: The Modern Researcher, New York, Harcourt, Brace and World Inc, 1970
25. Moorhead L: The occupational history. Am J Occup Ther 23: 329-334, 1969
26. Larrington GG: An Exploratory Study of the Temporal Aspects of Adaptive Functioning. Master's thesis. Occupational Therapy Department, University of Southern California, 1970

This paper is based on a thesis presented to the University of Southern California in partial fulfillment of the requirements for the master of arts degree. The work was supported in part by an Allied Health Professions Fellowship, U.S. Department of HEW.

Doing and Becoming:

Purposeful Action and Self-Actualization

Gail S. Fidler
Jay W. Fidler

While the critical nature of action to human existence and adaptation has been pursued by philosophers for many years, the characteristics of action transformed into purposeful doing and the meaning of human productivity have remained relatively unexplored in the behavioral sciences. This paper discusses several theoretical constructs in social and individual psychology that provide perspectives for understanding human action; defines doing as purposeful action that enables the nascent human to become humanized; and suggests, on the basis of these constructs, a prescription for doing for the development of performance skills and as a means for investigating the causes of psychopathology or dysfunction.

Gail S. Fidler, OTR, is a consultant in private practice.

Jay W. Fidler, M.D., is Clinical Professor of Psychiatry, College of Medicine and Dentistry of New Jersey, Rutgers Medical School.

Aristotle made the following observations: "Now we realize our being in action (for we exist by living and acting) and the man who has made something may be said to exist in a manner through his activity. — So he loves his handiwork because he loves existence. It is part of the nature of things. What is potential becomes actual in the work which gives it expression."

During the intervening centuries the behavioral sciences have contributed little to the elaboration of the relationship between handiwork and individual development. Belief in the value of activity for the mentally ill has nevertheless been sustained for many years and is reflected in the universal use of activity programs in community mental health and psychiatric hospital services. However, despite the historical use of activity experiences for patients, understanding it has remained limited. Human action and doing continue to be viewed as peripheral components of intervention. Motivation for such programming seems to be to avoid immobility, rather than for providing positive help. When aftercare programs emphasize medication, psychotherapy, and social service as having priority over the development and improvement of those functional skills that make it possible to achieve a sense of mastery of self and the environment, services remain tangential to mental health or human needs. Also, when services consist of activity programs characterized by single techniques such as art, dance, music, or poetry, a comprehensive perspective on human productivity is sacrificed.

If health professionals are to assume a major responsibility for designing environments and experiences for the prevention of illness, for the maintenance and restoration of health, they need to achieve a more sophisticated understanding of *doing*. The word *doing* is selected to convey the sense of performing, producing, or causing. It is purposeful action in contrast to random activity in that the action is directed toward the intrapersonal (testing a skill), the interpersonal (clarifying a relationship), or the nonhuman (creating an end product). *Doing* is viewed as enabling the development and integration of the sensory, motor, cognitive, and psychological systems; serving as a socializing agent, and verifying one's efficacy as a competent, contributing member of one's society.

All organisms are born to act. Although lower forms of animals come equipped with behavioral patterns enabling them to cope with the external world, humans are dependent upon their social and cultural environments for learning and developing the action patterns necessary for both survival and satisfaction. That action is essential to human existence has been known and pursued by philosophers for many years, although the fields of medicine and psychiatry, with few exceptions, have viewed action (in the sense of doing) as peripheral to the human condition. Today, developments in social psychiatry, ethology, brain research, and developmental psychology reflect a growing sophistication in understanding the relationship of mental activity to motor behavior. There is an accumulation of significant data to support the thesis that the drive to action, transformed into the ability to "do," is fundamental to ego development and adaptation.

Becoming—"I"

The ability to adapt, to cope with the problems of everyday living, and to fulfill age-specific life roles requires a rich reservoir of experiences gathered from direct engagement with both human and nonhuman objects in one's environment. *Doing* is a process of investigating, trying out, and gaining evidence of one's capacities for experiencing, responding, managing, creating, and controlling. It is through such action with feedback from both nonhuman and human objects that an individual comes to know the potential and limitations of self and the environment and achieves a sense of competence and intrinsic worth.

The play of childhood is a striking manifestation of the natural drive to action in the service of learning—of exploration and discovery about the body, the self, and the external world. Bruner's studies of perception and learning emphasize the need for on-going engagement with the world of reality as the means by which behavioral patterns and strategies for dealing with the environment are learned. His recent explorations into the meaning and uses of play (1) provide impressive evidence of the critical value of all aspects of play in individual development and evolution. Piaget's (2) observations about play and other exploratory behaviors led

him to define these as the processes by which the child assimilates experiences while accommodating to the world. His remarkable studies continue to expand the body of knowledge regarding adaptive human action in a world of objects. Reilly (3) views play as a "connectivity" phenomenon leading to competence and adult "workmanship." She makes some valuable observations about the development of adaptive function and productivity. Erickson continues to emphasize the value of *doing* in achieving a sense of mastery, personal integrity, and in successfully participating in one's external world. His psychoanalytic background and ego psychology orientation are reflected in his focus on the expressive aspects of play (4) and on *doing* in the process of self-actualization and acculturation. (5)

In his study of the nonhuman environment, Searles (6) convincingly argues that relatedness to nonhuman objects is a significant force in the development of the sense of self as human, as differentiated from the nonhuman. He describes how involvement with one's nonhuman environment is a means for learning about self and others, and for both symbolically and realistically dealing with one's affective states, needs, and ideations.

In another work, the authors (7) hypothesize that when an activity relates both realistically and symbolically to an individual's needs and personal characteristics, it is an agent for learning and growth. *Doing* within this context is seen as a means for communicating feelings and ideas, expressing and clarifying individuality, and achieving gratification. The authors and Edelson (8) emphasize that *doing* in this sense can mediate between one's inner and outer world, nurture the capacity to invest, teach realistic responses to

success and failure, provide concrete evidence of one's capacities and limitations, test the reality base of fantasy and perceptions, and validate the ability to achieve and influence one's environment.

The writings of John Dewey articulate the criticality of *doing* for developing a sense of "I" and in accumulating a store of action experiences essential for human functioning. Becker (9) explores how the sense of self is developed by and sustained in action. He adds dimension to Dewey's earlier hypothesis, emphasizing the significance of the inherent feedback loop process in *doing*. He views such action an essential for coming to know the realities of self and the world and for testing out the truth of one's perceptions and mental images. Becker's thesis considers schizophrenia and other psychiatric disorders as occurring when internal and external factors limit or preclude an individual's acting on— trying out—an idea or thought.

In defining "objective orientation," Black (10) states that the process of acting enables knowing or "taking account of" the presence of independent, material objects, and emphasizes that it is such action processes that make possible the distinction between reality and illusion.

Neurophysiologic theory seems to be converging on a similar description of behavior. In Karl Pribram's (11) intriguing use of the holographic paradigm, an organism perceives a reality, conceives an intended reality or goal, and learns what motor activity is needed to achieve the goal through a constant series of "tests" to define each increment of change in perceived reality.

A counterpoint to *doing* as the means for defining reality is made by Don Juan as he explains **not**-*doing* to Castaneda. The sorcerer discovers a separate or nonordinary reality by

* my swimming! * juggling!

freeing himself from consensual reality. Don Juan explains, "that a rock is a rock because of all the things you know how to do to it—I call that "doing."—A man of knowledge—knows the rock is a rock only because of "doing," so if he doesn't want the rock to be a rock, all he has to do is—"not-doing." (12, p 227)

In another context, each individual has personal evidence of the sense of well-being, the excitement of challenge, the satisfaction of achievement that comes, for example, from a particular job success: mastering the calculator, planting the garden, repairing the carburetor, "teeing off" in form, or painting a landscape. Whatever limitations there may be in the "artistry" of the end product from the viewpoint of the "expert," there is a keen satisfaction and sense of competence in having accomplished it from one's own resources. Such gratification, the joy of being a cause, can be understood within the context of the human being's innate drive to master the environment.

Robert W. White (13) for a number of years has articulated the thesis that there is an innate human drive to explore and master the environment and that this drive can best be understood as motivation toward competence. White views a sense of competence and efficacy as emerging from direct encounters with and mastery of the environment. He further suggests that gratification from such mastery is intrinsic "in the sense that strictly speaking it requires no social reward or ratification from others. The child acts on the intention, for instance, to climb a stone wall; the outcome of the ensuing struggle between his muscles, hard surfaces, and the law of gravity is brilliantly clear to him even if no one is around to pronounce upon it." (14, p 273)

White urges that the "helping" professionals become more knowledgeable about the phenomenon of competence and more alert to the patient's sense of competence. He suggests that to become "as sensitive to the client's feeling of competence as we are to anxiety, defensiveness, love and hate, would open a wide additional channel to being of help." (14, p 274)

When one's accomplishments, one's sense of competence is verified and given value by others, one's efficacy and value as a human being is confirmed. If, for example, climbing the stone wall has no relevance to the child's social group, the intrinsic gratification may be short lived, or limited as an exploratory learning experience. The meaning and worth of one's doing or mastery is appreciably determined by the views and values of significant others. Humans are inextricably dependent upon others for learning and thus for the feedback that verifies that something has been learned and that the new function has value to others. Self-esteem can therefore be understood as evolving from the intrinsic gratification of accomplishment and the feedback from others regarding the achievement.

The significance of doing and feedback from others in developing a realistic sense of competence and efficacy was illustrated in one of the author's experience with a patient group. The group was composed of patients who persistently refused any aspect of occupational therapy programming. With few exceptions, they acted out provocatively in the community and in the hosptial. Their actions were random. A decision was made to see them in a talking group and to move cautiously toward action with a purpose. It became evident that action planned toward productivity and achieve-

ment generated tremendous anxiety. Their nonverbal behavior in this setting and the groups' reflections on the experiences, strongly suggested that, "to do" was to risk verification of their incompetence, lack of control over self and the environment, inability to master the environment, and of their "nonhumanness." Subsequently, several members of the group were able to describe that. Their expectations were that what they produced, the "fruits" of their actions, would replicate what they were. Their appallingly limited "action-learning" experiences and the negative or nonexistent feedback from the environment had left them with few action alternatives.

Action leading to achievement is in contrast to random activity. Action is both the *product* of a mental image that sets the objective and the *creator* of a mental image. The mental image that is created includes the refinement of strategies for achieving the objective and an affective evaluation of the achievement. The actor builds a self-image as a competent actor, confronts the realities of the results of the action, finds the boundaries for reasonable objectives, and learns the social relevance of competent actions. When the motivation or ability to act on mental images or ideation is blocked or inhibited by forces in the environment or by sensorimotor deficits, coping behaviors and adaptive skills are not learned.

Becoming—"A Social Being"

Humanization, becoming part of human society, may be defined as the process whereby the individual, beginning life as a biologic organism, becomes a person whose primitive actions are gradually transformed into behavior that concomitantly satisfies individual needs as well as contributes to societal development. In this sense humanization can be viewed as the process of learning about self and one's world, of developing those perspectives and related performance skills essential to a functional society and a functional individual with satisfaction to both.

Mead (15) suggests that social roles are learned through the activity of play and games. Game playing teaches a perspective about the significant other and begins the process of internalization of social roles and values. Let us return again to White's child and the stone wall. As the child struggles to master the hard surface, the pull of gravity, the child is exploring, testing, and developing age-appropriate motor planning, physical skills, and agility. If peers share in the climbing experience, there is additional exploration and learning about "the significant other." If the activity becomes a game, it is reasonable to assume tht the rules for playing the game will be defined according to the cognitive, psychologic, and social learning needs appropriate to the developmental level of those participating and congruent with their culture. If significant adults applaud the achievement, then the efficacy of the action is reinforced and verified as socially significant.

The task-oriented groups described by one of the authors (16) are based on such hypotheses regarding doing, with the group providing consensual validation of the efficacy of action and interpreting social/cultural norms: the choices of tasks and the action process per se both reflect and meet the individual's developmental and learning needs.

Moore and Anderson (17) hypothesize that all societies have created "folk models" for dealing with the most critical features of their relationship with the environment. These models can be understood as games, the rules of which teach the necessary perspectives and skills. The authors identify first the nonrandom aspects of nature; second, the random or chance elements: third, interactional relations with others; and fourth, the normative aspects of group living. These are correlated with four types of games: puzzles, which teach a sense of agency, the joy of being a cause; games of chance, which teach a relationship to events over which one has no control; games of strategy, which teach the individual to attend to the behavior and motivation of significant others; and aesthetic entities, or art forms, which teach people to make normative judgments and evaluations of their experiences. Learning experiences planned from this folk model are thus structured to include activities that incorporate varying aspects and characteristics of these models, and are matched with the developmental level and personal characteristics of the learner.

As reviewed here, such perspectives about doing bring into focus two critical dimensions for determining the value of any activity for a given individual. First, the activity or doing must match the individual's sensory, motor, cognitive, psychologic, and social maturation, as well as their developmental needs and skill readiness. Second, it must be recognized by the social, cultural group as relevant to their values and needs.

The information that is available from the various social sciences for research is impressive. However, what is not known about doing and human productivity and what is not being investigated is even more impressive.

Constraints on Doing

Middle class values place great significance on verbal skills. Professionals frequently reinforce the priority of this value in both their educational and treatment orientations and practices regardless of what they know about learning and human functioning.

In mental health practice, there is the familiar problem posed by those patients who, with impressive verbal skill, can describe the psychodynamics of their difficulties and articulate the psychotherapeutic process, but are much less able to act on such cognitive awareness. These are most frequently the clients who disdain activity programs and view action and doing as irrelevant to their needs, problems, or life style. As community mental health programs have broadened the base of psychiatric services, practice has come to include those persons whose culture and learning experiences place a priority on action. These persons most frequently view talking as oblique to their needs, problems, and life style.

There is a need to pursue investigation into the neurological, perceptual, and social components of action in relation to mental health. Simultaneously, conscious efforts need to be made toward breaking down the stereotypes regarding priorities on introspection and talking in isolation of doing. Both the quality and variety of doing is critical for ego development and adaptation.

Social change and technological development have altered the interaction of the person and the world. Direct life-supporting and life-threatening contacts with flora and fauna are almost eliminated. Communication and information are dramatically extended. People hear of

---

Purposeful action enables humans to become humanized

→ no personal exp of yr actions/thots.

events immediately but do not interact with them. The accuracy of reality testing is always dependent upon one's neurological idiosyncrasies, perceptual distortions, the results of prior actions, and social responses. Contemporary psychopathology is fashioned by the current demands on all neurologic functions, on perceptual accuracy, on reduced opportunity for learning through action, and by the enlarged input of information and language.

One can, for instance, easily visualize the different possibilities in the world of John who lives on a farm near a wooded hillside with his parents, grandparents, three siblings, and an uncle. He is expected to be responsible for a number of chores to maintain the household. He is free to endlessly explore nature with all manner of physical skills. He gets direct and consistent response from several generations while also observing them in their work roles. He receives indirect response from family members reacting with value judgments to each other. Finally, he has the direct and indirect responses available to all children at school.

Compare John to Peter who lives in an apartment in a city with two working parents, a cat, and a neighborhood that holds personal threat during much of the 24 hours. He may have some chores but they may not be viewed as critical to the maintenance of family life. He is given very limited freedom to explore. He receives some direct response from two people whose work he does not observe except in the housework about which they complain. He gets vestigial, indirect response from his parents and many hours of passively received indirect response from television or radio. Finally, he has the direct and indirect responses available to all children at school. Once Peter has learned to manipulate his

predictable toys he is limited to exploring the behavior of his cat, which is limited in its own behavioral possibilities. A sense of mastery, especially for the new and unexpected, is difficult to achieve. A sense of value and social role identity is even more difficult. Feelings, actions, and meanings do not become integrated.

It can be hypothesized that the prevalence of senseless, purposeless violence by children and adolescents who show no remorse can be generated by hours of viewing television violence that has no relation to their behavior and that is not accompanied by action on their own part. When action does not follow thought, perception is distorted and the critical learning that comes from confronting the consequences of an act is precluded. This dissociation of thought, affect, and action so characteristic of schizophrenia can follow this process of "learning without action." Schizophrenic dissociation can occur when neurologic and perceptual deficits preclude action and when the nature of one's environment inhibits doing or does not support doing in a variety of contexts. The limited learning of functional, adaptive skills that occur when there is a paucity of opportunity for *doing* is emphasized by Winn (18). She discusses the faulty reality testing, loose distinction between illusion and reality, and the passivity of response evident in children whose daily hours are filled with TV viewing as opposed to psychomotor activity.

There is increasing evidence that limited action experiences are no less significant for the adult. Speaking to the role of activity in maintaining normal human functioning and the consequences of sensory deprivation, Bruner points out that "an immobilized human being in a sensorially impoverished environment soon loses control of his mental functions." (19,

p 7) Greenberg quotes Stainbrook commenting on thrill seeking as reflecting a search for individual mastery, "So much of our life has become sedentary, inhibitive action. There has been an over-emphasis on cerebration—thrill seeking behavior is expressing an almost desperate need for active, assertive mastery at something. We are programmed for action,—but where there is so much less adaptive behavior which requires physical action, there is an insidious anxiety about the concept of mastery. We need to restore a sense of physical mastery and assertion; a sense of control, of self doing rather than merely thinking." (20, p 21)

Prescribing Intervention

The complexities of a rapidly expanding, industrialized society make it imperative for the health professions to attend to those factors that preclude or inhibit *doing*. A reduction in *doing* generates pathology. When pathology is identified, *doing* must be used in the service of personality integration. If treatment is heavily biased toward verbal communication, and if treatment responds to symptoms rather than to performance skill development and reinforcement, then it will have a limited effect. Likewise, when activity programs fail to relate to the specific development of performance skills, their impact is more like random activity and much of their potential benefit is lost. The extent of carry over of learning and changes from the treatment setting to the *home* environment is frequently determined by the degree to which treatment modalities are relevant to the adaptive and performance skill demands and expectations of the *home* setting. *need this info from eval!*

Programming for the prevention of ill health or for the remedy of dysfunction must reflect an appreciation

(ie., the 4 unit!)

for and understanding of the interrelationship among internal and external systems in the generation and shaping of human behavior. Selective attention to one system, one skill area or component of coping, fragments the totality of the human being.

The question then is how to elaborate concepts about *doing* to create plans or prescriptions to enhance critical human functions? Different periods in the life cycle demand different configurations of skills, both those relating to the internal realities and those relating to the external realities. Performance can be understood as the ability, throughout the life cycle, to care for and maintain the self in a more independent manner, satisfy one's personal needs for intrinsic gratification, and contribute to the needs and welfare of others. The balance among these performance skill clusters, that is, the proportion of time, attention, and energy allocated to each, is critical in achieving and maintaining a way of life that is satisfying to self and others and is health sustaining.

The level and kind of skills and the balance among them at any one point are determined by age, developmental level, unique biology, and culture. For example, what is an adequate level of independent self care and what are appropriate self-care activities will vary in accordance with age as well as with cultural norms. Likewise, what is considered a healthy balance among caring for self, pursuing personal need gratification, and caring for others, changes with the different stages of life and varies according to one's culture.

Planning for intervention requires an initial assessment of the nature and level of the individual's intact skills, skill limitations, and balance among performance skill clusters.

Once such assessments have been made, it is necessary to identify those components or subsystems of performance that inhibit or prevent skill development. This description includes evaluations of the sensory, motor, psychologic, and social deficits as well as identification and assessment of those human and nonhuman factors in the environment that impact on being able *to do*.

Concepts regarding the components of *doing* make it possible to analyze activities or doing experiences in relation to skill acquisition. Planning therefore requires that activities be understood and analyzed in terms of the level and kind of motor skill requirements, sensory integrative components, psychologic meaning, cognitive requisites, interpersonal and social elements, and cultural relevance and significance. Such knowledge then makes it possible to match activity experiences to the individual's deficits, learning readiness, intact functions, and values. On the basis of such data and planning, *doing* can be designed to provide the action-learning experiences necessary for the development of the critical components of performance and for skill acquisition.

Each human action calls on some neurologic function. It is done within some social context and has various potential values and meaning. Understanding the nature and relevance of *doing* to human adaptation should make it possible to plan intervention programs to facilitate learning and change, increase the chances of helping others maintain a state of health, contribute to a better understanding of the basis of pathology or dysfunction and, thus, hopefully develop more effective prevention strategies.

Acknowledgment

This article is adapted from a paper presented to the Sixth International Congress of Social Psychiatry, Opatjia, Yugoslavia, October 1976.

REFERENCES

1. Bruner JS, Jolly A, Sylva K (Editors): *Play, Its Role in Development and Evolution,* New York: Basic Books, 1976
2. Piaget J: *Play, Dreams and Imitation in Childhood,* New York: W.W. Norton, 1962
3. Reilly M (Editor): *Play as Exploratory Learning,* Beverly Hills, CA: Sage Publications, 1974
4. Erickson EH: Play and actuality. In *Play, Its Role in Development and Evolution,* JS Bruner, A Jolly, K Sylva, Editors. New York: Basic Books, 1976
5. Erickson EH: *Childhood and Society,* New York: W.W. Norton, 1963
6. Searles HF: *The Nonhuman Environment,* New York: International University Press, 1960
7. Fidler GS, Fidler JW: *Occupational Therapy: A Communication Process in Psychiatry,* New York: MacMillan, 1964
8. Edelson M: *Ego Psychology, Group Dynamics and the Therapeutic Community,* New York: Grune and Stratton, 1964
9. Becker E: *The Revolution in Psychiatry,* New York: The Free Press, 1964
10. Black M. The objectivity of science. *Bull Atomic Scientist* 33: 55-60, 1977
11. Pribam KH: *Languages of the Brain,* Englewood Cliffs, NJ: Prentice Hall, 1971
12. Castaneda C: *Journey to IXTLAN,* New York: Simon and Schuster, 1972
13. White RW: Motivation reconsidered: the concept of competence. *Psychol Rev* 66: 297-333, 1959
14. White RW: The urge toward competence. *Am J Occup Ther* 25: 271-274, 1971
15. Mead GH: *Mind, Self and Society,* Chicago: University of Chicago Press, 1934
16. Fidler GS: The task oriented group as a context for treatment. *Am J Occup Ther* 23: 43-48, 1969
17. Moore OK, Anderson AR: Some principles for the design of clarifying educational environments. In *Handbook of Socialization Theory and Research,* D Goslin, Editor. Chicago: Rand McNally, 1968
18. Winn M: *The Plug-In Drug,* New York: Viking Press, 1977
19. Bruner JS: *On-Knowing—Essays for the Left Hand,* Cambridge, MA: The Belknap Press of Harvard University Press, 1962
20. Greenberg PF: The thrill seekers. *Human Behav* 6: 17-21, 1977

Toward a Science of Adaptive Responses *

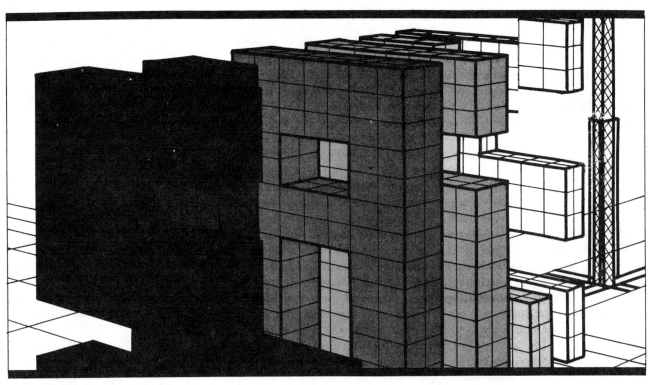

Lorna Jean King

Lorna Jean King, OTR, FAOTA, Phoenix, Arizona.

The 1978 Eleanor Clarke Slagle Lecture was presented by Lorna Jean King at the Annual Conference of the American Occupational Therapy Association on May 10, 1978, San Diego, California.

An "asset almost peculiar to occupational therapists is their high tolerance for puzzlement, confusion and frustration." (1) Ten years ago this was the opinion of Dr. J. S. Bockoven, one of our profession's most vocal admirers. Today one might argue about the tolerance, but who could dispute the puzzlement, confusion and frustration as we look back on a good many years of effort to define practice, to structure theory, and to build philosophies of occupational therapy.

Need for a Comprehensive Theory

And, as we look toward an era of increasing specialization, we are soberly aware that, without a unifying theory to insure cohesiveness, specialization could easily become fragmentation. In fact, back at the time when the profession's definition began "Occupational therapy is any activity, mental or physical, . . . ," (2) recreation, art, music, and dance all fell under the rubric of occupational therapy. The responsibility for the fact that these modality-based specialties have become separate professions can be assigned in large measure to the lack of unifying theory.

It seems readily apparent that splintering into small professions results in watering-down of job development effectiveness, the scattering of progressively scarcer financial resources for education, and the loss of political "clout." The economics of the health care delivery system will not indefinitely support professional proliferation and duplication of effort. To allow future specialization to result in further fragmentation might well be suicidal. Therefore, we need a framework that will give specialists the bond of a common structure.

We must also cope with the fact that today's consumers, far more sophisticated than in the past, expect to understand what they are paying for. They will no longer accept "on faith" what they are told. This underscores the need for a coherent theoretical model understandable, not just to the professional initiate, but also to the consumer. We may develop complex theories, but, in order to be really useful, they will need to be based on a straightforward structure that can be widely understood, and is clearly related to the client's life functions.

Difficulties in Constructing a Science of Occupation

As a prelude to an attempt to identify a usable theoretical framework, let us look at the roots of some of our difficulties in achieving a science of occupation. One of the difficulties is related to the fact that occupational therapy was born of common sense; and common sense is, by definition, "what everyone knows." Everyone knows that it is a good thing to keep busy. There is the old proverb, "The devil finds mischief for idle hands." Carlyle said it with great feeling, "An endless significance lies in work; in idleness alone is there perpetual despair." (3) One must reach far down on the evolutionary ladder to find organisms that are not active, that simply exist. Occupation, or employment, or activity, is quite literally bred in our bones. Occupational therapy, then, deals with purposeful behavior—with people *doing*. But isn't this what people are engaged in during most of their waking hours? It is hard to see what is significant about such a commonplace fact of life, and that is precisely the problem, or one of them—something so ever present is hard to grasp conceptually. Whitehead is credited with saying that the more familiar something is to us, the more difficult it is to subject it to scientific inquiry (4). As a commonplace example, consider how many eons must have gone by before Man even thought to wonder about the nothingness that surrounded him. A great many more eons probably passed before Man realized that it was *not* nothingness, and named it atmosphere. I am suggesting, then, that the very universality of the filling or occupying of time with purposeful behavior has made it difficult to form concepts that would help us to construct a theory or science of occupation.

Who has not had the experience of trying to explain occupational therapy to someone, only to realize that people think they know all about it because, of course, they have *experienced* occupation and activity.

They are thinking about it in everyday terms, and the therapist is, hopefully, thinking about it scientifically and analytically. So, although words are exchanged, frequently no communication takes place.

Another problem in constructing models is the difficulty that therapists sometimes have in communicating with each other because of the many levels on which purposeful behavior can be organized. One can talk about the effects of activity on the biochemistry of cells, or about its place as an essential component of neurodevelopment. Purposeful behavior is also basic to cognitive processes; and on the still broader scale of cultural anthropology, an individual's role in the cultural milieu can be thought of as determining purposeful behavior. Conversely, behavior may determine cultural roles. So, whether one looks at biochemical Man, psychological Man, social, economic or ecological Man, purposeful behavior is inextricably woven into the total fabric of human function. However, if one therapist looks at occupation solely in terms of its psychological implications, while another looks only at the cognitive issues, and a third describes chiefly the neurophysiological consequences, a situation results much like that of the blind men examining the elephant. One described the leg, another the ear, and another the trunk. Finally, they were convinced that they could not possibly be talking about the same creature. Certainly an outsider would be hard-pressed to find a principle unifying work simplification, sensory integration, hand splints, and acceptable outlets for aggression, to name just a few of the topics with which therapists may be concerned.

Naturally, attempts have been made to deal with this disparity of viewpoints. Development frameworks are appropriate for many clients, but are not particularly helpful with the normally developed adult who is suddenly faced with trauma or disabling disease. Other models deal with occupation in terms of chronic conditions or the sequelae of disease—a rehabilitative context. These are not readily applicable to developmental problems or acute, as contrasted with chronic, conditions. Few models that I am aware of have spelled out what it is that is peculiar to occupational therapy as contrasted with physical therapy or vocational counseling, for example. What *is* that factor which makes occupational therapy so uniquely valuable that, as Dr. Reilly says, if the profession were to disappear tomorrow, it would have to be quickly reinvented? (5)

General systems theory teaches that systems share common features, that large inclusive systems tend to recapitulate the features found in more specific units. As Laszlo says, "A system in one perspective is a subsystem in another." (6) It seems, then, that our task in finding a theoretical frame for occupational therapy is to identify a level of system that is not so specific as to shut out some of our areas of specialization, nor yet so general as to include a great many more areas than are applicable.

In short, in order to satisfy the profession's current needs, a theory or science of occupational therapy should provide:

1. a unifying concept that will apply to all areas of specialization;

2. a framework that will clearly distinguish occupational therapy theory and techniques from those of other disciplines;

3. a model that is readily explainable to other professionals and to consumers; and

4. a theory that is adequate for scientific elaboration and refinement.

Adaptation as a Unifying Concept

While mulling over some of these considerations, I read Konrad Lorenz's recent book, *Behind the Mirror, A Search for a Natural History of Human Knowledge* (7). Lorenz deals essentially with the evolutionary and individual processes of adaptation that are involved in Man's active acquisition of knowledge and techniques. I was struck with the implications of his work for occupational therapy. Then Kielhofner and Burke's recent review of the ideological history of occupational therapy (8) drew my attention to Dr. Ayres' phrase, "eliciting an adaptive response," (9) which seemed a succinct and accurate description of what an occupational therapist does. I was at this time going over the occupational therapy literature, and suddenly the words *adaptation* and *adaptive* seemed to leap out from almost every page. In fact, few of our professional articles fail to mention adaptation, regardless of the author's specialty or point of view. I was struck, like Cortez, with "a wild surmise" (10); could the *adaptive process* be an adequate synthesizing principle for our profession? Is it too nebulous a concept to be useful? Surely it is too simple an idea—or is it? Has its very familiarity, like that of the word *occupation* blinded us to its true significance?

Certainly the words *adaptation* and *adaptive* are well known to us. We advertise on bumper stickers that occupational therapists are adaptive; we have large investments in adaptive equipment; and assumptions about adaptation are implicit in our literature. Adolph Meyer began his treatise on "The Philosophy of Occupation Therapy," in 1922, by defining disease and health in terms of

adaptation (11). But I have not found evidence that we have rigorously analyzed the concept or used it consciously to explain our functions in any broad sense. Perhaps it is time that some of our implicit assumptions about adaptation be made explicit. Only when these assumptions are articulated can their validity be examined through research.

At the outset we must distinguish between adaptation as an evolutionary concept and the process of individual adaptation. Evolutionary adaptation refers to changes in the structure or function of an organism or any of its parts that result from the process of natural selection (12). Natural selection, in turn, is the process by which a differential survival advantage is transmitted to successive generations. The process of evolutionary adaptation is very slow, requiring at the minimum hundreds of thousands of years for significant changes in form or function to occur.

Individual adaptation refers to adjustments made by the individual that primarily enhance personal rather than species survival, and secondarily contribute to actualization of personal potential. Tinbergen says, "Adaptedness is a certain relationship between the environment and what the organism must do to meet it." (13)

The idea of using adaptation as a model in a health-related profession is reinforced by Dr. Rene Dubos in his book, *Man Adapting* (14). He says "states of health or disease are the expressions of the success or failure experienced by the organism in its efforts to respond adaptively to environmental challenges."

Rappaport, the general systems theorist, says "Science is clearly a systematized search for simplicity." He adds, "Seek simplicity, and distrust it." (15) I would invite you, then, to keep a healthy skepticism as we explore the concept, a relatively simple one, that the adaptive process constitutes the core of occupational therapy theory, and that specific attributes of adaptation are also the significant and characteristic attributes of occupational therapy. This will make explicit and specific and testable some of our heretofore unexamined assumptions.

Characteristics of the Adaptive Process

Initially, let us discuss four specific features of individual, as opposed to evolutionary, adaptation. The first characteristic of adaptation is that it demands of the individual a positive role. The adapting person is defined as "adjusting himself to different conditions or environments." (12) In doing this he is acting, not being acted upon. An adaptive response cannot be imposed, it must be actively created. To quote Nobel prize-winning ethologist Tinbergen again, "Living things do not move passively through the physical processes of the environment; they do something against it." (13) Active participation of the client in the treatment process has long been recognized as characteristic of occupational therapy.

Alexei Leontiev, Chairman of the Psychology Faculty of the University of Moscow, reminds us that "Even seemingly simple human functions develop as an interaction between sensory stimulation from the environment and the *person's own activity*." (16) (Italics by this author)

Even unprofitable or maladaptive adjustments to change are actively entered into. Withdrawal, for example, which is often considered a negative condition, is actually an active response, sometimes appropriate, sometimes maladaptive.

Secondly, adaptation is called forth by the demands of the environment. The challenge of something

the individual needs or wants to do—obstructed by change or deficit in the self or the environment—calls forth a specific adaptive response. We could say that occupational therapy consists of structuring the surroundings, materials, and especially the demands, of the environment in such a way as to call forth a specific adaptive response. Another way of saying this is that occupational therapy uses the demands of tasks or other goal-oriented activities in a specially structured environment to trigger the unfolding of a need adaptation.

Among the healing sciences, occupational therapy is unique in its utilization of the demands of the real-life environment. An adaptive response cannot truly be said to have occurred until the individual consistently carries it out in the course of ordinary activities. Thus an amputee may practice opening the hook of the prosthesis over and over, but has not truly adapted to it until the prosthesis is used habitually in a daily routine. The occupational therapist uses this knowledge by providing the amputee with many real-life activities in which to use the prosthesis. The therapist knows that pure exercise, no matter how repetitive, often does not generalize into daily activities, and therefore fails to be adaptive.

This brings us to the *third* characteristic of the adaptive response, namely that it is usually most efficiently organized subcortically, and, in fact, often can *only* be organized below the conscious level. Conscious attention to a task or an object permits the subconscious centers to integrate and organize a response. Dr. Yerxa, in her 1966 Slagle Lecture (17), gave an example that can hardly be improved upon. She said, "A year ago I helped evaluate a brain damaged client's function. She was asked to open her hand. No response

occurred, except that she was obviously trying. Next she was moved passively into finger extension while the therapist demonstrated the desired movement. This time the client responded with increased finger flexion. In frustration she cried, 'I know, I know.' Finally she was offered a cup of water. As the cup was perceived, her fingers opened almost miraculously to grasp it." It would be hard to overemphasize the importance of the therapist's using his or her cognitive powers to structure situations that will elicit a subcortical adaptive response from the client. We tend to rely too much on the client's cognitive processes.

Another example of the importance of subcortical adaptive learning is less familiar to the therapist, but popular with the sports enthusiast. It is to be found in such concepts as "inner tennis." Gallweg, author of *The Inner Game of Tennis* (18), says, "There is a far more natural and effective process for learning and doing almost anything than most of us realize. It is similar to the process we all used but soon forgot as we learned to walk and talk. It uses the so-called unconscious mind more than the deliberate "self-conscious" mind, the spinal and mid-brain areas of the nervous system more than the cerebral cortex. This process doesn't have to be learned, we already know it. All that is needed is to unlearn those habits which interfere with it, and then to just *let it happen*." This approach recognizes the frequently *dis*organizing effects of analyzing consciously what should be automatic sequences of movement.

I stress this point because it is another essential reason why occupational therapists use purposeful activity instead of exercise: namely, that tasks, including crafts, or other goal-directed activities, such as play (where the goal is fun), focus attention on the object or outcome, and leave the organizing of the sensory input and motor output to the subcortical centers where it is handled most efficiently and adaptively. I am suggesting, then, that the distinguishing characteristic of occupational therapy, derived from a similar truth about adaptation, is that *there is always a double motivation:* first, the motivation of the activity itself—catching the ball, creating the vase, making the bed; and the second motivation, recovering from illness, maintaining health, preventing disability—in short, adapting. Now no *animal* recognizes the need to "adapt." It sets out to do something specific—escape a pursuer, or find food. The immediate objective provides the motivation. Adaptation is a secondary and unrecognized goal. But in dealing with humans we need to recognize that the double motivation of therapeutic activity may or may not need to be brought to the client's awareness, depending on age, cognitive function, and so forth. The therapist should see to it, however, that other professionals and the client's family are made aware of *both* motivations, and of how the direct motivation of the activity subserves the indirect, but *primary* motive of therapy.

The implications of the foregoing definitions of the nature of occupational therapy practice are important in light of certain current problems. As mentioned earlier, the profession has been concerned with role definition—how to delimit the boundaries that separate our practice from that of physical therapy or other professions. In a recent report of an American Occupational Therapy Foundation board meeting, to which Washington area therapists were invited, concern was expressed about occupational therapists "infringing on" exercise, the territory of physical

therapy (19). And well may we be concerned, for it is *our* professional identity that will be diluted by this infringement, not theirs. Obviously all disciplines that are working with a client should work, together cooperatively, but it seems equally obvious that it is uneconomic if there is duplication of function. Exercise has its important place, so also does purposeful activity as a producer of adaptive responses, and this latter is the realm of the occupational therapist. We need to be able to explain in terms of the principles outlined above why purposeful behavior can elicit adaptive responses that exercise alone cannot. Defining our role in this way will be much more satisfactory than the old way of dividing the patient in the middle and giving the top half to the occupational therapist and the bottom half to the physical therapist.

The *fourth* characteristic of the adaptive response is that it is self-reinforcing. In animal behavior the reward for successful mastery of environmental demand is survival, and the penalty for failure is death. In humans the results are seldom so immediate and stark. Nevertheless, mastery of environmental demand is a powerful reinforcer and Maslow lists the drive to master the surroundings as one of Man's innate needs (20). Mastery of one demand is rewarding and serves as a stimulus for attention to the next necessary response at a higher level of challenge. This is the genius of occupational therapy—that, as the old adage has it, "nothing succeeds like success." As the occupational therapist plans and structures successful efforts, each success serves as a spur to a greater effort. Exercise, psychotherapy, behavior modification are all means to an end. But with purposeful activity, the activity itself is an end, as well as being a means to a larger end, ther-

apy or adaptation, hence the double motivation mentioned before.

To summarize the thesis thus far, I am implying that the essential purpose of occupational therapy is to stimulate and guide the adaptive processes through which an individual may best survive and develop. I have suggested that the basic characteristics of occupational therapy derive from the corresponding elements of adaptation; *first,* that it is an active response; *second,* that it is evoked by the specific environmental demands of needs, tasks and goals; *third,* that it is most efficiently organized below the level of consciousness, with conscious attention being directed to objects or tasks; and *fourth,* that it is self-reinforcing, with each successful adaptation serving as a stimulus for tackling the next more complex environmental challenge.

Having tried to identify the basic characteristics of the adaptive process from which the significant features of occupational therapy derive, let us look at some familiar aspects or categories of practice in the light of adaptation, and also at the adaptive process as an organizing principle in two newer or less familiar areas of practice.

In broad general terms we can divide individual adaptation, on the one hand, into the phase that is synonymous with developmental learning, and, on the other hand, the process of adjusting to change or stress.

Developmental Learning as an Adaptive Process

The organizing of sensory input into information, and the subsequent integration of an appropriate motor response, is a continuous adaptive process. As mentioned earlier, Leontiev suggests that human functions consist of the interaction of sensory input and individual activity. For example, we learn to see by seeing. The visual figure-ground skills of a child raised in the green leafy lights and shadows of the jungle will be different from those of the child raised in the clear light and great vistas of the Navajo reservation. Each child begins with similar, basic visual equipment, but the process of learning to see in each environment is a process of adaptation in which available stimuli, combined with active sorting and filing, produce patterned vision.

There are a number of theoretical frames for considering the adaptive processes of early childhood, and the occupational therapy profession can be proud of the several outstanding developmental theorists among its ranks. It is not the intention here to recapitulate developmental theories, but to emphasize the fact that "eliciting an adaptive response," in Dr. Ayres' apt phrase, is, in essence, eliciting goal-directed or purposeful behavior. This may be as basic as enticing an infant to lift its head to look at a toy, or more complex, such as suggesting to a child that he shovel sand into a wheelbarrow to trundle across the playground to a sand box. The child's goal is playing with the sand; the therapist's goal is stimulating co-contraction, heavy work patterns, and so forth, in the service of integrating and organizing sensory input and motor behavior.

The role of the occupational therapist in stimulating this sequence of integration and response appears deceptively simple to the consumer who cannot be expected to understand, without explanation, that it takes considerable knowledge and professional finesse to know which adaptive response is needed and to provide the proper setting and stimuli for a given action at the opportune moment when the individual's development makes it possible for him to make a successful response.

We have been considering the well-known field of developmental learning in children. However, it is not only in childhood that one must organize sensory data and respond appropriately. This process goes on throughout life. Afferent, or incoming impulses, particularly those characterized as proprioceptive feedback, play a crucial role in sensory integrative processes in adults as well as in children. The key concept is that sensory input is the raw material for adaptation at *any* age. If developmental adaptation does not take place normally in childhood, the adult will show various disabilities ranging, as an example, from mild motor planning problems to severe disabilities such as process schizophrenia. Recent studies, suggesting that the adult brain is relatively plastic, give some hope that even in adulthood developmental adaptations can be facilitated.

The role of sensory data in the adult has been strikingly illuminated in the last 25 years by a large number of sensory deprivation studies, which have, as a matter of fact, strengthened the theoretical base for sensory integration theory. However, the critical relationship between these studies and the health of the average citizen is just beginning to be appreciated. As an example, consider the scenario for an all too familiar tragedy that goes something like this. An elderly man, in somewhat precarious health, must undergo major surgery. As a precaution, he is kept somewhat longer than usual in the intensive care unit. When he is moved to a room, he is kept very quiet, sedated, curtains drawn, and visitors restricted. Somewhere between the third and fifth day, post-surgery, the nurse's notes show that the patient appears to be confused and disoriented. The following day he is halluci-

nating and has to be restrained because he is trying to get out of bed. There are no family members who are willing to care for him in his apparently deranged state, so he is transferred to a nursing home where he continues in a state of relative sensory deprivation, and his mental and physical condition deteriorates rapidly.

The tragedy is that this kind of occurrence is often preventable. And in the instances where confusion or disorientation occur in spite of precautions, it is important to note that it is often reversible if suitable sensory input is provided. Lipowski, whose studies (21) suggest the reversibility of deprivation-caused psychiatric symptoms, also warns that around age 55 vulnerability to the effects of sensory deprivation increases quite sharply. Thus it is apparent that it is not just the very old who are at risk.

It is also important to note that the effects of deprivation are cumulative, and that the more sensory modes that are understimulated, the faster confusion and disorientation result. One of Lipowski's most significant findings appears to be that immobilization is the most disabling form of deprivation, and that, if added to other sensory losses, is very likely to produce psychiatric symptoms in the vulnerable.

In terms of the emphasis of this discussion on adaptation, we may think of confusion and disorientation as *dis*-adaptation—failure of organization and response. Hallucinatory and delusional phenomena, on the other hand, represent *mal*-adaptation; the sensory data is organized, but incorrectly, and therefore, of course, the response seems inappropriate. So-called unpatterned stimuli are as bad or worse than complete absence of stimuli. "White noise," such as the constant hum of a motor, is an auditory example, while the test pattern on a television set is an instance from the visual domain. Kornfeld, Zimberg, and Malm, in a paper on psychiatric complications of open heart surgery (22), report that "The patient might first experience an illusion involving, for example, sounds arising from the air conditioning vent or the reflection of light from the plastic oxygen tent. Many experience a rocking or floating sensation. These phenomena were often not reported to the staff and could then develop into hallucinatory phenomena and associated paranoid ideation." Kornfeld and his group confirm the harmful effects of immobilization, noting that many patients interviewed after recovery remembered as one of their chief discomforts not being able to move. Let us emphasize again that *sensory input is the raw material for adaptation.* Without adequate sensory data, the individual's adaptive capacity is greatly curtailed.

Motivational loss is another aspect of hospital-induced sensory deprivation that is of critical importance in rehabilitation or therapy. Zubek, in a report on electroencephalographic correlates of sensory deprivation (23), reports that not only were alpha frequencies progressively decreased during 14-day deprivation experiments, but this was also accompanied by severe motivational losses. The abnormal encephalograms persisted for a week after the subjects returned to normal living conditions, *but the motivational losses lasted even longer.* These findings have profound implications for all medical personnel who are trying to motivate patients toward independence. Perhaps the cart has been ahead of the horse! Perhaps the first thing to do is to provide sensory stimulation, particularly of the proprioceptors, through whatever degree of mobility

is possible. Then motivation for independent behavior might follow more quickly and spontaneously.

I am indebted to Lillian Hoyle Parent for discussing with me some of the material on sensory deprivation, and, as she points out in her recent helpful summary of the deprivation studies (24), occupational therapists are better prepared than any other health care professionals to make use of this information. A dozen exciting research projects come readily to mind in reference to hospital-induced deprivation. For example, a control group receiving the usual post-operative care could be compared with an experimental group receiving systematic meaningful sensory stimulation under an occupational therapist's supervision. Comparisons could be made of number of hospital days post-surgery, incidence of complications, and amounts of pain and sleep medications.

We have suggested that sensory input and motor output are the essentials of individual adaptation as seen in the familiar field of developmental learning, and we have looked at the less familiar concept of sensory deprivation as a prime factor in *dis*-adaptation or *mal*-adaptation.

Therapeutic Adaptation to Change or Stress

The *second* general category of adaptive response is adaptation to change or stress. One aspect of response to change is represented by a very active current field of specialization in occupational therapy, namely the field of physical disabilities. This field concerns itself with the individual's adaptation to physical change.

Changes within the person can be of many kinds; what they have in common is they demand that the individual alter habitual responses. Ar-

thritis, heart disease, amputations, spinal cord injuries, stroke, blindness are a few examples. The use of adaptive equipment, work simplification, splinting, development of strength and skill in residual body segments are among the adaptive considerations in this area of practice. Sometimes the acquiring of appropriate adaptive responses may actually be a matter of survival, as with the cardiac client. More often adaptation means the possibility of actualizing potential that would otherwise be wasted.

While the concepts of adapting to physical change are very familiar to us as therapists, we have had less direct experience with the relatively new field of adaptation as it relates to stress medicine. The role of activity in adapting to or coping with stress is an old idea whose scientific time has come. Dr. Hans Selye, who is considered the "father" of stress medicine, comments, "The existence of physical and mental strain, the manifold interactions between somatic and psychic reactions, as well as the importance of defensive-adaptive responses, had all been more or less clearly recognized since time immemorial. But stress did not become meaningful to me until I found that it could be dissected by modern research methods and that individual tangible components of the stress response could be identified in chemical and physical terms." (25) Dr. Selye called this stress response the "general adaptation syndrome." Today few literate people are unaware of the fact he demonstrated: that any stimulus which appears to pose a threat to survival elicits a response that includes the secretion of the cortico-steroids which prepare the body for a fight or flight reaction. The heightened blood pressure, pulse, and respiration that follow a danger signal had a distinct survival value when the appropriate reaction was running, or climbing, or hand-to-hand combat. In our present culture, running, climbing, or fighting are seldom considered appropriate responses, and threats are often perceived as long continued, like the danger of losing one's job, or the daily stress of driving through rush-hour traffic. There are well-known stress diseases such as ulcers, high blood pressure, and heart disease, to mention the most common, that follow chronic stimulation of cortico-steroid secretion. The current vogue for jogging, marathon running, and other strenuous sports owes part of its very real usefulness as a health maintenance measure to the fact that exercise metabolizes and renders harmless the stress hormones that otherwise might accumulate and cause permanent damage to the body.

What is not so often considered is the effect of either subtle or overt stress on an already over-taxed system. A person who is already feeling ill is told he must enter the hospital. Whether it is for surgery or for tests, or for nursing care, everything about the experience spells danger: the strangeness, the uncertainty, the painful or uncomfortable procedures, but most of all the feeling of helplessness. Stress hormones are poured into a system that not only is already reacting to the stress of illness, but also has few opportunities for activity that might help to metabolize and dissipate the cortico-steroids. Stress hormones can make the sick person sicker and can retard recovery.

It is often assumed that *rest* is what is needed in the hospital, but, as Dr. Selye points out, unless the organism is completely exhausted, activity of some sort is much more appropriate to stress dissipation than too much rest. Many years ago an occupational therapist frequently stopped into a

hospital room and made available purposeful, goal-directed activities that allowed the patient an adaptive response to stress. If we had known then what we know now, we might have called it *stress management* or *stress reduction therapy*. Instead, someone used the word *diversional*, with the result that the whole area of human needs has been virtually abandoned, and the word *diversional* has become the equivalent of profanity. In fairness we must point out that few third-party reimbursement agents are willing to pay for something labeled *diversional*.

To turn to another aspect of this subject, before the stress hormones and their physiological effects had been identified by Dr. Selye, we often spoke of *tension,* and in the mental health field were able to recognize the usefulness of activity, even though the reasons were vague. Dr. Roy Grinker writes of the treatment of *battle fatigue* or *war neuroses* (26) and says, "In their free time physical activities are encouraged in order to dissipate accumulated tensions. Enforced idleness and rest are bad therapy for these states." Later he comments, "The patients are busy the whole day with physical and mental activities and various aspects of occupational therapy."

The high hopes held for the usefulness of the psychotropic drugs led to the serious curtailment of other forms of treatment such as those described by Grinker. Now that there is widespread disillusionment with the major tranquilizers, which seem to cause almost as many problems as they solve, perhaps the efficacy of what might be called *adaptational therapy* will be rediscovered.

The psychiatric disorders provide excellent examples of the interrelatedness of the various aspects of the adaptive process. In some instances, as in autism or in process schizophre-

nia, we are probably dealing with inadequate developmental adaptive learning and the attendant severe problems in perception and communication. These problems inevitably produce stress and the concomitant physical changes produced by the stress hormones. These, in turn, probably further derange the sensory-integrative processes. Many of the symptoms seen in the psychoses represent either disadaptations or maladaptive behavior. As the therapist is able to facilitate adaptive development, that is, sensory integration, coping behaviors improve. Activity also helps to metabolize stress hormones and thus increases the client's feeling of well-being. Though basic biochemical causes may ultimately be found for some of the major psychoses, there will probably always be a need for facilitating adaptive or coping skills in a society that seems increasingly stressful.

Psychologists Gal and Lazarus, it seems to me, have made the strongest case of activity as an adaptive response to stress. Their article, "The Role of Activity in Anticipating and Confronting Stressful Situations" (27), spells out the physiological correlation of activity with the reduction, or metabolism, of the stress hormones. They point out that while activity which is related to the cause of the stress is best, yet activity of any kind is better than none. Their useful analysis of the literature concludes with these words: "Regardless of the interpretation, it seems quite evident that activity during stressful periods play a significant role in regulating emotional states. We are inclined to interpret activity as being a principal factor in coping with stress. As has been repeatedly argued by Lazarus a person may alter his/her psychological and physiological stress reactions in a given situation simply by taking action. In turn this will affect his/her appraisal of the situation, thereby ultimately altering the stress reaction."

To summarize, we may divide adaptation in response to change or stress into three major components of concern to the occupational therapist:

1. adaptation to physical change (which includes a component of adaptation to stress because the physical changes are in themselves stressors); 2. adaptation to the stress of hospitalization or acute illness; 3. adaptation to reduce stress reactions in psychiatric conditions.

We have engaged in a lengthy exploration of stress and adaptation because it seems that in the foreseeable future coping with or adapting to stress is going to be one of the major health challenges facing humanity. Toffler, in his book *Future Shock* (28), makes a good case for the thesis that the extremely rapid rate of change in almost all of our cultural institutions is a significant cause of stress for large segments of humanity, certainly including our own. Ethologist Tinbergen warns, "The amounts of strain now imposed on the individual may well overstretch man's capabilities to adjust." (13) If it is true that stress is a major health problem for modern man, and if, as Gal and Lazarus propose, activity is of major importance in stress adaptation, then occupational therapy has a major role to play in health maintenance and disease prevention as well as in health restoration.

One of my colleagues (Roene Shortsleeve) once drew a cartoon that expressed this rather well. She drew a bearded figure in the white robes of a prophet. In his hand was a placard which read, "The world is NOT coming to an end; therefore, you had better come to occupational therapy and learn to cope."

Conclusion

I have attempted to demonstrate in this paper that the adaptive process can provide a theoretical framework for occupational therapy that meets the criteria suggested at the outset: that it can be applied to all the specialty areas as a unifying concept; that it will differentiate occupational therapy from other professions; that it is readily explainable to other professionals and to consumers; and that it is adequate in depth to allow for scientific elaboration and refinement.

The adaptive process is probably not the only tenable model for occupational therapy. If this paper spurs others to articulate a more suitable theory, it will have served its purpose.

Toffler, in concluding *Future Shock*, comments that, as yet, there is no science of adaptation. Is it too ambitious to suggest that occupational therapists are uniquely prepared to begin constructing *a science of adaptive responses?* It is a challenge worthy of our best.

REFERENCES

1. Bockoven JS: Challenge of the new clinical approaches. *Am J Occup Ther* 22: 24, 1968
2. Dunton WR: *Prescribing Occupational Therapy*, Springfield, IL: Charles C Thomas, 1947
3. Carlyle T: *Past and Present*, Boston: Houghton Mifflin, 1965, p 196
4. Thayer L: Communications systems. In *The Relevance of General Systems Theory*, E Laszlo, Editor. New York: Braziller, 1972, p 96
5. Reilly M: The educational process. *Am J Occup Ther* 23: 300, 1969
6. Laszlo E: *The Systems View of the World*, New York: Braziller, 1972, p 14
7. Lorenz K: *Behind the Mirror: A Search for a Natural History of Human Knowledge*, New York: Harcourt Brace Jovanovich, 1977
8. Kielhofner G, Burke JP: Occupation-al therapy after 60 years; An account of changing identity and knowledge. *Am J Occup Ther* 31: 657-689, 1977
9. Ayres AJ: *Southern California Sensory Integration Tests Manual*, Los Angeles: Western Psychological Services, 1972
10. Keats J: On first looking into Chapman's Homer. In *Century Readings in English Literature*, JW Cunliffe, Editor. New York: The Century Company, 1920, p 639
11. Meyer A: The philosophy of occupation therapy. *Arch Occup Ther* 1: 1-10, 1922
12. Stein J (Editor): *Random House Dictionary of the English Language*, Unabridged. New York: Random House, 1966
13. Tinbergen N, Hall E: A conversation with Nobel prize winner Niko Tinbergen. *Psychol Today*, March 1974, pp 66, 74
14. Dubos R: *Man Adapting*, New Haven: Yale University Press, 1965, p xvii
15. Rappaport A: The search for simplicity. In *The Relevance of General Systems Theory*, E Laszlo, Editor. New York: Braziller, 1972, pp 18, 30
16. Leontiev AN, cited by Cole M, Cole S: Three giants of Soviet psychology, conversations and sketches. *Psychol Today* 10: 94, 1971
17. Yerxa E: Authentic occupational therapy. *Am J Occup Ther* 21: 2, 1967
18. Gallweg WT: *The Inner Game of Tennis*, New York: Random House, 1974, p 13
19. The Foundation. *Am J Occup Ther* 31: 114, 1978
20. Maslow AH, Murphy G (Editors): *Maturation and Personality*, New York: Harpers, 1954
21. Lipowski ZJ: Delirium, clouding of consciousness and confusion. *J Nerv Ment Dis* 145: 227-255, 1967
22. Kornfeld DS, Zimberg S, Malm JR: Psychiatric complications of open-heart surgery. *New Engl J Med* 273: 287-292, 1965
23. Zubek JP: Electroencephalographic changes during and after 14 days of perceptual deprivation. *Science* 139: 490-492, 1963
24. Parent LH: Effects of a low-stimulus environment on behavior. *Am J Occup Ther* 32: 19-25, 1978
25. Selye H: *The Stress of Life*, New York: McGraw-Hill, 1956, p 263
26. Grinker R: *Men Under Stress*, 2nd edition. New York: McGraw-Hill, 1962, pp 30, 218
27. Gal R, Lazarus RS: The role of activity in anticipating and confronting stressful situations. *J Human Stress* 4: 4-20, 1975
28. Toffler A: *Future Shock*, New York: Random House, 1970

Four Concepts Basic to the Occupational Therapy Process

SANDRA WATANABE, O.T.R.*

The Setting

Home Treatment Service

For two years occupational therapy, sponsored by a National Institute of Mental Health research grant, has been an integral part of the Psychiatric Home Treatment Service at Boston State Hospital. During this time a new role has been evolving for the occupational therapist as a community mental health worker. To explore this role and distinguish it from that of other Psychiatric Home Treatment Service staff members—nurses, psychiatrists, and social workers, who provide similar services—both the clinical practice of the occupational therapist and the conceptual foundations for this practice have been of equal interest in the research.

As the clinical program developed, the core ideas were brought into focus by the research. The following aspects of the program influenced the direction of our thinking: a comprehensive interview evaluation in the home; treatment directly in the home and the community, making use of the patient's own life objects and not traditional clinic activities; a focus on natural treatment groups such as families, neighbors, community caregivers, and not on therapist-composed patient groups; collaborative and consultive programs in which the occupational therapist must be able to delineate her knowledge.

These factors highlight a crucial point: by treating a patient in his daily surroundings, the occupational therapist must make use of the objects and activities unique to each situation if treatment is to be meaningful to the patient and his family. However, to find the continuity in our treatment which earmarks it as occupational therapy, the objects and activities per se have taken second place to the reasoning behind their use. Hence, the identification of these underlying ideas about man in relationship with his environment have become imperative to our practice.

Out of this experience have evolved four concepts basic to the occupational therapy process: life space, mastery, responsibility and life tasks.

*Head Occupational Therapist, Home Treatment Service, Boston State Hospital, Boston, Mass.

These concepts, reflecting our understanding of man in relation to his world and what can go wrong in this relationship, also describe the dysfunction (i.e. constricted life space, insufficient mastery, etc.) we are treating. For example, a person medically labeled as schizophrenic is treated as an individual with dysfunctions in life space, mastery, responsibility and life tasks. (This conceptual framework, grounded in a developmental [the differentiation process] approach, is being further developed to include problem identification and creative problem-solving processes as the therapeutic correlates to the basic concepts.)

Concepts

Life Space

Life space is a fundamental life dimension intrinsically related to the other dimensions of life —energy and time. In our context life space is understood as the physical, perceptual, cognitive, psychological and socio-cultural realms of an individual. The development of life space is based on learning through experience about the spatial and temporal extensions of one's private world. Some people never develop or expand their life space sufficiently to provide substance and consistency to their self-concept or meet the demands of daily life; the stratum in which they function fringes on unreality where their life space does not take them beyond the front door, an overpowering delusion, or a fragmented self-identity.

Rollo May views psychiatric symptoms as the shrinking of the range of one's world to protect it from threat.[1] When a life space is thus restricted there develops little mastery over one's environment and control over one's life situation. As Kurt Lewin points out. . . . "only in a sufficiently free life space in which (there is) the possibility of choosing goals according to (one's) needs and in which, at the same time, (one) fully experiences the objectively conditioned difficulties in the attainment of the goal, can a clear level of reality be formed, only thus can the ability for responsible decisions develop . . . ."[2] (Lewin's basic concept of life space is concerned with the totality of forces in a given moment and hence is limited in time perspective and is without structure. This differs from our broader, more inclusive use of the concept which deals with both the continuity and specific aspects of time, space, human and natural resources and relationships.)

This concept of life space seems fundamental to all areas of occupational therapy. When treating physical disabilities and perceptual motor dysfunctions we are concerned with the patient's ability to utilize his life space comfortably and expand it to its realistic limits. In psychiatry, occupational therapists are basically concerned with the nature and extent of the patient's life space and how he utilizes it as an indication of his mental health and how it can be altered and expanded in treatment.

Robert, a nineteen-year-old man was referred to the Home Treatment Service by a sister with whom he lives because he was "vegetating". He had left school five years previous to referral and since then had been sitting in the house, going out only to play with children half his age.

Upon evaluation, the occupational therapist found that Robert had a very limited life space: he was familiar with his neighborhood only two blocks in one direction; knew nothing about his community, state or country beyond this two-block radius; had a distorted view of world geography and a morbid sense of world history; felt no sense of personal history and had an almost non-existent social sense, i.e., a sense of relationships, institutions, authority, etc. In treatment with the occupational therapist, the patient has been able to make considerable progress in expanding his life space. Key to this mobilization has been the shift of his life's "center of gravity" from the momentary present to the future.

By using this life space concept to guide the therapeutic approach, the therapist can help turn everyday situations into experimental learning situations for Robert. An example of this is seen in the development of his physical life space.

Together, Robert and I explored his neighborhood on foot, then on a map of the local area and finally with maps that placed "his territory" in perspective with the city, state and country. As his familiarity with the maps grew, so did his interest in exploring and incorporating these places into his "territory". And so his life space expanded as these new goals oriented him to the future. By Robert's realizing these goals, the use of buses and libraries, following directions and getting lost, developing ease with new people and new places, he moved from projective wishfulness to the stratum of reality.

Along with this development in his physical life, similar developments took place in his perceptual, cognitive and psychological and sociocultural spheres. Outstanding progress could be seen in his shaping of a social sense and a feeling of personal history, of a placement and continuity in time and space.

All of this would not have taken place if the therapist had simply provided Robert with experimental situations. The initial direction and structure must come from collaborative planning between patient and therapist; however, the motivation to make use of what he has learned about his extended world must come from within the patient himself. At this point our attention is directed from the concept of life space to its logical extension, the concept of mastery.

Mastery

Mastery is skill in comprehending and appropriately using one's human and non-human environment. The nature of one's mastery can be noted in the extent and use of the life space, the mechanisms used in coping with life situations and the ease in handling and integrating new experiences. Mastery then, is the ability to recognize the options that society offers and make choices appropriate to one's own needs and abilities, rather than a passive accommodation to situations.

The development of mastery is motivated by man's need to control what happens to him and around him. Robert White[3] postulates in his theory of competence motivation that man actively seeks experiences which challenge his ability to manipulate his environment. The research of White and others[4-8] indicates that man has an innate need to manipulate and explore, to stimulate himself by doing and thinking with no other goal than the development of mastery and achievement of success.

The development of mastery in an orderly fashion is necessary for keeping in step with one's reference group. John Arsenian deals with this issue in his theory of TEMPO, a cryptogram which "calls attention to the importance of flow, pace and timing in the life cycle, and a regulatory pressure of conformity in keeping up and getting along."[9]

The letters in TEMPO stand for the individual's "doing the right things at the right *T*ime, with the right *E*nergy (and *E*xpectancy), in the right *M*ode, in the right *P*lace, with the right *O*bjects."[9] Inherent in Dr. Arsenian's theory are the concepts of life space and mastery, for one must have a sufficient life space and skill in using it to negotiate the tempo of our society.

If a person's degree of mastery is insufficient or the attempted mastery inappropriate, he will not be able to handle the stress of daily living. Then he becomes more vulnerable to intrapsychic and interpersonal disorganization and cannot make effective use of his life space. Consequently he falls

Tempo— are you ē it? can you handle it?

24

out of TEMPO and will have increased difficulty in developing further mastery.

In practice occupational therapists are intuitively concerned with the patient's development of the mastery needed to handle his daily stresses whether he is suffering from cerebral palsy or a psychosis. Yet, without identifying it as a working concept, it remains on the periphery of our evaluation and treatment when, in fact, it is at the core of the occupational therapy process.

Consider Robert once again. Here is a young man who, at an early age, fell out of TEMPO and dampened his competence motivation, consequently diminishing his chances for developing his mastery. He had not been educated with his peers and so had no peer reference group. His experience in the society around him had been so limited that he really did not understand its expectations. Therefore, he had no expectations for himself.

Indeed, his level of mastery was so low that he was unable to stop children half his age from teasing and beating him; he had no manual or intellectual skill and no ideas whatsoever about his vocational future; he could not negotiate appropriate social encounters with peers, children or elders. In other words, he was unable to solve any problems within the context of society, for he had limited knowledge of and therefore limited use of his environment.

Robert rekindled his competence motivation and developed his mastery because the occupational therapist turned the problems posed by an increased life space into learning experiences. This began with: how do you find out how to get from one place to another, judge the time it will take, or ask a bus driver for directions; how do you know what store to go into to make which kind of purchases; what is an appropriate birthday present for a sister? His general problem-solving abilities have increased as his life space and mastery have increased.

He has been able to master the basic skills of woodworking and is currently learning production carpentry, the vocation of his choice. These experiences have given him his first opportunity in years to relate to peers. They are also teaching him how to make best use of relationships with teachers, work supervisors and employers.

Clearly, as his life space expands, he faces many new and often perplexing and frightening life situations. His increasing ability to handle these new experiences with satisfaction has grown out of the problem-solving approach taken during our sessions.

Responsibility

Life space and mastery are allied in treatment, interacting with each other to provide a continuity of growth. A third concept, that of responsibility, is also closely related, for without responsibility or the accountability of an individual for his own choices, decisions and actions, a life space would lack consensual meaning and mastery would be impaired. William Glasser has defined responsibility as . . . . . "the ability to fulfill one's needs, and to do so in a way that does not deprive others of the ability to fulfill their needs . . . . . ."[10]

Too often, in our therapeutic relationships, responsibility rests primarily with the therapist, for we do not share planning and goals with the patient or expect any commitments from him. Issues of decision-making, problem-solving and responsibility should not be left to chance, or taken over by the therapist, but be the fulcrum of therapy.

Occupational therapy provides excellent opportunities for evoking and fostering responsibility, for we do not put limbs through routine exercises or talk abstractly about living. We are involved with patients in active experiences where reality and the possibility of responsibility are essential. Because of its action orientation, occupational therapy has the potential to consciously and concretely put before the patient options for what, to what, or to whom he understands himself to be responsible.

Reflecting on Robert's situation we can see how the therapist's awareness of this youngster's need to develop a sense of responsibility has been translated into practical terms. To overcome his inertia, the occupational therapist has made use of the responsibility evoking experiences inherent in the occupational therapy process by bringing to Robert's attention the courses of action, the options available to him —leaving the decisions to him.

We began with the smallest, least complex of decisions—the hour of the visit. The therapist presented the choices to him directly, leaving no escape from the responsibility for the decision. From this simple beginning Robert was encouraged to increase his decision-making and problem-solving ability. The progressively complex and demanding issues have always been drawn from his current life situation.

To help him sort out the options and make the whole realm of responsibility decreasingly traumatic, the therapist has used discussion, visual techniques and role playing, graded to the patient's current level of responsibility. Through this method he has become accountable for keeping or cancelling our appointments, participating in planning his treatment program and evaluating his own progress.

As his awareness of his responsibilities in the therapeutic relationship has grown so has his awareness of his general responsibility for himself as a maturing young man. He has registered for the draft, makes and keeps medical appointments, wears clothes appropriate to the season and takes the lead in new friendships. He is developing a sense of financial responsibility and is beginning to sense his responsibility to his school and job.

For most of his life, Robert had rarely experienced himself as being a responsible person. Two factors which prohibited his development of responsibility were a constricted life space, experienced by him as a life vacuum, and his total lack of mastery, experienced by him as immobility in a fast-paced world. As these areas developed, possibilities for responsible action were continually before him. Through the active, graded occupational therapy process he has become able to recognize the choices, make the decisions and acknowledge his responsibilities.

Life Tasks

We have seen how life space, mastery and responsibility are related. The concept of life tasks complete this developmental sequence and is amplified by all of the preceding ideas.

Life tasks are the personal and social undertakings from which an individual derives satisfaction and to which he feels a commitment. Life tasks correlate with those general categories of activities which are considered vital in our society, such as: activities of daily living, a vocation, socializing, education, creative or avocational interests, family living, child-bearing and child-rearing.

While all are vital to the maintenance of our society, these categories are not rigid molds of the social system, for a variety of options or courses of action are available in each area. For each individual, then, his life tasks differ from his functional activities in that he chooses to make a particular investment in a life task and get singular satisfaction from it, while he performs his functions in an uncommitted, minimally gratifying manner.

For example, working is a life task for some, while for others it is a matter of functioning. For some, mothering or ironing or a hobby is merely a way of functioning, whereas for others it is a satisfying life task experience.

An individual's expectations about his personal life tasks and his specific choices of the options is based upon such factors as his inherent (biological) capabilities, his sub-culture's values, his own perception of the general culture, his socioeconomic position, his family experience, his emotional status, the extent of his life space and his level of mastery and responsibility. The categories from which one's specific life tasks are chosen are developmentally[11-14] and traditionally[15-18] associated with specific age groups. Individuals are expected to take the responsibility for choosing and meeting their life tasks at appropriate times in their lives.

Thus the choosing and meeting of life tasks are an integral part of keeping in TEMPO with society as well as a basic expression of those aspects of personality that make for inward unity, or what Gordon Allport terms the "proprium".[19] The distinguishing properties of the proprium are: (1) bodily sense (coenthesis), (2) self-identity (temporal, social and spatial awareness), (3) ego enhancement (self-seeking), (4) ego extension (objects of importance), (5) rational agent (in touch with reality), (6) self-image (phenomenal self), (7) propriate striving ("ego involved" motivation), (8) the knower (cognizing self). This is of importance when making a further distinction between life tasks and functioning.

Life tasks involve a propriate commitment to one's own choices, decisions and actions. They have special meaning as the basic expressions of an integrated individual making his place in the world. Functioning, then, becomes the mechanical, routine follow-through on the aspects of daily life which are not experienced as propriate but which none the less, are seen as necessary to do.

Our understanding of life tasks is grounded in an understanding of TEMPO and proprium, reflecting a concern with the balance in man's productivity—the balance between personal satisfaction and meaning and social viability and acceptability. It is felt that this concern is inherent in the occupational therapy process, as witnessed by our use of self-chosen graded activity and ADL instead of impersonal exercises.

The term "occupational therapy process" also connotes our concern with the evolutionary aspects of the life tasks, for the term is seen here as: the use of objects and activities in the process of becoming. This focus on becoming, on an individual's unique pattern of potentials for growth and change, marks an occupational therapist's active orientation to life tasks.

To turn this basic life task orientation into an actual therapeutic tool, a phenomenological approach[20] is useful with each patient we encounter. Rollo May describes an application of the phenomenological method as an . . . . ."endeavor to take (the) phenomena as given. It is a disciplined effort to clear one's mind of the presuppositions that so often cause us to see in the patient only our own theories or the dogmas of our own system, (an) effort to experience instead the phenomena in their full reality as they present themselves . . . . .".[21] This means a conscious, lived participation in the patient's world and the acceptance of and respect for things as they are experienced.

A characteristic of the phenomenological approach is that the technique changes according to the needs of the patient in his social context. For us to effectively facilitate change in unsatisfying or inappropriate life task patterns our techniques of motivating, confronting, developing problem-identification and problem-solving abilities and providing change-oriented experiences, must be flexible and mobile, directed specifically to the patient's evolving ability to meet his life tasks.

Returning to our young patient Robert, we can see this concept in practice. At the time of evaluation, Robert existed in a minimal life space, possessing little mastery or sense of responsibility. This put him so out of touch with the possible life task options that he had no framework for considering his life tasks let alone undertaking them. His typical reactions to the subject were: "I guess I might have to go to work when I'm old and tired—around thirty . . . ." "Me have a girlfriend or family someday?! Never! I knew a girl once when I was seven and she hit me . . . ." "What do I like to do? Be a kid I guess."

Soon after the therapist became involved with Robert, it was evident that he felt great discomfort by being so out of TEMPO, even though he could not identify it as such. He seemed to have little of the propriate development and mastery needed to alleviate this disturbing situation. This distress caused a freezing effect whereby he could not take any steps to alleviate the anguish, lest he cause a disaster—to maintain his present course was to be teased and beaten up by children half his age; to "grow up" was to plunge into a fearful unknown.

The anxiety he was experiencing was viewed as stemming from his feeling of separation from an unyielding, contingent world. "Anxiety" as used here is based on Rollo May's definition: . . . . ."the state of the human being in the struggle against that which would destroy his being." The discomfort it caused was the first leverage we had for treatment, for despite his inability to do anything about it himself, he wished the tension it caused to be reduced. He felt nervous and alone.

The phenomenological approach used to identify the nature of his anxiety has been carried throughout his treatment. We began by focusing on his life space, for this seemed the most fundamental area of deficit and, in a sense, the correction of this became his first life task. By beginning here, the therapist put herself into his existing life space, experiencing it with him; in turn, Robert experienced the presence of another person and had to deal with this new relationship.

With an increase in mutual experiences, communication and consensual validation found in this relationship, came the increase in his ability to act, for he saw that changes were possible

without disaster. A growing mastery over his enlarging environment followed, as did an evolving sense of responsibility. Relearning—and new learning—had begun to take place in a developmental order.

Within this framework he began to know enough about himself and society so that the life task options of a young adult became less frightening. With the challenge and support of his therapist, he could now examine these options and begin to make choices.

The area of work illustrates this focus on life tasks. Robert had had no work experiences as a youngster and the thought of that unhappy state, adult-job holder, literally gave him the shakes. He could not imagine himself working. To orient him to being productive and masterful we made simple projects for Christmas gifts. With the budding confidence this gave him he became involved in an extended pre-vocational evaluation with me and a male occupational therapy assistant skilled in woodworking, the one school subject about which Robert had any pleasant memories.

Our interests ranged from basic perceptual motor functioning such as eye-hand coordination, dexterity, and speed/accuracy to his ability to follow directions, relate to fellow workers and develop work tolerance. However, Robert's participation in the program went beyond just the "doing". He joined in the planning and periodic reevaluation sessions, and used the woodshop experiences as grist for our discussion mill, focusing on his continually increasing life space, mastery and responsibility and his improving abilities to identify and resolve problems.

Within three months he was able to work in the shop five days a week, six hours a day. He was actively choosing and planning his own projects and was consciously trying to relate to the occupational therapy instructor as a work supervisor, not grade school teacher.

In our weekly sessions the issue of work as a social and personal experience had also come into focus. Exploration of work as a life task had now begun. He asked about my job and my feelings about work, took field trips to places where work was going on, i.e., shoe repair shops and grocery stores, and tentatively approached the possibility of work for himself before the age of thirty.

But what could he do? He felt he knew too little to hold a job—a far cry from being unable to conceive of himself working at all. We both agreed he needed an education and approached the State Rehabilitation Commission to finance his training. With the help of the rehabilitation counselor assigned from the Commission, he enrolled in a private trade school. His instructor and I have been in close communication, collaborating on what the school terms his personal adjustment.

A major part of his program has been getting

out in the world on his own. For example, he has been in charge of getting the coffee order during coffee breaks and has applied for part-time jobs with only an address and brief directions from his instructor. However, the school feels it will take longer than usual before he can fully enter the work-world, for his general experience is so limited.

Whether he will ultimately become a carpenter is still uncertain, yet they are willing to put in the time and effort, just as his rehabilitation counselor is willing to underwrite him as long as we continue to collaborate and Robert continues to progress. Because this commitment to Robert comes from three sources, much time has been spent in consolidating our approach to him in order to insure the continuing development of his ability to meet his life tasks.

Similar growth has been noted in other life tasks that he sees as his own. The techniques used to mobilize him have been graded to match the level at which he is currently meeting his life tasks and designed to provide the impetus to move him to a more mature level. The objects and activities used in this ever-changing process are based on his present, here-and-now needs. In one year he has moved from total immobility to becoming a young man, responsible for his own actions and life tasks in a world less contingent and alien.

Summary

Although our profession is building a body of theoretical knowledge, many of the fundamental concepts of occupational therapy remain unarticulated. These are the concepts that underly the practice of occupational therapy and unify the divergent interests of occupational therapists. They also delineate areas of dysfunction which can be treated through the occupational therapy process.

What has been described in this paper are four of these concepts considered basic to the occupational therapy process: life space, mastery, responsibility, life tasks.

Life space is described as the physical, perceptual, cognitive and psychological and sociocultural realm of an individual. Its development is based on learning through experience about the spacial and temporal extensions of one's private world. The nature and extent of an individual's life space is reflexed in his self-concept, internal experience of time and space and the actual components of his physical world. Dysfunction related to an individual's life space can be treated effectively through the active occupational therapy process.

Mastery is viewed as skill in comprehending and appropriately using one's human and non-human environment. Its development is based on an innate need to explore and manipulate, to be competent. The ability to be masterful, to recognize the choices society puts forth and make appropriate decisions, can be developed or enhanced by graded occupational therapy geared to problem-solving and skill-building.

Responsibility is defined as an individual's accountability for his own choices, decisions, and actions. Occupational therapy holds real potential for developing responsibility through the use of reality-oriented experiences which are based on mutual planning between patient and therapist.

Life tasks are the personal and social undertakings from which an individual gains satisfaction and to which he feels a commitment. They are derived from the general catagories of activities considered vital to the maintenance of our society. Individuals are expected to take the responsibility for choosing and meeting their life tasks at the appropriate times in their lives in order to keep in tempo with society while fulfilling propriate needs.

Occupational therapy can effectively deal with life task issues by utilizing a phenomenological approach in the occupational therapy process. Phenomenology in this context is understood to be the active participation in the patient's lived-world with acceptance of and respect for things as they are experienced. This phenomenological approach is relevant not only to life task issues but underlies all of the evaluation and treatment described.

REFERENCES

1. May, Rollo, (ed.), *Existential Psychology*, N.Y., Random House (1963), p. 76.
2. Lewin, Kurt, *A Dynamic Theory of Personality*, N.Y. McGraw-Hill Book Co., Inc. 1945, p. 179.
3. White, Robert, "Motivation Reconsidered: The Concept of Competence," *Psychol Rev* (1959).
4. Atkinson, J. and McLelland, N., *A Theory of Achievement Motivation*, New York: J. Wiley (1966).
5. Hebb, D. O., "Drive and the C.N.S.," *Psychol Rev* (1955).
6. Hendrick, I., The Discussion of the "Instinct to Master," *Psychoanal Quart* (1943).
7. Kardnier, A. and Spiegal, H., *War Stress & Neurotic Illness*, N.Y., Hoeber (1947).
8. Piaget, J., *The Origins of Intelligence in Children*, (Trans. by M. Cook) New York: Inter. Univer. Press (1952).
9. Arsenian, John, "Life Cycle Factors in Mental Illness," *Ment Hyg* (1968), p. 3.
10. Glasser, William, *Reality Therapy*, N.Y.: Harper & Rowe (1965), p. 14.
11. Erikson, E. H., *Childhood and Society*, New York: Norton (1952).
12. Havinghurst, Robert J., *Developmental Tasks and Education*, 2nd ed., N.Y., David McKay Co., Inc. (1952).
13. Pearce, J. and Newton, S., *The Conditions of Human Growth*, N.Y., The Citadel Press (1963).
14. Sullivan, H. S., *The Interpersonal Theory of Psychiatry*, N.Y., Norton (1953).

15. Irelan, Lola, (ed.), *Low Income Life Cycles,* Washington, D.C., U.S. Gov't Printing Office (1966).

16. Langer, T. and Michael, S., *Life Stress and Mental Health,* London, The Free Press of Glencoe (1963).

17. Leighton, A., "My Name is Legion," *Foundation for a Theory of Man's Response to Culture,* Illinois, Basic Books (1959).

18. Parsons, T. and Boles, R., *Family Socialization and Interaction Process,* Glencoe, Ill., The Free Press (1955).

19. Allport; G., *On Becoming,* New Haven, Yale Univ. Press (1955), pp. 40 – 57.

20. May, R., Angel, E. and Ellenberger, H., *Existence,* N.Y., Basic Books, Inc. (1958).

21. May, Rollo, *Existential Psychology,* N.Y., Random House (1963), p. 26.

Human Development through Occupation:

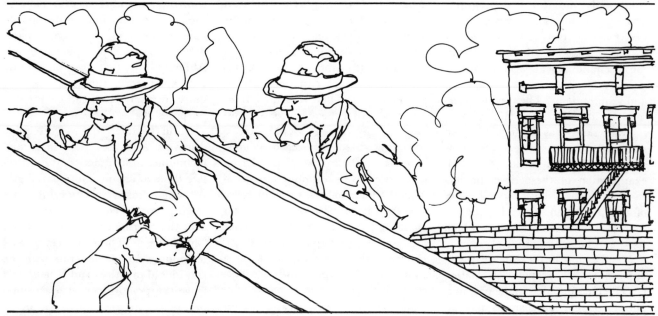

Theoretical Frameworks in Contemporary Occupational Therapy Practice, Part 1

Pat Nuse Clark

In 1968, the report of a conference sponsored by the American Occupational Therapy Association called for the development of an integrated theory of occupational therapy. A review of the practical problems faced by therapists today, contrasted with major developments in the art and science of the field during the past decade, suggests that this goal has not been attained. However, three major theoretical frameworks for therapy have evolved through the work of Fidler and Mosey, Wilbarger, and Llorens, who participated in the conference on theory. Reilly and associates developed a fourth framework of significance. Through analysis of theoretical constructs, generic concepts that

characterize occupational therapy can be identified. Theoretical constructs and research validation of the four approaches to occupational therapy are discussed in this article. A second article to appear in a subsequent issue of AJOT illustrates the use of the four theoretical frameworks to derive a philosophical basis for practice and a model of the practice process called "human development through occupation."

Pat Nuse Clark, MOT, OTR, is an Itinerant Occupational Therapist, Related/Support Services, Department of Special Education, Cobb County Public Schools, Marietta, Georgia.

What Are the Problems?

The scope and status of occupational therapy today is complex, changing, and often confusing. The explosion of knowledge and technology in the arts and sciences that support occupational therapy practice is sometimes overwhelming. Locales for practice have extended from medically based institutions to a seemingly infinite variety of community health, educational, and social service agencies. Trends in consumer rights, documentation and accountability of services, and Federal intervention in service delivery have made an impact on each service locale and provider.

These external influences have contributed to dynamic growth in the theory, practice, and critical issues of occupational therapy. It is equally apparent that therapists are continually initiating new programs and testing the parameters of practice. Even a cursory review of content in the discussions and literature of the discipline reveals a multitude of new service programs, approaches, and requirements. The task of determining, attaining, and maintaining relevant skills may be forbidding to students and experienced practitioners alike. However, a more thorough examination of these developments can help identify both the mandates of the profession, and also the resources and actions through which these can be achieved.

Membership in the American Occupational Therapy Association (AOTA) has doubled in the past decade. Each year four persons may apply for each available space in the basic professional curricula for occupational therapy. This growth may be caused by an increased interest in human service fields, and also to an agreeable job market in occupational therapy. Employment opportunities continue to open for new graduates and experienced therapists, and positions remain unfilled. Mandates for occupational therapy under Federal Medicaid and Education for the Handicapped programs are producing an even greater need for therapists and assistants, particularly for consultation and program development services.

In contrast, there are warnings that other professionals are usurping therapists' jobs because occupational therapy has been unable to clearly define its role, functions, and theoretical and research bases (1). Johnson (2) suggested that therapists have trained other service providers to use occupational therapy techniques, without demonstrating the broader range and value of their other serv-

ices. Yet the knowledge and research bases of the discipline have increased, if annual editions of *The American Journal of Occupational Therapy* (AJOT) and publications by therapists appearing in books and other journals are indicators.

Jantzen (3) and Acquaviva (4) made surveys of occupational therapy manpower. Their respective findings reveal that the average therapist devotes only three to four years in providing direct services to clients. Afterward, these therapists take on primary roles as administrators, educators, homemakers, or other roles. The shortage of positions for "master clinicians" in the traditional service facilities is well publicized (1,2). However, there also appears to be a shortage of therapists with the necessary inclination and clinical, educational, and research expertise for the many employment opportunities available in academic occupational therapy. An unfortunate result of the lack of master clinician positions and understaffed academic departments is the loss of potential research. Yet, research can justify the funding of master clinician positions.

There are recognizable contradictions among the strengths, weaknesses, and problems described thus far. These paradoxes suggest that the increase in both personnel and the literature, vital resources of the discipline, lack direction and organization.

Kielhofner and Burke (5) proposed that occupational therapy needs a new paradigm that can promote cohesiveness in the field and guide service and research. Their discussion was based upon the concepts developed by **Kuhn** in *The Structure of Scientific Revolutions* (6). Kuhn defined the paradigm of a discipline as its prevailing value system, which specifies for that discipline its theoretical assumptions, problem field,

methods to be used, and standards for problem resolution. He further described the process of paradigm construction and reconstruction over the course of time in four distinguishable phases: pre-paradigm, paradigm, crisis, and post-paradigm (6). Although the first two phases are self-explanatory, the latter two require further clarification for the purposes of this discussion.

Kuhn (6) stated that as a discipline discovers and uses new facts and techniques in its practice, it must relate these to its prevailing paradigm. Although many relationships are readily constructed and accepted, over the course of time there remain "anomalies." These concepts and techniques do not integrate with the traditional practices and beliefs, and leave the practitioner with a feeling of discomfort about what is being done and why. An example would be the therapist's use of the physical modalities of neuromuscular facilitation as a primary treatment program, with or without the accompaniment of a craft, recreational, or vocational activity.

These anomalies increase, either in number or in singular importance, as the discipline experiences a growing state of crisis. Eventually, the need for "retooling" becomes paramount and precipitates a search for a new way of approaching and doing things. Many schools of thought may develop and compete for construction of a new paradigm. Kuhn proposed that the crisis period is resolved in one of three ways. First, the old paradigm may ultimately handle the anomalies, and is not replaced. Second, no new schools of thought may be able to deal with an anomaly, so that it is set aside as a problem to be solved in the future. Third, a new and usable paradigm may emerge and gradually gain acceptance. The intradisciplinary conflict generated during the resolution of the crisis comprises the scientific revolution. Post-paradigm refers to the period of operation under the new paradigm (6).

Kielhofner and Burke (5) suggested that the new occupational therapy paradigm must be grounded in general systems theory and in the discipline's original concept of human occupation. These foundations would provide a holistic and dynamic view of humanity and related professional services. They also proposed that the new paradigm must allow for integration of the accumulated technology that developed through occupational therapy involvement with the rehabilitation movement. This would result in a system with linkages to those practices that have been found effective for dealing with specific remediative problems (5).

This writer believes that the elements of such a paradigm have been developed, but are obscured by the diversity of the practice and literature in occupational therapy today. A more visible organization is needed, one that documents the present art and science of occupational therapy, and that identifies the commonalities of resulting practices. The purpose of this paper (parts 1 and 2) is to attempt to meet that need. Special attention will be directed to those elements of theory and practice generated since 1967. This time period in particular represents a crisis phase in occupational therapy, as defined by Kuhn (6), and described by Kielhofner and Burke (5).

Functions of Theory in a Practice Profession. In 1967, a conference of occupational therapists was held in Albion, Michigan (7). This group (Fidler, Kovalenko, Llorens, Mosey, Overly, Wilbarger, and Mazer) served as the faculty of the AOTA Regional Institutes on Object Relations. Their task for the conference

"Biodevelopment"

was to develop a theoretical framework on human behavior that would be particularly relevant to occupational therapy. In their discussions considerable emphasis was placed upon the amount of time the group used to define mutual terms and concepts. They concluded that occupational therapy had fostered two theoretical routes for practice: the psychosocial (Man and his environment) and the neuro-behavioral (Man and his central nervous system) (7). Their conference report ("Toward an Integrated Theory of Occupational Therapy"), is a noteworthy effort to acknowledge the contributions of both approaches. In addition, three major conclusions of their report are pertinent to the present exploration of occupational therapy knowledge:

1. "This polemic separation (into two theoretical routes) has been disjunctive and is of questionable value in occupational therapy's movement towards professionalization . . ."

2. "Educators and practicing therapists must be provided with further opportunities . . . to truly integrate significant links between the numerous bodies of knowledge which impinge upon the occupational therapy experience . . ."

3. "Occupational therapy research must begin to search out the inter-relationships between seemingly parallel or even divergent theories as we test their validity for the occupational therapy process." (7, p 456)

Before the subsequent theoretical developments in occupational therapy are examined, it is useful to clarify the nature and functions of theory from several perspectives. First, what purpose does a theory serve for any field of study? Second, what are the special requirements of a theory for a practice-oriented discipline? And finally, how may theory be useful for occupational therapy practice in particular?

Black and Champion (8) postulated that *a theory provides a systematic way of thinking about data.* They defined a theory as a "set of systematically related propositions specifying causal relationships among variables." (8, p 56) In addition to including propositions, a theory will also include definitions and specify how its concepts may be applied. It is generally agreed that the components of a theory must be internally consistent, interrelated, and must be exhaustive in attention to the general range of variations within a given subject matter. This latter requirement determines the applicability of the theory. Finally, the variables and propositions of the theory must lend themselves to testing by research methodology (8, 9). In turn, the usefulness of data accumulated through research is determined by their conformation to accepted theory. It may be concluded that a field of study gains its credibility through its use of research methodology to test its theory, and its use of theory to test its methods and findings.

Agyris and Schon (9) have detailed requirements for theories that are used to guide professional practice. They stated that effective theories of practice must be able to guide the actions of the practitioner and also to predict the results of such actions. Practice was defined by Agyris and Schon as "a sequence of actions undertaken by a person to serve others,

"Occupational Behavior"

who are considered clients." (9, p 6) Thus, a theory of practice is a set of interrelated theories of actions, which will deliberately explain, control, and predict behaviors. Agyris and Schon suggested further that the effectiveness of a professional practice is dependent upon the congruence and consistency of its *espoused theories of actions* (what it thinks should be done) and its *theories in use* (what it does in fact) (9).

In his discussion of professional intervention, Maier (10) stated that all practice and research must have a theoretical foundation, but that the applicability of any theory will be determined by the nature of the service situation to which it is applied. This leads into consideration of the use of theory by occupational therapy. It seems apparent that, because of the diversity of client problems and locales for practice encountered by therapists, no one theory can be expected to guide all professional actions. Instead, a therapist must knowledgeably select and use those theories appropriate to a specific practice situation (9, 10).

In 1968, Mosey stated that the therapist's behavior is based upon the knowledge of cause and effect relationships and an understanding that the therapist's behavior follows those laws as well (11). Therefore, she concluded that a theory must identify four interrelated sets of phenomena for the practitioner. First, the theory must specify the *focus of interven-*

tion, or "that which the therapist seeks to alter." (11, p 6) Second, the desired outcome of intervention, or *state of function*, must be described. Third, the theory must enable the therapist to identify a *state of dysfunction*. Finally, the theory must prescribe and define the therapist's *actions* with the client (11).

More recently, Shapiro and Shanahan (12) discussed the teaching and use of theories in occupational therapy. They stated that the ability to use a theory-based approach to practice is what qualifies and differentiates such practice as professional. This includes the ability to "see a relationship between a client's need and a theoretical principle, and then to apply a technique on the basis of skilled prediction." (12, p 218)

In light of this discussion, it may be concluded that the development and use of theory and theory-testing in practice can and will define the validity of occupational therapy as a professional service. The theories developed for and through practice may be evaluated in terms of their capacity to define and describe that practice, including actions and technology; and their predictive value for the outcome of practice. The first two functions may be examined through Mosey's four sets of phenomena, which were described previously. The predictive value of an occupational therapy theory must be determined by its validation through research. For the purposes of this paper, the descriptive nature of theory is used to define the art of occupational therapy, and the predictive value will define its science.

Elements of the Art. It is appropriate to begin consideration of the growth of occupational therapy during the past ten years by considering the productivity of several Albion Conference members. Fidler and Mosey, Wilbarger, and Llorens to-

day represent three major theoretical approaches to human service delivery expressed as occupational therapy. A fourth approach, generated by Reilly, will also be discussed. Each of the four theoretical bases will be presented as it relates to the general scope of occupational therapy practice. To describe the approach only within the context with which a therapist is most associated may limit examination of its theoretical constructs. These constructs will be discussed as they have developed over the years, and are condensed in Table 1.

Adaptive Performance. In this paper, the work of Fidler and Mosey has been integrated to represent one major theoretical approach. The term *adaptive performance* was chosen to designate the common areas of study and often concurrent development of ideas that characterize the work of these two theorists.

Fidler's early work on refinement of the psychodynamic approach to occupational therapy (13) provided the foundation for a more general view of humanity and model for intervention. Continued study of the influence of sociocultural environments on human behavior led to a broader focus on ego functions, learning, and adaptive skills (14). This was illustrated in Fidler's use of the task-oriented group. In 1969, she discussed the goals and functions of these groups in occupational therapy:

The intent of the task oriented group is to provide a shared working experience wherein the relationship between feeling, thinking, and behaviors, their impact on others, and on task accomplishment can be viewed and explored . . . . The nature of the occupational therapy setting, which effects active involvement in doing, provides a microcosm

Table 1. Analysis of Four Theoretical Frameworks for Occupational Therapy

	Art of Occupational Therapy				Science of Occupational Therapy
Theory	**Focus of Intervention**	**State of Function**	**State of Dysfunction**	**Actions**	**Research Validation**
Adaptive Performance *Fidler* *Mosey*	Adaptive skills of doing Self-care Intrinsic gratification Service to others	Balance between skills and subskills promotes competence and efficacy	Imbalance due to influence of internal processes or external environment causes subskill deficits and problems of doing	Identify levels of functions in skills and subskills Provide shared learning experiences in life-work situations Promote subskill development	Descriptive Analytical Criterion-referenced measurements program plans
Biodevelopment *Ayres*	Developmental sequence of human biological processes	Integrative use of biological processes promotes adaptive skills\ Conceptualization Manipulation Socialization	Impairment of ability to process and act upon information received from the environment	Identify process deficits Use developmentally sequenced sensory motor activities, special techniques and equipment to normalize biological processes	
Facilitating Growth and Development *Llorens*	Physical, social, and psychological parameters of human life roles, tasks, and relationships	Mastery of tasks and relationships necessary to engage in life roles	Stress, trauma, or disease affect performance or achievement of necessary behaviors	Role of change agent Controlled use of purposeful activity to stimulate role behaviors Developmental analysis of problems	Quasi-experimental Descriptive/ Analytical Criterion-referenced measurements Standardized measurements Program plans Program modalities
Occupational *Behav.* *Reilly*	Acquisition and performance of work and play behaviors	Self-directed achievement of role requirements	Internal and/or external forces impair capacity for participation and adaptation	Promote exploration and competency of role requirements through identification and development of functions, habits, skills, and task performance	Descriptive/ Analytical Criterion-referenced measurements Program plans

of life-work situations which can be seen and explored as they occur rather than in retrospect. (14, p 45)

Until recently, the continued development of Fidler's concepts has been partially obscured by their presentation through the official literature of the AOTA. For example, her theoretical framework has weighed heavily in the construction of the "occupational performance" model, definitions and standards for practice and service reimbursement, and other official statements issued by the AOTA through the mid-70s. The subtle influence of Fidler's theory in current practice and education is estimable.

Fidler's major premise is "doing is being" (personal communication, 1976). *Doing* is defined as action with a purpose and serves as the focus of intervention. The random actions of an infant are replaced by purposeful, directed action through the mediation of the humanization process. Maturation and acculturation are the factors that influence this change. Fidler (15) identifies the three critical skill areas of *doing* as self-care, intrinsic gratification, and service to others. In a state of function, *doing* meets intrinsic needs for a sense of competence, and the needs of the environment by establishing the efficacy of the individual. Balance among the three performance skill areas varies according to age and culture. A skewing of the normal ranges of balance, due to the influence of the internal processes or external environment on subskills, leads to performance dysfunction. Occupational therapists deal with people who have problems of *doing* (15). The discipline is unique in that it has traditionally examined human behavior through the totality of a person's motor actions, and provided services through the modalities of

doing. Fidler has stated that therapists analyze and choose activities that "duplicate, simulate, or represent" the range of daily activities (personal communication, 1975).

Shortly after the Albion Conference, Mosey began to publish her theoretical framework for occupational therapy practice. She expanded concepts developed through study with Fidler into "recapitulation of ontogenesis." (16) Mosey stated that "the occupational therapist is concerned with assisting individuals to develop adaptive skills: those learned patterns of behavior which enable man to satisfy human needs and meet environmental demands." (11, p 65) The recapitulation framework presented a sequential developmental schedule for seven sets of subskills (both psychosocial and neurobehavioral), which broadly support adaptive skill development. Her premise was that occupational therapy actions would identify a client's levels of functions within subskill areas and facilitate that client's progression through the sequence of subskill development and integration to age-appropriate or environmentally required adaptive capacities (11, 16).

In concert with increased movement of the profession from medical facilities into the broader health community, Mosey looked further into the basic health needs of the individual. These were defined in 1973 (17) based upon the traditional hierarchy of Maslow, but with recognition of the additional literature supporting innate drives for excitation and activity. She then called for a reorientation of the organizational frame of reference for health service delivery. Rather than acquiescing to the constraints on practice imposed by alignment with the medical or public health models, she proposed that the profession define its service delivery system according to its edu-

cational roots in the biological, psychological, and social sciences (18). The biopsychosocial approach to health care, first mentioned by Reilly in 1969 (19), was defined further by Mosey to emphasize "man as a biological entity, a thinking and feeling person, and as a member of a community of others." (18, p 40) This describes the ideal state of function, and again, adaptive skill performance requirements to achieve and maintain this state serve as the focus of intervention. It becomes the role of the therapist to work with clients in a teacher-learner situation to solve problems in living (18).

Biodevelopment. Wilbarger, in cooperation with Ayres and others, has continued to investigate the effects of basic human biological functions on activity performance. This neuro-behavioral approach represents the second major knowledge base and practice orientation seen in occupational therapy today. Other primary practitioners associated with this theoretical framework during the past decade include Rood, the Bobaths, King, Moore, Huss, Farber, and Fiorentino. The term *biodevelopmental* is used here to integrate the variety of sensory-integrative, neurodevelopmental, neurobehavioral, and kinesiological theories and methods represented by these and similar authors. The biological processes serve as the main focus of intervention, and the therapist's actions are guided by the developmental sequence of these processes.

The theoretical premise is that normalization of sensory and motor patterns, and their integration for interaction with the environment, will promote adaptive development of conceptualization, manipulative, and social skills (20, 21). The actions specified by the biodevelopmental approach include the use of basic

"General Systems Theory"

sensorimotor activities, and special techniques and equipment that inhibit or excite the neural mechanisms. A state of dysfunction may be defined as the inability of the body to process or correctly act upon information received from the environment in an efficient, appropriate way (20). The theory base of the biodevelopmental approach has been derived from the neurosciences, ethology, the cognitive psychology of Jean Piaget, physiological psychology, and other experimental branches of the behavioral sciences (21). Moore has made numerous contributions to the art of this approach through publications that relate new evidence from the sciences to observable human function and dysfunction (22-24).

Facilitating Growth and Development. Llorens has continued to work toward an integrative model of occupational therapy practice that addresses the human life span from birth to death. In her 1969 Eleanor Clarke Slagle Lecture, she proposed that occupational therapists focus on the physical, social, and psychological parameters of human life tasks and relationships. Within this context, the therapist would look at individual functions and their integration, both during specific periods of life (horizontal development), and over the course of time (longitudinal development). The therapist's role is that of a change agent, facilitating the growth and development of the client (25).

In subsequent work, Llorens designed and described a systematic approach to the occupational therapy process, based upon the horizontal-longitudinal model of development. Through analysis of the life roles and expectations of the individual, and the potential effects of stress, trauma, or disease, on performance or achievement of necessary behaviors, one is able to identify consumer service needs (26, 27). The Developmental Analysis provides a self-connecting, self-correcting model for planning assessments, program goals, and methods (27). This model has recently been developed further to include a problem-oriented method of recording and evaluating the intervention process (28). Llorens described the art of the occupational therapy process as "learning to combine appropriate information from the basic science fields with knowledge of sensorimotor, developmental, symbolic, and daily life activities, and interpersonal relationships to help individuals to solve problems in their abilities to function." (27, p 1)

In recent unpublished work, Llorens explored the meaning of activity in the occupational therapy process. She suggests that the actions of the therapist involve the use of purposeful activity for organized, controlled stimulation of adaptive role behaviors in the client. Llorens hypothesized that direct and indirect stimulation of the central nervous system and other body systems can be controlled by the therapist through the activity process. Activities must be analyzed and selected for their relation to normalizing both the physical, psychological, and social components of individual task performance, and to the totality of life role performance (personal communication, 1977).

Occupational Behavior. In the theoretical framework of occupational behavior developed by Reilly and colleagues, it is proposed that the profession's most unique view of humanity, and therefore its focus of intervention, is through the acquisition and performance of those categories of human activities that occupy time, energy, interest, and attention. Reilly's initial proposal called for a return to the Meyerian categories of occupation in work, play, rest, and sleep (29), with a most concentrated examination of work and play behaviors (30).

Through extensive research of the literature relating to work and play, Reilly and associates have defined solid concepts of the components and sequential development of the functions, skills, habits, and tasks necessary to engage in occupational roles. Matsutsuyu stated that occupational behavior is grounded in the "sociological concept of role and socialization and by the psychological theories of achievement motivation, problem-solving, and personality development." (31, p 292) The occupational behavior framework is also allied to the general systems theory philosophy. In essence, this states that Man is a goal-directed creator of his own world, or culture (32), adapting through time and space (33, 34). The actions of the therapist are guided by Reilly's classic premise "that man, through use of his hands, as they are energized by mind and will, can influence the state of his own health." (35, p 2)

Basic to the occupational behavior approach is the client's exploration, competency, and achievement of occupational role requirements (36). Heard (37) proposed that occupational therapists work with clients who are chronically disabled. Chronic disease refers to "the presence of any physical, mental, or social handicap that disrupts or lessens man's

"Ontogenesis"

capacities for participation in and adaptation to his environment." (37, p 243) The actions of the therapist will enable the client to try out the tasks of different role requirements within situations structured to enhance the adaptive capacity of the individual and the adaptable nature of the task (37). Florey (38) developed the concept of intrinsic gratification as a determinant of task performance that must be stimulated by the therapist. Kielhofner (33) suggested that the therapist must consider the client's concepts and adaptive use of time in planning and performing tasks. Finally, Dunning (34) stressed the influence of environmental requirements and constraints on task performance, indicating that the therapist must enable the client to function outside of the service setting.

Elements of the Science. In his discussion of paradigms and scientific revolutions, Kuhn stated:

Few scientists will easily be persuaded to adopt a viewpoint that opens again to question many problems that have previously been solved . . . . The new candidate (for paradigm) must seem to resolve some outstanding and generally recognized problem that can be met in no other way. Second, the new paradigm must promise to preserve a relatively large part of the concrete problem-solving ability that has accrued to science through its predecessors. (6, p 169)

Perhaps it is these two requirements of a paradigm that have prevented occupational therapy from wholeheartedly endorsing any one of the four theoretical bases described. Two major problems of the profession were identified earlier as lack of a substantive research base to support its premises; and lack of a cohesive set of premises that organize its technological advances. Therefore, the general problem-solving ability and predictive value of the four theory bases need to be considered.

In general, the theories lend themselves to comprehensive analyses of human behavior and the activity process. Through examination of articles published in the *AJOT*, from 1967, two categories of content are prevalent. The first category identifies behavioral components that should be considered by the therapist, and describes how to recognize and grade these components with one or more client populations. Unfortunately, normative information is rarely included. In the second category, specific activity programs the therapist can use and adapt for designated client populations are proposed. Whether or not the activity program is truly meaningful to the client and effective in the client's life environment may not always be subjected to thorough analysis and measurement. A third type of paper, which would seem to meet the critical needs of the discipline, is noticeably scarce. This would be the analysis and testing of a theoretical approach through a total intervention process, using valid, reliable measurements and control or comparative groups.

In examining the science of the four theories, the biodevelopmental therapists appear to have made the greatest effort to document and evaluate the application of concepts through both measurement and programming. Examples of such research may be found in the series of reports on sensory integration research with various populations edited by Price, Myers, and Gilfoyle (39). Other comprehensive studies include Ayres' comparison of performance test scores with Gesell scores (40) and analysis of the relationships between test score clusters and program effectiveness (41), as well as Norton's study of biodevelopmental programming with severely retarded children (42). Measurement instruments have been standardized in varying degrees and program results have been tested. Although the results are not always statistically significant, at least this information is available to other therapists for use in decision making.

It seems fair to state that the adaptive performance and occupational behavior frameworks have generated comprehensive evaluation and program planning methods. There is less evidence of the relative value of data gathered, of the tested value of program plans, and of modalities used to implement planning. Reports of programs are generally descriptive, and are confined to one subject or group of subjects (14, 15, 30, 33, 37). Quantitative data and use of control or comparative groups are generally not reported. Although the value of descriptive research is not questioned, the need for other types of measures is apparent.

Llorens' early research in design, implementation, and evaluation of programs for children with behavioral and learning problems lends credibility to the theoretical constructs developed later (43, 44). Her recent work with Schuster in documenting program sequence and results (28) goes one step further and should produce valuable data in years to come.

Although the theoretical constructs of the four frameworks have potential for application with many populations encountered by therapists, the reported testing of such constructs has been with limited populations. There is little information about the tested use of adaptive performance and occupational behavior programs with clients who manifest physical dysfunctions as primary problems. Also, minimal information is available about the effectiveness of programs designed to facilitate the growth and development of adult clients. Although the biodevelopmental approach has been tested and reported with a variety of age and diagnostic groups, because of the focus of intervention, researchers have often failed to report on changes in performance of life roles and tasks.

Discussion

Occupational therapy is a discipline that has produced and adopted a considerable amount of theoretical content and technology, but has yet to pull these together in a scientifically meaningful way. For example, changes in scar tissue formation on burned clients following the use of special occupational therapy technology have been documented (45). However, there is no information about subsequent changes in that client's life style and body image, which are visibly altered by the treatment modalities used. Rather than the two approaches to practice found in 1967, there are now at least four. One can observe evidence of conflict, cultism, and bias among the four approaches, particularly on the part of the advocates of the different theorists. This would indicate that occupational therapy is indeed in a state of scientific revolution and has been unable to integrate its content through one generally acceptable paradigm.

One such attempt deserves recognition. During the 1970s, the conceptual model called "occupational performance" evolved through the official functions and literature of the AOTA (46). It was an attempt to present a uniform language base and practice focus to the general public. The areas of performance pertinent to occupational therapy were identified in this model as play-leisure, work, and self-care. Performance of these activities is dependent upon the integrated development of six performance component functions: sensory-integrative, motor, cognitive, social, psychological, and cultural/economic. The term *life space* was used to designate the temporal, physical, and cultural mileau of the client. These terms have been used extensively in defining roles and functions of occupational therapy personnel, as well as in standards for practice, education, and legislation. The weaknesses of the occupational performance model are that it is basically a collection of terms and it has no visible, organized theoretical base to support its use. This limits its ability to address the thinking and technology of the field in a consistent manner that spans age and diagnostic groups. In addition, testing the model in practice has not been reported.

Summary

This first of two papers was concerned with the art and science of contemporary occupational therapy. Examination of the resources, issues, and atmosphere of current practice revealed some perplexing contradictions in the strengths and weaknesses of the field. It determined that much of the confusion resulted from a fragmentation of occupational therapy personnel and literature during a time of tremendous growth in the theory and technology that support

service delivery. The two critical problems of occupational therapy were identified as the lack of a substantive, disciplinary research base, and the lack of a cohesive set of disciplinary premises to organize the technology used by therapists. Despite the recommendations of a group of occupational therapy theorists in 1968 (7), the growth of theory and research since then has lacked collaborative effort. Underlying much of the fragmentation and areas of conflict in the discipline is the need for an acceptable paradigm that can organize and support the scope of occupational therapy practice.

Four significant theoretical frameworks for occupational therapy were readily identified through a review of literature. Fidler and Mosey described concepts of occupational therapy that promote the "adaptive performance" of clients. Llorens defined the practice of therapy as "facilitating growth and development." A group of "biodevelopmental" theorists studied the neuromotor components of task performance. Reilly and associates defined and described "occupational behavior" as the focus of practice.

The functions of theory in the description and prediction of professional practices were reviewed, and a model for the analysis of a theory was selected. This analytical model, developed by Mosey, identifies four sets of phenomena: the focus of intervention, the state of function, the state of dysfunction, and the therapist's actions (11). The four theoretical frameworks were summarized according to these constructs, and their validation through research and problem-solving ability was critiqued.

The next article will describe the combination of generic and bridging concepts from the four theoretical frameworks into a philosophy of practice for occupational therapy. It is proposed that occupational therapy subscribes to a belief in "human development through occupation." Through systematic use of the theoretical and philosophical bases, a conceptual model of the occupational therapy process was derived and will be presented. Practical application of the derived model in client programs, education, and research will be discussed.

REFERENCES

1. American Occupational Therapy Association: Report of the Mental Health Task Force. *Am J Occup Ther* 30 (9):6-7, 1976
2. Johnson JA: Delegate Assembly Address: Commitment to action. *Am J Occup Ther* 30: 135-148, 1976.
3. Jantzen AC: Some characteristics of female occupational therapists, 1970, Part II. Employment patterns of female occupational therapists. *Am J Occup Ther* 26:67-77, 1972
4. Acquaviva FA: AOTA Human Resources Project, IV. The member data survey—demographic characteristics of occupational therapy personnel. *Am J Occup Ther* 29:426-432, 1975
5. Kielhofner G, Burke JP: Occupational therapy after 60 years: An account of changing identity and knowledge. *Am J Occup Ther* 31: 675-689, 1977
6. Kuhn TS: *The Structure of Scientific Revolutions*, Chicago: University of Chicago Press, 1970 (second edition)
7. American Occupational Therapy Association: Conference Report: Toward an integrated theory of occupational therapy. *Am J Occup Ther* 22:451-456, 1968
8. Black JA, Champion DJ: *Methods and Issues in Social Research*, New York: John Wiley and Sons Inc, 1976
9. Agyris C, Schon DA: *Theory in Practice: Increasing Professional Effectiveness*, San Francisco: Jossey-Bass Publishers, 1974
10. Maier H: *Three Theories of Child Development*, New York: Harper and Row, 1965
11. Mosey AC: *Occupational Therapy: Theory and Practice*, Medford, MA: Pothier Brothers Inc, 1968
12. Shapiro D, Shanahan PM: Methodology for teaching theory in occupational therapy basic professional education. *Am J Occup Ther* 30:217-224, 1976
13. Fidler GS, Fidler JW: *Occupational Therapy: A Communication Process in Psychiatry*, New York: Macmillan Co, 1963
14. Fidler GS: The task-oriented group as a context for treatment. *Am J Occup Ther* 23:43-48, 1969
15. Fidler GS, Fidler JW: Doing and becoming: purposeful action and self-actualization. *Am J Occup Ther* 32:305-310, 1978
16. Mosey AC: Recapitulation of ontogenesis: a theory for the practice of occupational therapy. *Am J Occup Ther* 22: 426-438, 1968
17. Mosey AC: Meeting health needs. *Am J Occup Ther* 27: 14-17, 1973
18. Mosey AC: An alternative: the bio-psychosocial model. *Am J Occup Ther* 28: 137-140, 1974
19. Reilly M: The educational process. *Am J Occup Ther* 23: 299-307, 1969
20. King LJ: A sensory-integrative approach to schizophrenia. *Am J Occup Ther* 28: 529-536, 1974
21. Ayres AJ: *Sensory Integration and Learning Disorders*, Los Angeles: Western Psychological Services, 1972
22. Moore JC: *Neuroanatomy Simplified: Some Basic Concepts for Understanding Rehabilitation Techniques.* Dubuque, IA: Kendall/Hunt Publishing Co, 1969
23. Moore JC: *Concepts from the Neurobehavioral Sciences,* Dubuque, IA: Kendall/Hunt Publishing Co, 1973
24. Moore JC: 1975 Eleanor Clarke Slagle Lecture: Behavior, bias, and the limbic system. *Am J Occup Ther* 30: 11-19, 1976
25. Llorens LA: 1969 Eleanor Clarke Slagle Lecture: Facilitating growth and development: the promise of occupational therapy. *Am J Occup Ther* 24: 1-9, 1970
26. Llorens LA: The effects of stress on growth and development. *Am J Occup Ther* 28: 82-86, 1974
27. Llorens LA: *Application of a Developmental Theory for Health and Rehabilitation*, Rockville, MD: American Occupational Therapy Association, Inc, 1976
28. Llorens LA, Schuster JA: Occupational therapy sequential client care recording system: A comparative study. *Am J Occup Ther* 31: 367-371, 1977
29. Meyer A: The philosophy of occupation therapy. *Am J Occup Ther* 31: 639-642, 1977
30. Reilly M: A psychiatric occupational therapy program as a teaching model. *Am J Occup Ther* 20: 61-67, 1966
31. Matsutsuyu J: Occupational behavior: a perspective on work and play. *Am J Occup Ther* 25: 291-294, 1971
32. Von Bertalanffy L: *General System Theory: Foundations, Development, Applications*, New York: George Braziller, 1968 (revised edition)
33. Kielhofner GW: Temporal adaptation: A conceptual framework for occupational therapy. *Am J Occup Ther* 31: 235-242, 1977
34. Dunning H: Environmental occupational therapy. *Am J Occup Ther* 26: 292-298, 1972
35. Reilly M: 1961 Eleanor Clarke Slagle Lecture: Occupational therapy can be one of the great ideas of 20th century medicine. *Am J Occup Ther* 16: 1-9, 1962
36. Reilly M: An explanation of play. In *Play as Exploratory Learning: Studies in Curiosity Behavior*, M Reilly, Editor. Los Angeles: Sage Publications, 1974, pp 117-149
37. Heard C: Occupational role acquisition: A perspective on the chronically disabled. *Am J Occup Ther* 31: 243-247, 1977
38. Florey LL: Intrinsic motivation: the dynamics of occupational therapy theory. *Am J Occup Ther* 23: 319-322, 1969
39. Price A, Gilfoyle E, Myers C (Editors): *Research in Sensory-Integrative Development*, Rockville, MD: American Occupational Therapy Association, Inc, 1976
40. Ayres AJ: Relation between Gesell developmental quotients and later perceptual-motor performance. *Am J Occup Ther* 23:11-17, 1969
41. Ayres AJ: Cluster analyses of measures of sensory integration. *Am J Occup Ther* 31: 362-366, 1977
42. Norton Y: Neurodevelopment and sensory integration for the profoundly retarded multiply handicapped child. *Am J Occup Ther* 29:93-100, 1975
43. Llorens LA, Rubin EZ: *Developing Ego Functions in Disturbed Children*, Detroit: Wayne State University Press, 1967
44. Rubin EZ, Braun JS, Llorens LA et al: *Cognitive-Perceptual-Motor Dysfunction: From Research to Practice*, Detroit: Wayne State University Press, 1972
45. Larson DL, Absten S, Evans EB, et al: Techniques for decreasing scar formation and contractures in the burned patient. *J Trauma* 11: 807-823, 1971
46. *A Curriculum Guide for Occupational Therapy Educators*, Rockville, MD: American Occupational Therapy Association, Inc, 1974

(A list of related readings is available upon request from the author.)

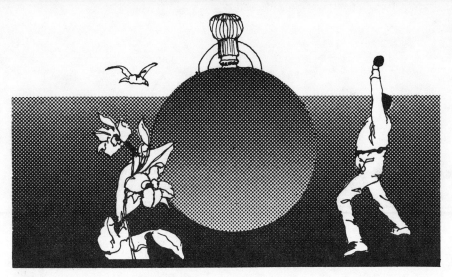

Human Development through Occupation: A Philosophy and Conceptual Model for Practice, Part 2

Pat Nuse Clark

The development of a philosophy of practice called "human development through occupation" is described in this paper. This philosophy was developed through study and identification of generic concepts in four major theoretical frameworks for occupational therapy described in a preceding article. The philosophy of practice proposes a view of Man, a view of human health, and a view of the profession. These theoretical and philosophical resources are then used to construct a conceptual model of the content and sequence of the occupational therapy practice process. It is believed that the four theoretical frameworks, philosophy of practice, and conceptual model detailed in these two papers can provide direction for general practitioners and specialists in service, education, and research. Examples of application are included, together with suggestions for further investigation.

Pat Nuse Clark, MOT, OTR, is an Itinerant Occupational Therapist, Related/Support Services, Department of Special Education, Cobb County Public Schools, Marietta, Georgia.

In the first of two articles, a review of practical problems faced by contemporary occupational therapists was contrasted with major developments in the art and science of the field during the past decade. In 1968, a group of theorists identified two prevalent approaches to practice as the psychosocial and neuro-behavioral, and called for the development of an integrated theory of occupational therapy through collaborative research efforts (1).

In the review of subsequent literature, it was determined that four distinguishable theoretical approaches now dominate occupational therapy practice. These were identified as the "adaptive performance" theory of Fidler and Mosey; the "biodevelopmental" framework of Ayres, Wilbarger, and others; the Llorens approach known as "facilitating growth and development," and the "occupational behavior" framework developed by Reilly and associates. The operational constructs of these four theoretical frameworks were reviewed, and the testing of constructs through research methodology was critiqued.

In the conclusions of the first article, it was stated that occupational therapy has produced and adopted a considerable amount of theoretical content and technology, but has yet to pull these together in a scientifically meaningful way. Underlying much of the fragmentation and areas of conflict in the discipline today is the need for a unifying value system, or paradigm, that can organize, support, and delineate the scope of occupational therapy practice.

Silva (2) suggested that the first step in developing a curriculum for occupational therapy is the statement of the philosophy upon which service is based. This would include

Figure 1
Conceptual model of the philosophy of practice

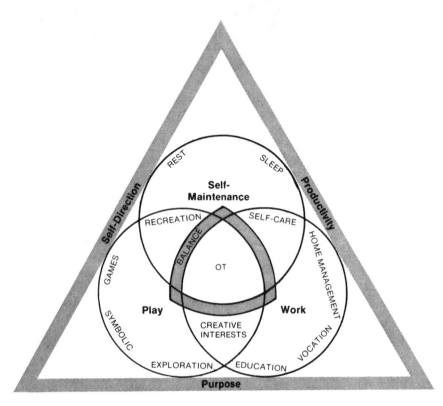

a view of Man (as broadly representative of human beings), a view of health (or focus of intervention), and a view of the profession. This philosophy should be derived through study of what is known and valued in a field, and should clarify the content of the curriculum (2). Silva's suggestion can be applied to the practice of occupational therapy as a whole. The philosophy of occupational therapy described by Meyer in 1922 remained the primary resource for many of the theoretical constructs described in the first article, and recently attracted new attention through a second publication (3). Although it still provides a breathtaking sense of recognition, Meyer's philosophy does not account for the cultural, theoretical, and technological changes that have taken place in Man, health care, and the profession since it was first published.

It is proposed that the philosophy for practice in occupational therapy needs to be updated and restated. This can lead to identification of the necessary paradigm for the field today, and therefore clarify the content of occupational therapy practices in service, education, and research. The purposes of this paper are to state a philosophy of contemporary occupational therapy practice, and to present a conceptual model for the practice process derived through use to the stated philosophy and the four theoretical frameworks. A conceptual model is defined as an abstract representation of a process, which is communicated through written, spoken, or pictorial form (4). The conceptual model will then be related to service, education, and research functions in occupational therapy.

The first task in describing a philosophy of practice is to identify what constructs are of importance to the field (2). This was done through the analysis of the four theoretical frameworks, and examination of the occupational performance conceptual model of the American Occupational Therapy Association (AOTA) (5). Although areas of disagreement exist among these four theories, it is the identification of the areas of agreement that is critical. A connecting concept found between the four theoretical approaches is that the occupational therapy view is of Man as an adaptive creator. This provides the starting point for the proposed philosophy by "human development through occupation." (This philosophy derived its name from the title of a course developed by the author at Towson State University. Credit for the title is extended to the Towson State College Occupational Therapy Curriculum Planning Committee.) In its total presentation of philosophy and conceptual model for the practice process, "human development through occupation" has a character that is different from any of the four theoretical frameworks discussed because it is derived from all. Names of supportive references are deleted from the philosophy for a smooth presentation of statements.

Philosophy of Practice
View of Man

Human adaptation is distinguished by Man's capacity to purposefully effect his own world of self, culture, and environment. The unique richness of this creative function is the product of two biological characteristics: the ability of the human brain to formulate and symbolize concepts, (6,7) and the ability of the human hands to translate concepts into action (8,9). Man's awareness of these abilities promotes the will for purposeful activities (8,10).

Purposeful activities are further described as the goal-directed use of a person's resources, time, energy, interest, and attention (9,11). Related to this concept is another: that Man spends most of his time occupied in certain types of purposeful activities. There is a recognized sequence to the emergence and primary engagement of such occupying activities (12). This includes the development and use of:

Self-Maintenance. Including self-care, sleep, rest, recreation, and other activities directed toward preservation of the self and the species (3, 13), and preparation for play and work.

Play. As the anticipator and facilitator of subsequent goal-directed activities. Play includes sensorimotor exploration, symbolic activities such as drawing and dramatics, and games. The behaviors acquired through playful exploration of the self, culture, and environment serve as the bridge to adult competence and creative achievement (7).

Work. As the economic function of Man in his world, and the healthy state of Man the achiever (7, 13). Work includes educational, vocational, and home-management activities (see Figure 1).

View of Health

Man's ability to direct and effect his own purpose in life may be seen as a most unique and primary indicator of his general well-being, or health. Man maintains health through a flexible balance of work,

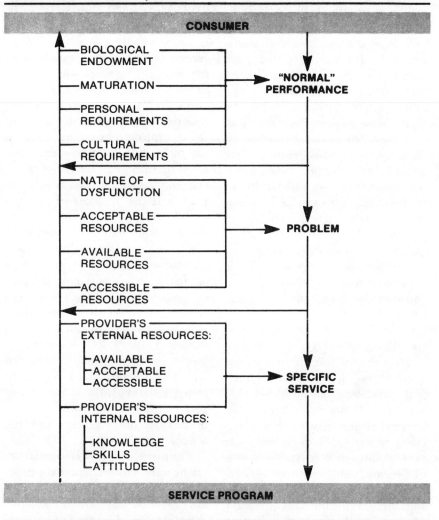

Figure 2
A continuum of health and dysfunction

play, and self-maintenance activities, which develop and change throughout the life span (3, 8, 13).

In a healthy state, the individual is able to adapt and achieve a satisfying life, function adequately in chosen personal, sexual, and occupational roles, and enjoy a sense of well-being (14, 15). Role performance involves the use of selected purposeful activities, including the various skills, habits, tasks, and relationships acquired through the acculturation of the individual (8, 11, 16). The healthy performance of

roles is influenced by four major factors. First, the person's basic *biological endowment*, which includes the various body systems, functions, and genetic capacities, provides the individual with the potential to develop and learn a variety of skills. Second, there is a hierarchical *maturation* of these basic components, as the individual grows and accommodates to changing environments, assimilating new experiences, and learning. Together, these physiological characteristics account for a foundation of sensory-integrative, motor, and cognitive functions that permit the development of adaptive skills (7, 8, 11, 17, 18).

The interaction between the individual and cultures, physical space, and other environmental elements becomes increasingly complex throughout the life span. Therefore, task performance must change and adapt as it is influenced by the third factor group of *cultural, spatial, and temporal requirements*. The individual must learn to effect a satisfying balance between meeting internal needs and adapting to external influences. The emergent *personal* requirements change in concert with the three other factors and are the fourth determiant of one's "normal" performance. The human processes that develop through the interaction of these internal and external forces provice a foundation of psychological and social functions (7-11, 16, 17, 19-21).

Throughout life, the individual encounters physiological, social, and psychological problems that may or may not impede performance of various roles. Analysis of the effect of the problem on adequate performance and critical elements of development is both qualitative and quantitative (22). Several questions arise. Is the individual capable of resolving the problem, adapting to, or coping with it independently? Or, is the nature of the problem such that it threatens to disrupt, delay, or impair functions or life role skills, or both? If the problem is sufficient to cause dysfunction in the individual's performance and balance of daily tasks and roles, what resources are available, acceptable, and accessible to the individual? (see Figure 2)

View of the Profession

It is the heritage and concern of occupational therapy that the aware-ness of Man's special need for both purpose and balance in living be applied to health service delivery (8, 9). Occupational therapy may be viewed as an applied health service concerned with the quality and satisfaction of daily living from birth to death (22). The scope and delivery of such service may be as complex and varied as the nature of human occupation (23). It is the belief of the discipline that "man, through use of his hands, as they are energized by mind and will, can influence the state of his own health" (9, p 2). It is the mandate of occupational therapy to provide services that facilitate man's achievement of health through occupation in purposeful activity (3, 3, 11, 13). Inherent in this mandate is a second: that occupational therapy must be relevant to the time, cultures, and environments of the consumer's health needs (13, 18, 22, 24). Accordingly, service programs must be designed and implemented that use goal-directed, meaningful, and age-appropriate activities to influence quality of human development and life adaptation.

The therapist's role is to assist the client with those adaptation processes necessary to promote a balanced, satisfying, and productive life style (23). The core of occupational therapy service delivery is the therapist's use of activity analysis and adaptation processes. Both analysis and adaptation of the activity are determined by the functional components and developmentally antecedent skills required for task performance. The intervention process will require attention to the enhancement and integration of sensory-integrative, motor, cognitive, psychological, and social functions *as these relate to performance* of daily activities. The outcome of occupational therapy service deliv-ery is determined by the client's mastery of tasks and relationships necessary to actively engage in play, work, and self-maintenance (22).

The occupational therapist may work with consumers in varied age and diagnostic groups, in the broad spectrum of health care, educational, and social service settings. Services provided include assessment of the client's performance of play, work, and self-maintenance tasks, and the design, execution, and evaluation of client-specific, goal-directed activity programs. The goals of occupational therapy intervention (23) are always related to:

1. The *development* and *maintenance* of functions and skills necessary for performance of desired and/or required activities;

2. *Prevention* of inadequate development, deterioration, and/or loss of those functions necessary to engage in play, work, and the various self-maintenance activities;

3. *Remediation* or rehabilitation of dysfunction that impairs acceptable performance of daily activities;

4. *Facilitation* of the consumers' adaptive capacity to influence and change their own health status through each successive stage of life; and

5. *Collaboration*, communication, and cooperation in the planning and achievement of goals with the client and significant others in the client's life, including family and other service providers.

**Conceptual Model of the
Occupational Therapy Process**

In essence, the practice of occupational therapy must be directly related to each client's overall mastery of occupational roles, and also support achievement of goals and balance in the broader scope of personal/sexual and social roles. There-

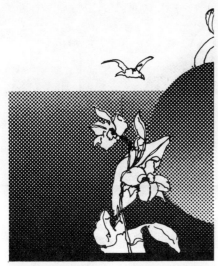

fore, the therapist must be familiar with the human development process, its functional and skill components and sequence, and must relate these to the needs generated by an individual's status within a continuum of health and dysfunction (23). Figure 2, which depicts the statements of the "human development through occupation" view of health, also represents the process through which a consumer might encounter occupational therapy services.

Similarly, the components of the philosophy of practice and its theoretical foundation may be used to construct a conceptual model of the occupational therapy intervention process (also known as practice process). Figure 3 illustrates the general content, sequence, and service functions of the process, which will be described in further detail. This model was originally adapted from Llorens' Developmental Analysis (25) but has been expanded and subjected to considerable language revision.

The constructs of "human development through occupation" suggest there are modalities and processes that are generic to the occupational therapy process. The processes are *activity analysis and adaptation*. The modalities include the use of selected *occupational activities, relationships, special adaptation techniques, tools, materials,* and *equipment*. Occupational activities are selected from the play, work, and self-maintenance categories described earlier, based upon

the analysis of functional components, developmentally antecedent skills, and relevance to the role requirements of the client. The therapist can also structure and make use of the human and object relationships inherent in the activity situation. The activity itself can be adapted using concrete and abstract techniques to be discussed later. The tools, materials, and equipment of goal-directed activities are also subject to analysis and adaptation. These modalities may be used both to assess and enhance the performance of the individual, throughout the occupational therapy process.

Assessment

The initial contact between the therapist and client serves as a General Performance Screening. It is necessary to determine *whether* a client has problems in play, work, and or self-maintenance behaviors. Also, referral to additional disciplines and resources may be neccessary for effective problem identification and resolution. The therapist must determine whether occupational therapy intervention would help or hinder.

These decisions are usually based on data from a variety of resources, and a General Problem Analysis. Several basic assessment methods may be used by the therapist. First, the therapist will *observe* the client, preferably within an uncontrived activity performance situation. Skilled observation requires that the therapist carefully use all senses, and record data objectively. Whenever possible, the therapist will conduct short *interviews* with the client, significant members of the family and/or associates, and others on the service delivery team. The components of a good interview were described by Gillette as care-

fully structured, open-ended questions; unbiased observing, listening, and feedback; and objective recording of data (26). Next, a *performance-based screening test* may be administered to the client to identify developmental level, general performance capacities and weaknesses. Use of a standardized developmental evaluation is recommended, since it will provide a normative baseline for continued assessment as well as descriptive information that may be used for program planning.

General Problem Analysis, adapted from Llorens (22, 25), is a thought process used by the therapist to guide preliminary planning. As described in the view of health section, the therapist will consider the client's age and life roles, critical elements of development for the age and task/role requirements, and compare these with the potential effects of the presenting problem on the client's performance functions and skills. The therapist may then evaluate data collected in the screening process with relation to the potential effects on performance predicted by the General Problem Analysis.

This preliminary part of the assessment process can begin to determine what the client needs to be able to do that he or she cannot do in order to satisfy self, family, and society. Results of screening and general problem analysis will also guide the design of further evaluation as the therapist seeks to determine the more exact nature and degree of a client's functional capacities and performance skills, as well as program goals. Comprehensive Assessment includes:

1. *Life Space Data Collection* (5). Through *history-taking, interviews,* and *field observations,* the therapist defines the client's life roles and

environmental, cultural, and performance requirements. External resources, alternatives, and barriers to performance are identified.

2. *Evaluation of Component Functions of Behavior.* Formal and informal measures of functional capacity are used to determine *why* a client has performance problems. This information may be collected directly by the therapist through observation, interviews, and administration of *standardized and criterion-referenced tests of performance.* Data may also be collected from other service providers and resources through use of record review and *consultation.* Interpretation of the assembled data will provide a picture of the client's capacities and deficits in the five component functions (see Figure 3, Short-term Program).

3. *Evaluation of Occupational Role Performance.* Concurrently, the therapist will measure the client's ability to perform specific activities required in daily self-maintenance, work, and play roles. The variety of assessment methods used remains the same, but with focus on total task performance. Evaluations of performance of these activities will be both qualitative and quantitative, and will also identify the appropriateness of balance between the three role activity categories in the client's daily schedule. For example, can the client put on a shirt without assistance within a reasonable time period?

Program Development and Evaluation

Through the assessment process, the therapist will determine client-specific performance dysfunctions and problems: what areas and type of activity performance require intervention and why. The client's program goals can then be devel-

oped through consideration of the person's capacities and personal expectations, prognostic analysis of the effect of the problem(s) upon goal-achievement, and the availability of occupational therapy and other services. Program goals will be consistent with the general goals of occupational therapy, as described previously and shown in Figure 3. Program goals may be general in nature, but, when combined with the assessment data, will allow for the construction of specific objectives that the client may achieve. Llorens (27) suggested that these objectives should be measurable and specify what tasks the client will perform in order to demonstrate goal achievement.

Next, a therapy program is designed to meet those objectives, based upon the therapist's use of the activity analysis process with generic modalities. Program activities may be adapted to facilitate goal-achievement if inadequate function or skill development interferes with performance. Adaptation techniques include modification of activities according to the position of the body or work surface, as well as the choice of tools, materials, techniques, or equipment used in activity performance. The therapist may manipulate the activity process itself, breaking a task down into simple-to-complex, step-by-step progression. Another type of activity adaptation takes place when the therapist works with the client and significant others to alter expectations for independence in a specific task.

Most frequently, the initial, short-term goals and program will be directed toward improving basic capacities of the five component functions (see Figure 3). This practice is supported by the theoretical frameworks presented in the pre-

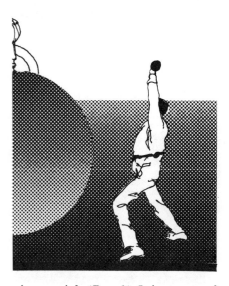

vious article (Part 1). It is proposed that most programs should begin with attention to the physiological components (sensory-integrative, motor, and cognitive functions) because research reports support the effectiveness of this approach in early programming (28-30). The long-term program and objectives are concerned with promoting acceptable performance in required role activities. At different intervals throughout the process, the therapist will retest and reassess the performance status of the client and program effectiveness. Goals and objectives of programming must maintain relevance to the changing needs of the client. A two-directional review of the intervention process, as outlined in Figure 3, may be used to check relationships between and within components of assessment data, program goals and objectives, and program modalities.

The theoretical frameworks and philosophy suggest that, throughout the intervention process, the therapist is concerned with development, integration, adaptation, competence, and initiative in task performance. Therefore, therapy is directed toward providing opportunities to enhance the individual's preparedness to deal with the requirements of daily living. The tools of the occupational therapist are the activities of daily living in the broadest sense (23). The processes of activity analysis and adaptation are the core functions of the occupational therapist. Together, these tools and processes of the discipline

Figure 3 Conceptual model of the occupational therapy process

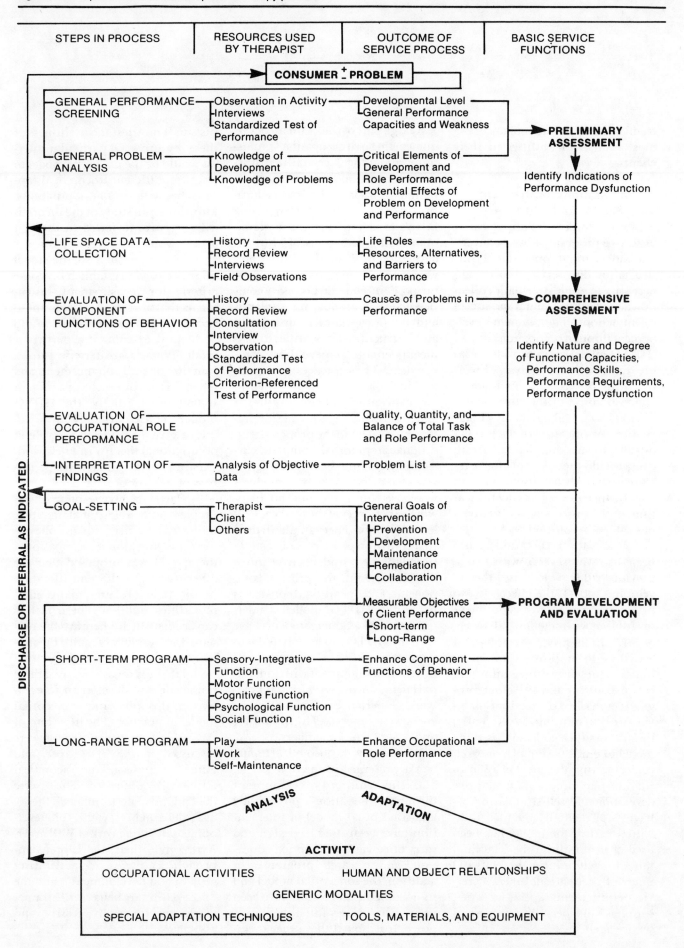

| STEPS IN PROCESS | RESOURCES USED BY THERAPIST | OUTCOME OF SERVICE PROCESS | BASIC SERVICE FUNCTIONS |

CONSUMER ± PROBLEM

GENERAL PERFORMANCE SCREENING
- Observation in Activity
- Interviews
- Standardized Test of Performance

- Developmental Level
- General Performance Capacities and Weakness

PRELIMINARY ASSESSMENT

GENERAL PROBLEM ANALYSIS
- Knowledge of Development
- Knowledge of Problems

- Critical Elements of Development and Role Performance
- Potential Effects of Problem on Development and Performance

Identify Indications of Performance Dysfunction

LIFE SPACE DATA COLLECTION
- History
- Record Review
- Interviews
- Field Observations

- Life Roles
- Resources, Alternatives, and Barriers to Performance

EVALUATION OF COMPONENT FUNCTIONS OF BEHAVIOR
- History
- Record Review
- Consultation
- Interview
- Observation
- Standardized Test of Performance
- Criterion-Referenced Test of Performance

- Causes of Problems in Performance

COMPREHENSIVE ASSESSMENT

Identify Nature and Degree of Functional Capacities, Performance Skills, Performance Requirements, Performance Dysfunction

EVALUATION OF OCCUPATIONAL ROLE PERFORMANCE
- Quality, Quantity, and Balance of Total Task and Role Performance

INTERPRETATION OF FINDINGS
- Analysis of Objective Data
- Problem List

GOAL-SETTING
- Therapist
- Client
- Others

- General Goals of Intervention
  - Prevention
  - Development
  - Maintenance
  - Remediation
  - Collaboration

Measurable Objectives of Client Performance
- Short-term
- Long-Range

PROGRAM DEVELOPMENT AND EVALUATION

SHORT-TERM PROGRAM
- Sensory-Integrative Function
- Motor Function
- Cognitive Function
- Psychological Function
- Social Function

- Enhance Component Functions of Behavior

LONG-RANGE PROGRAM
- Play
- Work
- Self-Maintenance

- Enhance Occupational Role Performance

DISCHARGE OR REFERRAL AS INDICATED

ANALYSIS ADAPTATION

ACTIVITY

OCCUPATIONAL ACTIVITIES   HUMAN AND OBJECT RELATIONSHIPS

GENERIC MODALITIES

SPECIAL ADAPTATION TECHNIQUES   TOOLS, MATERIALS, AND EQUIPMENT enable therapists to enhance the most human of abilities in their clients.

Implications for Research, Service, and Education

In order to develop any research or service program, a basic conceptual model and its operational constructs for that service process are necessary to guide systematic collection and analysis of data, and subsequent actions. The "human development through occupation" model (HDTO model) does provide a usable framework for analysis of relationships between its components and evaluation of the effectiveness of a total occupational therapy intervention. Application of the HDTO model with any one client or group can provide the elements for a research study within itself, through its sequence of problem-identification, problem-solving, and analysis of problem-resolution.

To date, the HDTO model has been used in several ways. In a previous study, which used the developing model, the effects of two programs on adaptive development of children with cerebral palsy were compared. One program emphasized activities to improve component functions of sensory integration and motor control, and the other program emphasized play and self-maintenance skill training (30). Recently, the author and a colleague used the model to guide design of a research project testing the effect of a sensorimotor play program on adaptive developmental self-stimulating behaviors of mentally retarded individuals. Also, the model has been used of determining the focus and range for determining the focus and range of occupational therapy service requirements, space, facilities, supplies, and personnel in several service agencies.

A large part of the "human development through occupation" philosophy and model crystallized during preparation of a curriculum design for basic professional education in occupational therapy. Using Silva's model of curriculum development (2), constructs of "human development through occupation" were used to identify curriculum purpose and content, necessary competencies of graduating students, and the appropriate learning theory and instructional modalities to enable students to achieve those competencies. The sequence of the occupational therapy process shown in the conceptual model (Figures 2 and 3) generated a sequence for presenting content in the proposed educational program. Although the curriculum design has not been tested yet, several of its content modules were used in academic and fieldwork experiences at the Medical College of Georgia. For example, in their first course on principles of occupational therapy, students were introduced to the practice process, components, and operational constructs using the HDTO model. Undergraduate and graduate students have used the HDTO model and its documentation record for case study and program development with individual clients during level I and II fieldwork experiences. These experiences were supervised by the author and other faculty members.

In summary, the theoretical frameworks presented in the first article, and the "human development through occupation" philosophy and conceptual model of intervention have been used to design and carry out a variety of service, education, and research programs. In addition, the conceptual model and its documentation record have been used by associates for similar purposes. It is hoped that other therapists will now test the usefulness of these resources. Of particular interest would be the use of the model to test the different theoretical approaches with similar populations. More in-depth study of the theoretical references reviewed in the first article would be necessary for any such investigation. Also, the model might be used to establish outcome criteria for measurement instruments that are specifically useful to occupational therapists. It would be helpful to know if a particular modality has a greater effect upon function or skill enhancement, and when, in the course of a program, it is best used. Finally, the HDTO model, conscientiously applied, might give direction to the role of occupational therapy in a new work situation, and validate the usefulness of services provided.

In Part 1, a review of practical problems and professional literature indicated the need for a cohesive force and direction in occupational therapy. It was proposed that the diversity of practice and literature in the field obscures many commonalities, but that generic factors can be identified. These articles presented an overview of major theoretical frameworks found in occupational therapy today, and used these frameworks to develop an integrative philosophy and conceptual model of practice. The functions of theory for a practice profession were discussed in the first paper, and guided analysis of the theoretical frameworks presented. These were the "adaptive performance" theory of Fidler and Mosey; the "biodevelopmental" framework of Wilbarger, Ayres, and others; the Llorens approach known as "facilitating growth and development"; and the "occupational behavior" framework developed by Reilly and associates.

Summary

"Human development through occupation" is proposed as the philosophy that unites and is derived from the four theoretical frameworks discussed in Part 1. The HDTO philosophy suggests a model of the occupational therapy process that demonstrates the integrated sequence of actions suggested by generic constructs of the four frameworks.

Theoretical constructs were selectively applied through different portions of the "human development through occupation" philosophy and conceptual model. The designated categories of occupational activities that serve as the focus of intervention relied heavily on occupational behavior theory. The influence of the adaptive performance concept is most evident in the philosophy of practice and in the language of the conceptual model. The basic structure of the conceptual model is derived from the Developmental Analysis proposed by Llorens (22, 25). Finally, the research findings of the biodevelopmental theorists have guided the sequencing of program objectives and modalities in the conceptual model.

Examples of the use of these frameworks, philosophy, and conceptual model were described. It was proposed that these resources can be used by other therapists in service, research, and education settings to guide assesment, program development, and program evaluation. Suggestions for application of the "human development through occupation" resources by other therapists were included.

Acknowledgments

Appreciation is extended to generous friends, colleagues, and teachers, through whom concepts were developed and clarified. The assistance of Leslie Dessauer and Shirley Esenther in construction of graphic materials is gratefully acknowledged. Parts of these papers were developed during work on a joint publication with Stella Gore Lansing (23) and others in partial fulfillment of graduate course requirements of the Occupational Therapy Departments of the University of Florida and the Medical College of Georgia.

REFERENCES

1. American Occupational Therapy Association: Conference Report: Toward an integrated theory of occupational therapy. *Am J Occup Ther* 22: 451-456, 1968
2. Silva D: Components in program development. *Am J Occup Ther* 30: 586-575, 1976
3. Meyer A: The philosophy of occupation therapy. *Am J Occup Ther* 31: 639-642, 1977
4. Conte JR, Conte WR: The use of conceptual models in occupational therapy. *Am J Occup Ther* Ther 31: 262-265, 1977
5. *A Curriculum Guide for Occupational Therapy Educators*, Rockville, MD: American Occupational Therapy Association, Inc., 1974
6. von Bertalanffy L: *General Systems Theory: Foundations, Development, Applications*, New York: George Braziller, 1968, revised edition
7. Reilly M: An explanation of play. In *Play as Exploratory Learning: Studies in Curiosity Behavior*, M Reilly, Editor. Los Angeles: Sage Publications, 1974, pp 117-149
8. Fidler GS, Fidler JW: Doing and becoming: purposeful action and self-actualization. *Am J Occup Ther* 32: 305-310, 1978
9. Reilly M: 1961 Eleanor Clark Slagle Lecture: Occupational therapy can be one of the great ideas of 20th century medicine. *Am J Occup Ther* 16: 1-9, 1962
10. Florey LL: Intrinsic motivation: the dynamics of occupational therapy theory. *Am J Occup Ther* 23: 319-322, 1969
11. Llorens LA: 1969 Eleanor Clark Slagle Lecture: Facilitating growth and development: the promise of occupational therapy. *Am J Occup Ther* 24: 1-9, 1970
12. Matsusuyu J: Occupational behavior: a perspective on work and play. *Am J Occup Ther* 25: 291-294, 1971
13. Reilly M: A psychiatric occupational therapy program as a teaching model. *Am J Occup Ther* 20: 61-67, 1966
14. Bertrand AL: *Social Organization: A General System and Role Theory Perspective*, Philadelphia: FA Davis Co, 1972
15. Pelligrino E: Preventive health care and the allied health professions. In *Review of Allied Health Education I*, J Hamburg, Editor. Lexington: The University of Kentucky Press, 1973, pp 1-18
16. Heard C: Occupational role acquisition: A perspective on the chronically disabled. *Am J Occup Ther* 31: 243-247, 1977
17. Mosey AC: Recapitulation of ontogenesis: a theory for the practice of occupational therapy. *Am J Occup Ther* 22: 426-438, 1968
18. Moore JC: 1975 Eleanor Clark Slagle Lecture: Behavior, bias, and the limbic system. *Am J Occup Ther* 30: 11-19, 1976
19. Moore JC: *Concepts from the Neurobehavioral Sciences.* Dubuque, IA: Kendall/Hunt Publ Co, 1973
20. Kielhofner GW: Temporal adaptation: A conceptual framework for occupational therapy. *Am J Occup Ther* 31: 235-242, 1977
21. Dunning H: Environmental occupational therapy. *Am J Occup Ther* 26: 292-298, 1972
22. Llorens LA: *Application of a Developmental Theory for Health and Rehabilitation*, Rockville, MD: American Occupational Therapy Association, Inc., 1976
23. Lansing SG, Carlsen PN: Occupational therapy. In *Interdisciplinary Approaches to Human Services*, P Valletutti, F Christoplos, Editors. Baltimore: University Park Press, 1977, pp 211-236
24. Mosey AC: Meeting health needs. *Am J Occup Ther* 27: 14-17, 1973
25. Llorens LA: The effects of stress on growth and development. *Am J Occup Ther* 28: 82-86, 1974
26. Gillette N: Occupational therapy and mental health. In *Occupational Therapy*, HS Willard, CS Spackman, Editors. Philadelphia: JB Lippincott Co, 1971, Fourth Edition, pp 51-131
27. Llorens LA, Schuster JA: Occupational therapy sequential client care recording system: A comparative study. *Am J Occup Ther* 31: 367-371, 1977
28. King LJ: A sensory-integrative approach to schizophrenia. *Am J Occup Ther* 28: 529-536, 1974
29. Norton Y: Neurodevelopment and sensory integration for the profoundly retarded multiply-handicapped child. *Am J Occup Ther* 29: 93-100, 1975
30. Carlsen PN: Comparison of two occupational therapy approaches for treating the young cerebral-palsied child. *Am J Occup Ther* 29: 267-272, 1975

(A list of related readings is available upon request from the author.)

Psychiatric Occupational Therapy:
Search for a Conceptual Framework in Light of Psychoanalytic Ego Psychology and Learning Theory*

KAREN DIASIO, M.A., O.T.R.†

Kurt Lewin once said "There is nothing so practical as a good theory." Reflecting upon the truth of that remark for psychiatric occupational therapy, we find it easier to understand the growing efforts being made to link theory with practice. In addition to providing the cornerstone upon which to base our professional mandate, theory guides our efforts in organizing isolated bits of information into a meaningful mosaic which can be used in framing strategies for treatment. It also ensures that useful observations and strategies will not be lost to future practitioners, and it provides the soil which nurtures our budding efforts to do research.

This paper explores two broad aspects of theory which are especially important to the practice of occupational therapy. FIRST, what *motivational constructs* are most relevant to the concerns of occupational therapy, since motivation provides the wellsprings of and antecedents to the behaviors with which we must deal, and upon which we must draw in energizing our patients' efforts in their own behalf. The problem of motivation is intrinsically interwoven with the problem of development, as Thompson and Schaefer have pointed out,[1] and particularly merits our study when behavioral difficulties such as schizophrenia and perceptual-motor deficits are thought to reflect a faulty developmental process. SECOND, any theory relevant to occupational therapy must deal with *the role that the environment plays in influencing man's behavior,* since the *manner* in which we energize our patients' efforts consists in providing or structuring environmental stimuli to promote beneficial change.

* Presented at the 47th Annual Conference of the American Occupational Therapy Association, Boston, Mass., October 15-21, 1967.

This paper was written during the tenure of a VRA graduate traineeship in psychology, Columbia University Teachers College. It contains extended references for the many who had particularly expressed interest in them.
† State University of New York, Downstate Medical Center, Brooklyn, N.Y.

In order to highlight the manner in which these dimensions are relevant to occupational therapy, the paper contrasts two approaches which attempt to chart the theoretical grounds from which our practice springs forth. The first of these approaches is perhaps most extensively set forth by the Fidlers. Stating in their book that "without a sound understanding of the unconscious, the concept of occupational therapy can be neither realized nor understood,"[2] they have stressed the importance of object relationships, including persons and things. They state:

A thing must be identified as that with which an instinctual impulse is gratified. It is this feature of instinctual gratification that gives it importance as a diagnostic or therapeutic tool. . . . With development of speech and ability to form abstract concepts, the individual learns to search with increasing effectiveness for objects to gratify instinctual needs and reduce tension.[3]

As an example, they describe how for one patient, the making of a pottery vase can represent genital instinctual gratification or for another it may represent oral or anal gratifications. They state that a knowledge of psychoanalytic dynamics "makes it possible to guide the patient toward gratification of needs and/or toward healthier, more constructive, sublimation."[4] Gradually, the patient moves toward activities less symbolic of the original needs.

In treatment, which is separated from mental health processes and rehabilitation, they state "utilization of real and symbolic significance of object relations and action marks the major contribution. . . . Emphasis on process rather than end product is of prime importance."[5] Their book makes little or no reference to problem-solving, learning or goal-direction apart from the analytic paradigm described above.

A different orientation has been suggested by Reilly and others, who focus more specifically upon the productive role of the individual as the modal point around which occupational therapy will center its appraisal and its treatment efforts. Reilly states that the capacity for productivity

> proceeds along the path of growth as man learns to intermesh his motor and his intellectual functions and adapt this integration to the tasks of his life which satisfy his need to control his environment. The focus is on the meaningful involvement in problem-solving tasks or creative performances. . . . The goal of the (occupational therapy) process is to encourage active, open encounter with the tasks which would reasonably belong to his role in life.[6]

Reilly sees psychoanalytic theory as focusing too exclusively on subjective reality and too little on objective, problem-solving reality. Stein, critical of the use of arts and crafts for sublimation such as the use of clay as an "outlet for hostility," thinks that we should more appropriately equip our patients with adaptive skills such as those provided by prevocational activities.[7] Jones focuses specifically upon the vast store of occupational therapy practices which can be more adequately understood in terms of learning theory.[8] Diasio and Jones discuss the work adjustment process, giving examples of the means by which we facilitate the acquisition of new behavioral repertoires and intervene into faulty ones.[9]

There are differences in the approaches which are worth-while examining more closely. The first draws heavily from some traditional psychoanalytic concepts, whereas the second stresses adaptive learning. The procedure was, after identifying the theories to which these models refer, (1) to examine their assumptions regarding motivation and environmental influences, and (2) to see if there were any converging trends which may lead to a fruitful synthesis between them by relating them to developments in other fields of psychology. This paper first examines Freudian theory, then its extension by the ego analysts and finally, therapy based on learning theory, for their conceptions of motivation and environment. Then it examines other trends in psychology which may lead to convergence between them, along with the implications and meaning they may hold for occupational therapy.

Freudian Psychoanalytic Theory

In the Freudian psychoanalytic movement, Freudian theory assumes that man is impelled to reduce tension or anxiety produced by instinctual drives. The infant adapts to reality only because it is necessary to do so to reduce drive states induced by a thwarting environment. Throughout life, behaviors are selected because they ultimately lead to *drive reduction.* Thus the purpose of thought or cognition, for example, was the control of motor behavior in order to both ensure instinctual gratification and avoid negative consequences.

Freud stressed mainly the defensive, rather than the adaptive, nature of the ego, which served the "three harsh masters" of id, superego and environment in an effort to avoid anxiety. As Ford and Urban have commented, "If this is true, life is considered to be one constant defensive battle."[10] Indeed, Freud once said that it was saddening to "know" that the contributions of society had come at the expense of the instincts.[11] Although the environment provided gratifications for the instinctual drives, Freud focused primarily on its restricting or frustrating aspects. Drives assume motivational primacy; the environment does little but mold behavior in various directions.

Freud's notion of ego has been expanded in recent decades by certain of his followers. Theoreticians such as Rapaport and Hartmann have stressed that man is capable of guiding himself in his environment through adaptive as well as defensive capacities. Concepts such as conflict-free ego sphere, and ego autonomy, have clearly enlarged the range of human abilities operating apart from libidinal or destructive drives.[12] It also seems clear, however, that the notion of instinctual drive is *basically* retained when Hartmann says that ego autonomy derives from neutralized sexual and aggressive impulses[13] and refers extensively to sublimation,[14] and when Rapaport states that thought processes are cathected.[15] These concepts seem only to highlight, as Baldwin puts it, "the basic assumption that all types of behavior, thoughts, feelings and other psychological processes, conscious or unconscious, are ultimately motivated by instinctual drives."[16]

It is in the formulations of Hendrick that we can see a significant departure from the psychoanalytic drive reduction model of motivation. Specifically, Hendrick postulated the existence of the *work principle,* which is "that primary pleasure is sought by the efficient use of the central nervous system for the performance of well-integrated ego functions which enable the individual to control or alter his environment."[17]

In concentrating upon defensive mechanisms, Hendrick states, psychoanalysis has neglected the study of the executant functions by which man perceives, appraises and manipulates his environment, and has generally assumed that once interpsychic conflict is resolved, work ability is "automatically restored." He says that "the functional use of minds and hands and tools is a primary pleasure and that its derivation from the 'need to master' is a more reasonable hypothesis than the assumption — implicit or otherwise — that work is always primarily a sublimation of sexual fantasies."[18]

The motivating force, therefore, is not drive reduction leading to quiescence, but rather the *efficient utilization of the individual's ability to control his environment* — a concept similar to that pro-

51

posed by Adler decades ago.[19] Hendrick's ideas, however, seemed not to have gained widespread acceptance in analytic circles. Instinct theory seems to have remained intact, although modified and given a considerably different emphasis by the ego analysts. Rapaport, for example, saw the instinctual drives as serving to *prevent* man from "being molded like putty by environmental forces."[20] Thus man is no longer seen as driven by instincts; instead he is conceived of as being a "pilot" over the environment precisely *because* of instinctual drives.

How then do the ego analysts view the role of the environment? Hartmann concedes that the social structure has a bearing on the frustrations and possibilities of sublimation available to the individual, but goes on to say that

the effect finally seen is on the most superficial layer of the personality. These effects one does not see on the psychic structure nor on the ways conflicts are resolved, etc., but merely on the choice of rationalizations, the conceptual language, certain psychic contents, and so on.[21]

Shortly before his death, Rapaport conceived of man's need for "stimulus nutriment" to ensure the ego's autonomy from the id, in light of Piaget's work and sensory deprivation studies,[22] but he was never to expand on this concept. By and large, it has been conservatively interpreted in treatment terms, such as face-to-face contact and more active intervention methods with certain patients.[23] Thus, although some analysts have begun to develop the theory to account more adequately for environmental influences in shaping man's development, translation into treatment practices based on theory has been rather limited.

This is reflected even in Searles' book, *The Nonhuman Environment,* one of the most extensive explorations yet into defining the contribution of non-human and subhuman objects in man's development.[24] Although specifically wishing to close an acknowledged gap between occupational therapy and psychoanalytic theory, he focuses his work mainly upon the need for empirical observation rather than the formulation of innovative treatment techniques stemming from the patient's interaction with environment.

It is significant that the concept of stimulus nutriment and man's adaptive ability has led some ego analysts to question the effect of hospitalization on the individual.[25] Although greatly enlarged since Freud's day, the role of the environment, or stimulus situation, remains an underdeveloped area in psychoanalytic theory. Many are also critical of psychoanalytic conceptions of motivation, as mentioned earlier in this paper, centered exclusively on notions of drive reduction. Holt has stated that "the concept of the passive nervous system whose function is to rid itself of stimulation . . . is

demonstrably wrong and constitutes the part of (psychoanalytic) theory that is most glaringly in need of revision.[26]

Neff, for example, reviewing the vast psychoanalytic literature, located only a handful of articles dealing with the topic of work[27] — with most explaining it in terms of sublimation.[28] These inadequacies account for some of the discomfort we have felt due to the lack of "fit" between psychoanalytic theory and the basic assumptions inherent in the occupational therapy experience.

Behavior Therapy and Learning Theory

We shall turn now to an analysis of motivation and environment in learning theory, the parent theory of that intriguing newcomer to the therapeutic scene, behavior therapy. A cursory review of the literature in behavior modification would convince most occupational therapists that the principles utilized in behavior therapy are similar to many of the unlabeled techniques we have used over the years. Furthermore, research evidence is accumulating that behavior therapy can be effective even with chronic schizophrenics who are totally mute and withdrawn.[29] Advocates of behavior therapy are critical of psychoanalytic therapy for stressing insight over actual behavior change, and for reifying "underlying" causes and disease concepts while ignoring the importance of current behavior and "symptoms," and how they are maintained by present environmental conditions.

In stimulus-response learning theory, the environment assumes the leading position in the causality of behavior. Man is considered a product of his learning experiences; given specific stimuli, man must automatically respond. Patterns of behavior are seen to be "increased, shaped, and maintained through reinforcement."[30]

Over the years, however, there has been an evolution in learning theory toward a recognition that central processes, or "intervening variables" as Tolman called them,[31] mediate between stimulus and response in order to explain many goal-directed behaviors. A growing group of neobehaviorists, including Berlyne, [32,33] Hebb,[34] and others, have been increasingly absorbed in what goes on in the "black box" *between* stimulus and response in the form of cognitive processes.

Before elaborating on motivational concepts in this form of cognitive behaviorism, it is important to recognize that the thrust of behavior therapy has inherently buttressed the position of occupational therapy as a treatment modality. The emphasis on the importance of analyzing the "demand characteristics" of the environment and its central role in initiating and maintaining behavior,[35] its use of specific stimuli, presented in small, graded steps in real-life situations, and the recognition that old problems explored do not fully answer the need for new modes of behavior to be learned and mastered through action — all these are congruent with occupational therapy assumptions, and they are impactful contributions to psychosocial therapy.

Our inquiry into motivation, however, has not yet been adequately covered because drive reduction has held sway in learning theory, although some behavior therapists, especially proponents of the Skinnerian operant conditioning paradigm, have questioned this. Therefore, let us turn now to the developments in experimental and cognitive psychology (mentioned earlier) which give rise to the clearest picture yet of the motivational forces relevant to occupational therapy, and which may eventually link some currently diverse elements in psychoanalytic and learning theories.

Other Psychological Developments

Psychologists began to turn their attention to the fact that man does not passively await stimuli, to which he automatically or invariably responds, as in traditional stimulus-response theory, nor is he impelled by drives to rid himself of stimulation, as in Freudian theory. Rather, recent experimental evidence clearly shows that both humans and animals actively seek out stimulation from the environment and will go to some lengths to obtain it — as perhaps any parent has wearily observed. White points out that rats will cross an electrified grid merely for the privilege of exploring new terrain,[36] and Harlow, Butler, Welker, and others have shown that monkeys can be rewarded by access to visual stimulation, or will for hours busy themselves with manipulating and exploring latches, locks, or other stimuli which may be novel, surprising, incongruous, or complex, quite apart from physiological needs such as hunger or sex.[37]

Furthermore, there is ample evidence that there are certain critical periods in the developmental timetable when stimuli are needed to activate physical and mental systems, their lack producing severe deficits.[38] The sensory deprivation studies confirm the fact that man, even when fully developed, is in constant need of stimuli and cannot maintain himself totally apart from the physical environment.[39] Studies of impaired or delayed feedback testify as to our dependence on stimulation for maintainance of our developed abilities such as speech and motor tasks.[40,41]

The aforementioned curiosity-exploratory studies intermesh well with the theory that we seek an optimal level of stimulation from our environment.[42] If there is too much stimulation, we seek to reduce it; if there is too little, we seek to increase it. This emphasis on the self-regulating nature of man's behavior as he adapts to his environment fits well into the larger picture provided by the information-processing and communication approach

used in behavioral cybernetic theory. Here the focus leads away from the deterministic views either of the primacy of man's drives or of environmental stimuli in directing behavior.

Instead, our attention is drawn to a study of the mutual transactions and communications which occur between them and which affect both, and for the moment there is no better practical example of this approach than the transactional analysis used by Berne in *Games People Play*.[43] You can recognize that this theoretical approach differs from both traditional psychoanalytic and stimulus-response motivational concepts, while retaining the ego analysts' notion of man unbound by "stimulus slavery" and capable of adapting himself effectively to his environment, and retaining from learning theory the profound importance of the environment in influencing man's actions. In this theoretical formulation, man, through his actions, acquires information about his environment in order to control what happens to him.

Smith and Smith state that *sensory feedback mechanisms* define the interaction between individual and environment. Progressive changes or transformations in feedback pattern through maturation and learning lead, they state, to an "elaboration of man's ability to exercise symbolic control over himself and over other people and environmental events."[44] The environment is of central importance for informational input or stimulation and therefore for the determination of the appropriate response, which is "defined by the tools and equipment, symbol systems, institutional structures and materials of consumption of contemporary society."[45]

Hunt calls the mechanism of motivation inherent in information-processing and action *intrinsic motivation,* whereby cognitive processes develop through interaction with the environment — as Aquinas, Montessori, Piaget, Hendrick and others have observed.[46] Guilford states that "the hypothetical role of motivation intrinsic within the operation of the eyes and ears in psychological development gives new meaning to the notion of organism-environment interaction and points to a radically changed conception of the role of experience in the development of both intelligence and motivation."[47] Furthermore, he says, "It would seem that the best hope at present for putting purposive or goal-seeking aspects of motivation into scientifically respectable form is through an application of the kind of thinking demonstrated by . . . cybernetics."[48]

One of the best illustrations of this view is the theme of the magnificent film shown at the New York World's Fair, "To Be Alive!" It contrasts in a most moving way the hustle of modern living — those extrinsic but adaptive behaviors in which we all must engage as we push through the subways and crowds — with the quiet joy of a child exploring the awesome beauty of the world around him through a prism glass, a world that turns wondrously as he pumps his swing into daring arcs or flies down the path in a scooter, a world revealing its surprises and complexities and yielding to his efforts at exploration and mastery.

Intrinsic motivation means that man has an innate need to manipulate and explore, to stimulate himself by doing and thinking. It is here that occupational therapy may some day best define its contribution to man's well being. A most important contribution has been made by Robert White to integrate these motivational concepts with psychoanalytic theory by proposing *competence motivation*.[49] Noting, as did Piaget, that young children give their closest attention to objects upon which it is possible through their own action to produce large effects, he proposes that the energy behind this force be referred to as *effectance,* and the relating affect the *sense of effectance.* Effectance leads to an accumulating knowledge of the effects of action upon the environment, and he states that "the inanimate environment, while it is not as important as the human one, clearly takes the lead as a means of reality testing."[50]

White states that *competence* may be regarded as the cumulative result of the history of interactions with the environment, with the *sense of competence* referring to the subjective evaluation of one's consciously felt competence, or self-esteem, in dealing with the environment. He proposes that independent ego energies, rooted in neurophysiological mechanisms, are the source of competence motivation, and that this conception allows for an integration of our knowledge concerning learning, skill acquisition, concept formation, and neurophysiology, with psychoanalytic theory.

Turning to social learning theory, we find that White's sense of competence is very similar to Julian Rotter's *control expectancy* concept, which refers to the person's feeling that he possesses or lacks the control, by means of his own behavioral repertoires, to obtain desired goals from the environment.[51] It is also similar to Atkinson and McClelland's *achievement motivation* theory, which has investigated the person's desire to achieve success and avoid failure.[52,53] Lefcourt has reviewed at length research generated by Rotter's internal-external control of reinforcement concept.[54] Internal control of reinforcement refers to "the perception of positive and/or negative events as being a consequence of one's own actions and thereby under personal control." On the other hand, external control of reinforcement refers to "the perception of positive and/or negative events as being unrelated to one's own behaviors in certain situations and therefore beyond personal control."

It is rather significant that this concept is virtually identical to sociologists' definition of alienation.[55] Responses of individuals who have external control scores paint a revealing and familiar portrait — of persons who find it difficult to evaluate their own skill but easy to resort to failure-avoidant strategies, who do not expect success in taking risks or in performing tasks but instead prefer immediate gratifications, who do not utilize available information for their own gain and participate minimally in effecting social change on their own behalf. If they are schizophrenic, they prefer structured situations over those which require autonomy.[56]

Implications for Occupational Therapy

This portrayal of the attitudes and behaviors of patients could serve as an example of the kind of baseline observations we make of patients in occupational therapy. The fact that these observations can be adequately rooted in theory, rather than that they stand apart from the "psychodynamics" of a case, represents a real advance for the position that occupational therapy can be a prime modality in psychosocial treatment. This is particularly true in a society that demands so much and rewards so heavily for competence and achievement.

It is further suggested in research by Lefcourt and Ladwig, showing that behavior based on a low estimate of effective control can be changed through the new self-conceptions gained through competence and mastery of skills.[57] We have all seen patients gain hope and show reawakened self-esteem as they begin to take some risks in exposing themselves to uncertainty or failure in proportion to the successes they have experienced through forming clay, typing a first letter, or successfully completing a task earlier viewed with apprehension.

Over time, we try to reawaken that intrinsic motivation which may have ben suffocated in the collision of environmental stress with individual deficit, or which for one reason or another the environment may never have allowed to develop. We encourage a pride in mastery which comes from a task well done, even if relatives or society may take it for granted. Initially, extrinsic motivation such as money, food, social reinforcement or its withdrawal, may be necessary to bring the patient to engage in an activity, but evidence shows that once he is engaged, self-reinforcement from intrinsic motivation can take over[29,58]—that ephemeral "sense of accomplishment" to which we so often refer.

As Bruner points out, "one *teaches* readiness or provides opportunities for its nurturance, one does not wait for it."[59] Readiness, comprised of mastery of simpler skills gained first through manipulation and actions and leading to the development of symbolic processes from perception to conceptual categorization, enables the person to establish self-reward sequences as he realizes that "learning one thing permits him to go on to something that was before out of reach."[60]

The sequence leading from action to categorization and conceptualization unfolds in human development and is true even of adult learning. This sequence adds support to the belief, found in the structural-functional and interactional schools of social psychology,[61] that behavior change precedes or can beget attitude change. For certain patients, unable to participate meaningfully in verbal insight therapy where attitude change is presumed to precede behavioral change, occupational therapy might be the treatment of choice because it echoes this developmental sequence leading from the concrete to the abstract. Indeed, French and Alexander once observed that insight seems more a result than a cause of behavior change.[62]

In occupational therapy, consequences of action are concrete and tangible as well as immediately available for evaluation and categorization. This can facilitate feedback and the adoption of new strategies through which competence is gained. The graded interchange of information, some verbal and some non-verbal, which is set into motion by the therapist's and patients' participation together in an action setting, becomes a vehicle which facilitates feedback and problem-solving.

As therapists we can help the patient in seeing the implications and consequences of his present actions — and what he may be gaining or giving up in the process. It may be that an optimal amount of incongruity or novelty caused by the therapist's values, behaviors in reaction to the patient, or definition of the situation — say, as we engage in a meaningful relationship with him or praise him on the accomplishment of a sheltered workshop activity he regarded as worthless — may facilitate change.

Indeed, the emphasis on cognitive processes in this approach has helped us realize that cognitive dissonance,[63] conceptual conflict,[32,33] or incongruity[46] are important determiners of behavior in their own right and can be utilized by the therapist to effect change. The therapist's or group's shaping and reinforcement of behavior appropriate to and adaptive in social roles, developmental tasks, and the acquisition of competence in light of environmental demands, further facilitates feedback so that the patient attends to stimuli and enlarges his repertoire of skills in areas he may have previously ignored.

One of the distinguishing features of occupational therapy, as previously mentioned, is its con-

scious emphasis and insistence that, in addition to man's need for meaningful engagement with his environment, there are *therapeutic properties inherent in the environment which may be structured for treatment purposes.* These properties include not only the structuring of the patient-therapist relationship, but in structuring the physical and complex social role environments as well. An information processing approach makes it easier to assign a place in theory to the environmental structuring and manipulation which the therapist provides.

In occupational therapy, it is necessary to provide more than one setting, in order to provide for quite different needs of patients based on a knowledge of their level of competence and the kind of developmental tasks and roles facing them. Different occupational therapy settings are provided, in collaboration with the patient, when emerging skills and needs dictate. The rationale for moving the patient along a continuum in occupational therapy is embedded in the theory of providing the optimal amount of stimulation from the environment to increase readiness or the competencies needed for the next step in the adaptation process.

Concluding Remarks

It is a somewhat disconcerting realization that the theoretical ground in which our practice can best be understood is at the very frontier in the science of human behavior, and that there is no "bible" standing ready to provide all the answers. Behavioral cybernetics, however, does hold promise in developing into an important theory relevant to occupational therapy. It may serve as a link between cognitive-phenomenological and behaviorist emphases in therapy, and it is useful in explaining both very large and very small units of human behavior, ranging from the behavior of groups[44] and nations,[64] to neurophysiological mechanisms.[34]

Instrumental or operant learning seems particularly compatible with a cybernetic learning approach, especially if the term reinforcement (which broadly means that behavior is selected by its effects or consequences) is expanded to include feedback control or knowledge of results. The idea that man can regulate his own behavior through an appreciation of the consequences of his actions is consonant with new approaches in therapy advocated by London[65] and Glasser[66] which stress moral behavior and responsibility as important dimensions overlooked in other therapeutic approaches.

Furthermore, it is particularly relevant to the rationale for an action-based therapy. It underlines our need to understand communication processes, both verbal and non-verbal, in both their temporal and spatial aspects. It demands extensions of our current activity analysis approach, so that the therapist may more effectively enable the patient to assume a productive role in society.

It gives focus and direction to our efforts to enlarge curriculum offerings in the behavioral sciences and neurophysiology, and provides a unifying framework from which to view our contribution in physical, perceptual-motor, and psychosocial dysfunction. It suggests that the skills we impart to our patients are important therapeutic agents in themselves, not merely the means by which to form a relationship, and that these skills might be better related to sociocultural demands and contexts than they are at present.

Finally, as a theory, it could provide an arena where some synthesis is possible between learning theory and psychoanalytic theory. The well-known analyst Franz Alexander suggested just such a synthesis in a paper written a few years ago.[67] In the meanwhile, Shands,[68] Breger and McGaugh,[69] and others are exploring the implications of a cybernetic or information-processing approach for psychotherapy, Kephart,[70] Llorens[71] and others the implications for perceptual-motor training, and Jordaan the implications for exploratory vocational development.[72]

We all need to know much more, to read extensively in these areas, to integrate the observations we make in our daily practice. We will then be able to develop hypotheses on the implications for occupational therapy, and then test them. Our reward may be greater vision of the contribution occupational therapy can make in harnessing the healing forces in man and nature.

REFERENCES

1. Thompson, W. and Schaefer, T., "Early Environmental Stimulation," *Functions of Varied Experience,* Fiske, D. and Maddi, S. (eds.) Homewood, Ill.: Dorsey Press (1961).

2. Fidler, J. and Fidler, G., *Occupational Therapy,* N. Y.: MacMillan Co. (1963) p. 22.

3. *Ibid.,* p. 32.

4. *Ibid.,* p. 74.

5. *Ibid.,* p. 118.

6. Reilly, M., "Occupational Therapy Can be One of the Great Ideas of 20th Century Medicine," *Amer J Occup Ther,* XVI, 1 (1962), 1 – 9.

7. Stein, F., "Ego Functioning in Schizophrenia." Paper read at the Fourth International Congress, World Federation of Occupational Therapists, London, 1966.

8. Jones, M., Unpublished manuscript, 1965.

9. Diasio, K. and Jones, M., "The Role of Prevocational Services in the Rehabilitation of the young Adult Psychiatric Patient." Paper read at the Fourth International Congress, World Federation of Occupational Therapists, London, 1966.

10. Ford, D. and Urban, H., *Systems of Psychotherapy.* N. Y.: Wiley and Sons (1963), p. 143.

11. *Ibid.,* p. 178.

12. Hartmann, H., *Ego Psychology and the Problem of Adaptation.* N. Y.: International Universities Press (1958).

13. Hartmann, H., "Comments on the Psychoanalytic Theory of the Ego," *Psychoanalytic Study of the Child,* 5: 74 – 96. N. Y. International Universities Press (1950).

14. Hartmann, H., "Notes on the Theory of Sublimation," *Psychoanalytic Study of the Child,* 10: 9 – 29. N. Y.: International Universities Press (1955).

15. Rapaport, D., Cited in Ford and Urban, *op. cit.,* pp. 196 – 201.

16. Baldwin, A., *Theories of Child Development,* N. Y.: Wiley and Sons (1967).

17. Hendrick, I., "Work and the Pleasure Principle," *Psychoan Quart, 12* (1943), p. 311.

18. *Ibid.,* p. 319.

19. Ansbacher, H. and Ansbacher, R., *The Individual Psychology of Alfred Adler.* N. Y.: Basic Books (1956).

20. Rapaport, D. and Shakow, P., "The Influence of Freud on American Psychology," *Psychological Issues* (1964), 13, N. Y.: International Universities Press, p. 134.

21. Hartmann, H., "Psychoanalysis and Sociology," *Psychoanalysis Today,* S. Lorand (ed.). N. Y.: International Universities Press (1944), p. 331.

22. Rapaport, D., "The Theory of Ego Autonomy: A Generalization," *Bull Menninger Clin* (1958), 22, pp. 13 – 35.

23. Cited in Searles, H., *The Nonhuman Environment.* N. Y.: International Universities Press (1960), p. 50.

24. *Ibid.*

25. Rapaport, D., Cited in Ford and Urban, *Ibid.*

26. Holt, R., "Ego Autonomy Revisited," *Int J Psychoanal 46* (1965) pp. 145 – 165.

27. Neff, W., "Psychoanalytic Concepts of the Meaning of Work," *Psychiatry, 28* (1965), pp. 324 – 332.

28. Menninger, K., "Work as a Sublimation," *Bull Menninger Clin, 6* (1942) pp. 170 – 182.

29. King, G., Armitage, G. and Tilton, J., "A Therapeutic Approach to Schizophrenics of Extreme Pathology: an Operant-Interpersonal Method," *Case Studies in Behavior Modification,* Ullman, L. and Krasner, L., N. Y.: Holt, Rinehart and Winston (1966), pp. 99 – 110.

30. Ullman and Krasner, *op. cit.,* p. 24.

31. Tolman, E., "Principles of Purposive Behavior," *Psychology: A Study of a Science,* vol. 2. S. Kock (ed.), N. Y.: McGraw-Hill (1959), pp. 158 – 195.

32. Berlyne, D., *Conflict, Arousal and Curiosity,* N. Y.: J. Wiley (1960).

33. Berlyne, D., *Structure and Direction in Thinking,* N. Y.: J. Wiley (1965).

34. Hebb, D., "Drive and the C.N.S. (Conceptual Nervous System)," *Psychol Review, 62* (1955), pp. 243 – 254.

35. Ulmann, L. and Krasner, L., *op. cit.,* p. 29.

36. White, R., "Motivation Reconsidered: The Concept of Competence," *Psychol Review 66* (1959), pp. 297 – 333.

37. Fowler, H., *Curiosity and Exploratory Behavior,* N. Y.: The MacMillan Co. (1965).

38. Fiske, D. and Maddi, S. (eds.), *Functions of Varied Experience,* Homewood, Ill.: Dorsey Press (1961).

39. Kubazansky, P., "The Effects of Reduced Environmental Stimulation on Human Behavior: a Review," *The Manipulation of Human Behavior,* Biederman, A. and Zimmer, H. (eds.). N. Y.: J. Wiley (1961), pp. 51 – 95.

40. Held, R., "Plasticity in Sensory Motor Systems," *Scientific American, 213* (1963) 5, pp. 85 – 95.

41. Smith, K. and Smith, M., *Cybernetic Principles of Learning and Educational Design,* N. Y.: Holt, Rinehart, and Winston (1965) Ch. 14, pp. 353 – 381.

42. See particularly Leuba, C., "Toward Some Integration of Learning Theories: the Concept of Optimal Stimulation," *Psych Rep 1,* (1955) pp. 27 – 33.

43. Berne, E., *Games People Play,* N. Y.: Grove Press (1964).

44. Smith, K., and Smith, M., *op. cit.,* p. 471.

45. *Ibid.*

46. Hunt, J. McV., "Intrinsic Motivation," *Nebraska Symposium on Motivation, 1965,* Lincoln: Univ. of Nebraska Press, p. 230.

47. Guilford, J. P., "Motivation in an Informational Psychology," *Nebraska Symposium on Motivation, 1965,* Lincoln: Univ. of Nebraska Press, p. 270.

48. *Ibid.,* p. 320.

49. White, R., *op. cit.*

50. White, R., "Ego and Reality in Psychoanalytic Theory,": *Psychological Issues, 3,* N. Y.: International Universities Press (1964).

51. Rotter, J., *Nebraska Symposium on Motivation, 1955,* Lincoln: Univ. of Nebraska Press, pp. 245 – 269.

52. McClelland, D., Atkinson, J., Clark, R. and Lowell, E., *The Achievement Motive,* N. Y.: Appleton Century Crofts (1953).

53. Atkinson, J. and Feather, N. (eds.), *A Theory of Achievement Motivation,* N. Y.: J: Wiley (1966).

54. Lefcourt, H., "Internal v. External Control of Reinforcement: A Review," *Psychol Bull, 65* (1966) pp. 206 – 220.

55. See Dean, D., "Alienation; Its Meaning and Measurement," *Amer Sociol Rev 26* (1961) pp. 753 – 758. Also, Seeman, M. and Evans, J., "Alienation and Learning in a Hospital Setting," *Amer Sociol Rev 27* (1962) pp. 772 – 782.

56. Lefcourt, *op. cit.*

57. Lefcourt, H. and Ladwig, G., "The effect of Reference Group upon Negroes' Task Persistence in a Biracial Competitive Game," *J Pers Social Psychol 1* (1965) pp. 668 – 671.

58. Peters, J. and Jenkins, R., "Improvement of Chronic Schizophrenics with Guided Problem-Solving Motivated by Hunger," *Psychiat Quart Supp, 28* (1954), pp. 84 – 101.

59. Bruner, J., "Education as Social Invention," *J Social Issues, 20* (1964), pp. 21 – 37.

60. *Ibid.,* pp. 26 – 27.

61. See Watson, G., especially Ch. 5, "Structure-Process-Attitude," *Social Psychology: Issues and Insights.* N. Y. Lippincott (1966), pp. 189 – 214.

62. Alexander, F. and French, T., *Psychoanalytic Therapy: Principles and Application.* N. Y.: Ronald Press (1946).

63. Festinger, L., *A Theory of Cognitive Dissonance,* N. Y.: Row (1957).

64. Deutsch, K., *The Nerves of Government,* N. Y.: Free Press (1963).

65. London, P., *The Modes and Morals of Psychotherapy.* N. Y.: Holt, Rinehart Winston (1964).

66. Glasser, W., *Reality Therapy,* N. Y.: Harper and Rowe (1965).

67. Alexander, F., "Dynamics of Psychotherapy in Light of Learning Theory," *Amer J Psychiat, 11* (1963) pp. 235 – 244.

68. Shands, H., *Thinking and Psychotherapy: An Inquiry into the Process of Communication,* Cambridge, Mass.: Harvard Univ. Press (1960).

69. Breger, L. and McGaugh, J., "Critique and Reformulation of 'Learning Theory' Approaches to Psychotherapy and Neuroses," *Psychol Bull, 63* (1963) pp. 338 – 358.

70. Kephart, N., *The Slow Learner in the Classroom,* Columbus, Ohio: Merril (1960).

71. Llorens, L. and Rubin, E., *Developing Ego Functions in Disturbed Children: Occupational Therapy in Milieu.* Detroit, Mich.: Wayne State Univ. Press (1967).

72. Jordaan, J. P., *Career Development: Self Concept Theory,* Super, D. et al. N. Y.: College Entrance Examination Board (1963) pp. 79 – 95.

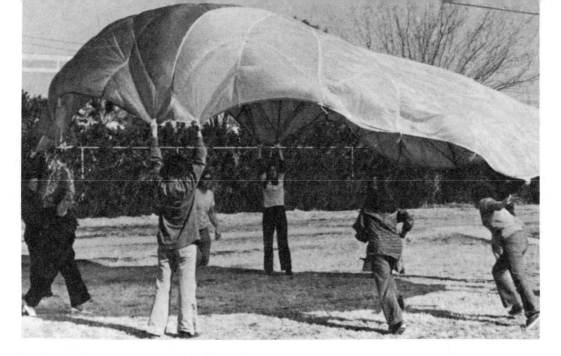

Parachute provides varied sensory experiences

A SENSORY-INTEGRATIVE APPROACH TO
SCHIZOPHRENIA

Lorna Jean King

Beginning with observations of posture and movement, patterns typical of process schizophrenia are identified and an empirical treatment program is described. Research growing out of the observed phenomena is described as indicating that the neurophysiological theories of Ayres provide a unified model which satisfactorily links Schilder's observations with current studies. It is hypothesized that defects in proprioceptive mechanisms result in lack of sensory integration. This in turn is said to result in lack of perceptual constancy, poor body image, inadequate motor planning, and fatigue-producing postural patterns. These handicaps are hypothesized to result in severe emotional stress and also to predispose to hallucinatory phenomena. Corticalization of movement is mentioned as a common attempt at compensation. Treatment principles are discussed and implications for preventive programs are noted.

"In our research we have purposely avoided any attempt to pursue therapy. Since rational treatment can only evolve from a firm knowledge of etiology, we believed that this is where our scientific efforts should be initially expended." With these words, Doctors Ritvo and Ornitz introduce a recent paper dealing with

Lorna Jean King, O.T.R., F.A.O.T.A., was director of rehabilitative therapies, Arizona State Hospital, Phoenix, from 1966 to 1974. She is presently a consultant in private practice.

their research into the etiology of childhood schizophrenia and infantile autism.[1]

Most clinicians, including occupational therapists, however much they may agree with this statement, still feel impelled to "do something" by way of treatment for the schizophrenic patient. The fact that therapeutic efforts have not been based upon solid knowledge of etiology has worried but not deterred them. Occupational therapists have been consoled by the knowledge that everyone, psychiatrists included, is standing on the same shaky ground.

To the widespread disillusionment with psychoanalysis as a "cure" has been added disappointment with the psychotherapeutic drugs that suppress symptoms but do not cure. These drugs produce side effects which may lead many patients to abandon them as soon as possible. Individual reactions vary greatly and many chronic schizophrenics, who comprise the backbone population of state hospitals, do not respond significantly to medication.[2] There seems to be a widespread tendency to abandon hope of treating the chronic schizophrenic and to turn instead to management in boarding homes as being an economical solution.

Occupational therapists may be among the last to give up hope of effective treatment since most have experienced tantalizing glimmers of improvement in their chronic patients from time to time.

This framework of frustration was a motivating factor six years ago when personnel at

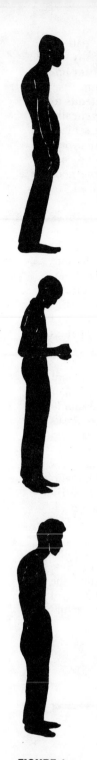

FIGURE 1
Process schizophrenic postures

the Arizona State Hospital, rehabilitative therapies department, decided to take a fresh look at the chronic schizophrenic population. The first rule of the scientific method is to begin with careful observation of what is actually seen, not what is inferred because of education and other biases.

It soon became clear that chronic schizophrenics have several highly visible postural and movement features in common: 1. a pronounced head to toe *S* curve posture (figure 1); 2. a shuffling-gait—inability to lift the feet and walk with a normal heel-toe pattern; 3. an inability to raise the arms above the head to anything approaching a vertical line; 4. an immobility of the head and shoulder girdle which is manifested by an inability to rotate the head on the vertical axis or to roll the head to the side, forward, or back—most marked is the inability to tip the head back, which was observed to be uncomfortable and anxiety-producing to most patients; 5. a tendency to hold arms and legs in a flexed, adducted, and internally rotated position both sitting and standing; 6. a lack of normal hand function that involves the thumb held in adduction, atrophy of the thenar eminence, ulnar deviation at the wrist, and also a weakness of grip, often limited to 10 to 15 pounds on the dynamometer, whereas the normal grip ranges from 40 to 150 pounds.

Is this characteristic limitation of movement and typical posture the result of chronic schizophrenia, or is it the result of years of institutionalization? Comparison with other long-term patients demonstrates that only the chronic nonparanoid schizophrenics exhibit this particular configuration of posture and limited movement. The fact that the chronic paranoids do not show this postural syndrome seems to eliminate the likelihood that it is caused by medication, since no differentiation between paranoid and nonparanoid is made in prescribing medication. Young, recently hospitalized process schizophrenics show the same postural configurations as the older patients, although not to the extreme.

To what degree can this pattern of posture and movement be changed? If it is changed, will there be corresponding changes in psychic organization? A group of 15 chronic schizophrenics was selected and a program of physical activity was instituted based upon extending range of motion, increasing amount of spontaneous movement, and improving posture.

Since these patients lacked any motivation to work or exercise, the activities were couched in terms of noncompetitive games that began with a circle of people tossing a ball back and forth. A ball thrown to a person almost forces some kind of response to catch it, duck, or bat it away. Kicking the ball around the circle brought attention to the poor balance of these individuals. Some patients literally could not balance on one foot long enough to kick.

Marching to music, stepping over ropes, ducking under the volleyball net, passing the ball backward over one's head around the circle, and trying to jump over a rope two or three inches off the ground were among the noncompetitive activities.

After two to three weeks, interesting changes in the group were visible and participation was more active and less sluggish. Patients began meeting staff at the door instead of having to be rounded up. Therapists noticed a marked increase in the amount of verbalization; patients who had scarcely spoken for years began to take part in conversations. Attention to grooming improved, and smiles began to appear on hitherto expressionless faces. These changes were in addition to improved mobility in the restricted areas outlined above.

The results of this initial physical activity program were gratifying and thought-provoking enough to stimulate a search for the neurophysiological meaning of the observations. This was the beginning of a spiral of observations leading to reading and formulation of hypotheses which led in turn to additional program designs, more observation, and more study. This process is still going on, and anything that is written today is tentative.

Theoretical Formulations

Working first with the meaning of our observations, it was acknowledged that it is scientifically acceptable to reject the model of a mind–body dichotomy in favor of a unitary view of man as a single organism, highly complex and completely unified. Thus, events that affect the organism affect the entire organism. Anything that affects the body will inexorably affect the mind and vice versa. With this postulate as a base, an hypothesis of the etiology of schizophrenia is stated, supported, and elaborated: *Some individuals have defective proprioceptive feedback mechanisms, the vestibular component in particular being first underreactive, and second, underactive in its role in the sensorimotor integration process. This defect, whether genetic, developmental, or the result of trauma, constitutes an important etiological or prodromal factor in process and reactive schizophrenia.*

Because this statement is limited to process and reactive schizophrenia, it is necessary to define and differentiate these two categories from paranoid schizophrenia.

The Subclassifications of Schizophrenia

The subclassification of schizophrenia is important when investigating etiology. If, as Hoskins[3] suggests, schizophrenia is like headache and may be a symptom of diverse conditions, it is as important to distinguish one kind of schizophrenia from another as it is to distinguish a migraine headache from a hypertensive headache.

Two main patterns of subclassification appear most commonly in the current literature, the paranoid–nonparanoid paradigm and the process–reactive continuum. Most of the literature on the process–reactive model leads the reader to assume that paranoid symptomatology occurs throughout the process–reactive grouping. Kantor and Herron,[4] however, postulate that the earlier the developmental age at which significant loss occurs, the more malign the illness, the greater the amount of personality disorganization, and the more severe the perceptual abnormalities. This indicates that the paranoid is in the reactive or less severe end of the continuum since he is developmentally more advanced.

The paranoid–nonparanoid model, on the other hand, seems to indicate a fundamental difference between the paranoid personality style and the process–reactive continuum. This view assumes that the words process and reactive describe severe and mild manifestations of an essentially similar disorder, where paranoid describes a separate entity.

Sullivan[5] categorized reactive schizophrenics as those who have functioned with at least marginal adequacy in life to a point where severe or recognizable stress was encountered. The psychotic break was in response to stress and tended to be temporary. Other authors[4,6] subsequently reported that such individuals respond well to medication and other treatment whether the psychotic break is an isolated episode or one of a recurring series.

Sullivan labeled as process schizophrenic the individual who from childhood had been *different,* who gradually and almost imperceptibly slipped deeper into psychosis until hospitalization was necessary. This patient usually does not respond dramatically to medication and does not show significant improvement in response to most treatments.[6] The process schizophrenic, therefore, tends to comprise a large segment of the chronically hospitalized population. The reactive schizophrenic roughly corresponds to the *good premorbid* schizophrenic, where the process schizophrenic may be equated with the *poor premorbid* schizophrenic as described in papers by Fowles et al.[7]

The paranoid schizophrenic usually does not suffer the degree of personality disorganization and perceptual abnormality observed in reactive or process schizophrenia[8] and is characterized chiefly by delusional patterns of a persecutory or grandiose nature. In the community it may be difficult to distinguish between the paranoid personality and the psychotic paranoid because of the relatively intact general functioning of both categories.

The observations of posture and movement described in the introduction to this paper seem to favor the logic of the paranoid–nonparanoid subclassification system. Treatment results also differ between these two groups. While relatively few studies have attempted to differentiate physiologically between the paranoid and nonparanoid classification, some differences do emerge as fairly reliable. If one accepts the idea that the paranoid is seldom found in the process end of the process–reactive continuum, and that the paranoid syndrome is at the higher or more normal end of the reactive continuum, one would have a scale emerging in which the process schizophrenic is at the lower or most deviant end, next higher is the reactive schiz-

TABLE 1

A Comparison of Selected Physiological Patterns
in Paranoid and Nonparanoid Schizophrenia

Physiological Patterns	Paranoid	Process and Acutely Ill Reactive	Research Source
Reaction Time (latency)	Normal	Slow	King H E[9]
Conditioning Pattern	Normal to Slow	Conditioning-Rapid, Extinction-Slow	Mednick S[10]
Scanning	Hyperscanning	Hyposcanning	Silverman J,[11] Spohn H, Thetford P, Canro R[12]
Muscle Tone	Normal	Hypertonic Phasic Groups Hypotonic Tonic Groups	Raush H L[13]
Resting Arousal Level (galvanic skin resistance, blood pressure)	Normal to Low	High	Funkenstein D H, Greenblatt M, Solomon H C,[14] Venables P, Wing J[15]
Posture	Normal	Head to Toe S-Curve- Flexion; Adduction and Internal Rotation of the Extremities	Observed at Arizona State Hospital

ophrenic and, higher still, is the paranoid.

Physiological differences between paranoid and nonparanoid schizophrenia as recorded in literature and observed at Arizona State Hospital are briefly summarized in table 1.

It seems possible that the often equivocal and inconsistent results of perceptual testing of schizophrenics may be caused by the frequent failure to separate the paranoid group from the process–reactive group. Two or more dissimilar syndromes, which have little in common other than the term schizophrenia, are treated as if these were the same syndrome. This point is discussed by Lipton,[16] Hoskins,[3] and others. Physiological differences are the primary clue to the divergent nature of these conditions and, of these, posture is the most readily observable factor.

Sensory-Integration Theory Related to Schizophrenia

The riddle of the paranoid syndrome remains obscure but the sensory-integration theory as delineated by Ayres[17–19] appears to offer some useful insights into organizing some of the diverse research on schizophrenia into a partial understanding of the etiology of the process–reactive syndrome.

Ayres set forth the critical role of vestibular and tactile input in organizing and integrating sensory stimuli primarily, but not solely, at the brainstem level. Integration of auditory, visual, and other sensory input is essential to the development of visual size and form constancy, reliable localization of auditory stimuli, and other sensory constancy. The lack of perceptual constancy caused by faulty sensory integration may be the mechanism that produces hallucinations. Constancy or reliability of perceptual information is essential to all kinds of learning. The infant can learn or relate only if objects and people look, sound, and feel the same each time he encounters them.

Two separate and long-known concepts about schizophrenics can be linked through the theories of sensory integration. It has long been accepted that schizophrenics suffer from perceptual distortion.[13,20] Chapman[21] has established loss of visual size and form constancy as one of the earliest symptoms of schizophrenia. One might theorize that the reactive schizophrenic *loses* perceptual constancy where the process schizophrenic or autistic child has never developed it. Sechehaye presents a compelling subjective account of loss of size and form constancy in *Autobiography of a Schizophrenic Girl.*[22]

Vestibular Underreactivity and Constancy

Paul Schilder[23] noted 40 years ago that schizophrenics are markedly underreactive to vestibular stimulation as measured by postrotational nystagmus. Research by Angyal, Blackman, and Sherman,[24,25] at Worcester State Hospital in the late 1930's and early 1940's, confirmed statistically that schizo-phrenics as a group were hyporesponsive to vestibular input, although there were wide variations between individuals.

Recently Ritvo and Ornitz[1] confirmed the absence or underreactivity of vestibular response with schizophrenic children, again with postrotational nystagmus used as the index of reactivity. The children, who did not show nystagmus in a lighted room, did react with nystagmus when rotated in the dark and photographed by infrared light. Ritvo and Ornitz hypothesize an inability to process both the visual and vestibular stimuli at the same time. This in turn implicates the integrative or processing centers in the brainstem. In a 1960 study,[26] Leach confirmed adult schizophrenic vestibular underreactivity and refers to it as "an integrative neural deficit."

It seems plausible that abnormalities of vestibular reactivity may reflect defective brainstem processing, which may be a *cause* of the lack of perceptual constancy characteristic of the schizophrenic population. The tendency of autistic and schizophrenic children to whirl, rock, and shake their heads, may be the organism's attempt to obtain the needed vestibular stimulation. These self-stimulating activities are also seen in adult patients.

Studies of monozygotic twins discordant for schizophrenia show that the twin susceptible to schizophrenia is more vulnerable at birth. He is lighter in weight, shorter, and more likely to have been cyanotic.[27] These factors would inevitably predispose the organism to minimal brain damage and would make the developmental delays and deficits readily explainable. Vestibular capabilities, being basic to other responses, would logically cause the severest results if impaired.

Vestibular Factors in Posture

Linking vestibular system abnormalities with posture and limitations of movement observed in the chronic (process) schizophrenic requires consideration of basic reflex patterns. The labyrinthine reflex is one of the most primitive reflexes and is evoked by a sensation of falling. In the prone position the infant reacts to the sensation of falling by going into a ball position of flexion, adduction, and internal rotation. This labyrinthine position has primitive survival value, according to Feldenkrais,[28] in that it puts the infant in the best possible posture to survive a fall.

Ayres noted that many learning disability children exhibited a persistence of the labyrinthine reflex pattern with associated inability to assume and hold the pivot-prone position of hyperextension.[18] The chronic schizophrenic also is unable to assume or hold this position. This is not unexpected in view of the postural picture of flexion, adduction, and internal rotation previously noted. Tension in these phasic muscle groups and hypotonicity in the opposing or tonic groups recorded in the literature also is a reflection of the persistence of the pattern characterizing the labyrinthine reflex.

Feldenkrais suggests the pattern by which inadequacy of vestibular responses may become part of a vicious circle. He believes that all anxiety generalizes or is conditioned from man's innate fear of falling. Noting that any part of a conditioned response will trigger the whole sequence, he suggests that anxiety by conditioning will trigger the autonomic and muscular reactions to the fear of falling. Thus, any anxiety will trigger the tightening of flexor, adductor, and internal rotator muscles, the sinking sensations in the pit of the stomach, sweating, and loss of tone in the extensor muscles. The antidote to these uncomfortable feelings is to remain quiet, preferably in the ball or labyrinthine reflex position. If balance is poor and a child falls often, movement may produce anxiety and lead to less movement. Lack of movement slows development of the vestibular system because of inadequacy of vestibular input, which sequentially leads to inadequate development of perceptual constancy, creating further anxiety and unsteadiness of movement. Being laughed at or scolded because of clumsiness produces a cumulative emotional impact in addition to that which began as a developmental deficit.

A feeling of security is subject to the day to day dependability of what the senses tell us about the environment. Perceptual inconstancy may be the key link in the chain that leads to the development of schizophrenia.

Vestibular Stimulation and Pleasure Response

Vestibular stimulation is a basic and important source of pleasure to the normal human. Babies laugh when tossed up in the air, little children whirl spontaneously and love to swing; in fact, almost all playground equipment involves vestibular stimulation. Many adults seek out roller coasters, Ferris wheels, and other carnival rides. Skiing, surfing, motorcycling, driving cars, all are pleasurable and have strong movement-through-space components.

Heath[29] notes that the pleasure response functions of the septal area are "in intimate relationship with certain sensory relay nuclei, especially those concerned with somatosensory function (particularly proprioception) and special sensory functions (levels of awareness and expression of feeling both psychological and physiological)."

Experience with patients at Arizona State Hospital showed that simple vestibular stimulation, such as whirling in an office chair, or being whirled by the elbow, will produce smiles and laughter in withdrawn and unresponsive patients; they often seek a repetition of the experience in days following.

Corticalization of Movement

An important corollary of the schizo-phrenic's postulated lack of sensorimotor integration is corticalization of movement. This may represent an attempt at compensation. Chapman[21] reports that one of the earliest complaints of schizophrenics is the need to think about moving. They can no longer walk or do other common activities automatically but instead must *think* every movement as they carry it out. This could account for the psychomotor retardation which is a hallmark of schizophrenia. It may also account for some of the characteristic disruptions of speech patterns, and perseverations in thought, speech, and motor behavior. While verbal response is cortical, the motor process of speech is automatic or subcortical. Speech can be disrupted by delaying the auditory feedback a fraction of a second.[30] Cortical attention to the motor process of speech could disrupt the act of speaking, especially if auditory inconstancies are experienced concurrently.

The attempt to think movement as a means of compensating for poor sensorimotor integration is costly in terms of energy expenditure. Rood[31] points out that the phasic muscles, which are largely responsible for willed or cortically directed movement, require nine times as much energy as the tonic or subcortically directed muscles. It is understandable that the schizophrenic complains of fatigue; he is expending relatively large amounts of energy on minimal amounts of movement.

Holtzman[30] in his careful review and analysis of research in this field suggests that "the feedback stage of the perceptual act, that is, that stage of perception which involves proprioceptive and automatic functions in response to sensory input, may indeed be disrupted and play a crucial but as yet undetermined role in the unfolding of the schizophrenic syndrome."

Associational and Emotional Aspects of Proprioception

Gellhorn[32] in turn implicates lack of proprioceptive feedback in bizarre or insufficient associational processes and also in flattened or inappropriate affect. Proprioceptive input, says Gellhorn, has a tuning effect on the reticular-activating system. Only when this system is tuned or in a state of tension are incoming perceptions carried high enough or through enough reverberating circuits for abstract associational processes to take place. Without this tension or tone in the reticular system, the associational process is slow or dull, and thinking tends to be limited to the concrete. Concrete associations, inability to think in abstract terms, and bizarre associations are characteristic of the cognitive patterns found in schizophrenia.

Reluctance to move or an inadequate amount of movement suppresses vestibular reactivity and makes it less likely that other forms of proprioceptive input will occur, such as jumping, running, or walking. These are examples of activities which result in input from joints and tendons traveling to the brainstem and exerting their toning or tuning effect.

It is possible that individual thresholds for the firing of convergent neurons may vary. An adequate amount of input for one person may be inadequate for another. Various influences may raise or lower thresholds and, although little is known about these factors, it appears from treatment experience that if large amounts of vestibular and other proprioceptive inputs are given, the threshold often is lowered slowly so that eventually less stimulation is needed.

Gellhorn, in *Motion and Emotion,*[33] states the case for the proposition that movement and posture can affect emotion. Feldenkrais[28] makes the point that the mask-like face frequently seen in the schizophrenic is a result of tension in the facial musculature caused by anxiety. Peturssen[34] has also documented high levels of muscle tension and other signs of anxiety seen in the chronic schizophrenic. Gellhorn further points out that the less mobility there is in the facial muscles, the less emotion will be experienced through the thalamus to the cortex. Mobility of the facial muscles, readily induced through laughter, increases affect; the reception in the thalamic area of pleasurable impulses from the laughter helps to reduce the chronic anxiety.

Body–Mind Interactions

The above is a summary of the basis of the formulation of the hypothesis: "some individuals have defective proprioceptive feedback mechanisms, the vestibular component in particular being underreactive and underactive in its role in the sensorimotor integration process. This defect . . . constitutes an important etiological factor in process and reactive schizophrenia."

To postulate this etiologic role for defective sensory-integrative development is not in conflict with the growing evidence for biochemical factors in the predisposition to schizophrenia.[35-37] While chemical abnormalities, such as thyrotoxicosis, or deficiency diseases such as pellagra, have been demonstrated to alter movement behavior and thought processes, it is also true that movement behavior and thought processes can alter biochemical states. This is one of the essential thrusts of Selye's widely accepted stress theory of disease.[38] In the last 30 years there has been much more emphasis in popular literature on psychosomatic illness than on somatopsychic dysfunction. Rather than an either–or view of causality, however, a circular or spiral model seems more accurate. In this view an event at one point of the circle leads inexorably to every other point. This model, it would seem, applies not only to etiology but also to treatment. Although we cannot be sure which chemicals to alter, or in what direction,

we can intervene in the motor behavior of the individual with the knowledge that there will be affects upon the thought processes and upon biochemistry. If improved adaptive responses and thought processes emerge, we may assume that the interventions have been effective.

Applications to Treatment

An empirical approach was used in the work described in this paper; activities were chosen first on the basis of attempts to counteract or normalize patterns of excessive flexion, adduction and internal rotation, and to increase the range of joint motions. As the therapeutic team studied the research implicating vestibular and proprioceptive feedback abnormalities, the applicability of Ayres' sensorimotor-integration theories became apparent. This led in turn to the incorporation of the activities suggested by Ayres, the scooter board, increased tactile input, and others. Rood[31] suggested complementary activities such as those involving heavy work patterns for the tonic muscle groups. Results appeared to validate the usefulness of these techniques. Patients have been the source of treatment ideas; it is hard to overemphasize the value of taking cues from movement patterns that patients initiate or seem to enjoy.

Ayres,[18] Barsch,[39] and others pioneered in demonstrating the usefulness of developing sensorimotor integration in children with learning disabilities and other developmental deficits. Ayres and Heskett[19] presented a case study of a schizophrenic child treated with sensory-integrative techniques. However, psychological folklore has long held that the central nervous system is relatively fixed after the ages of 10 or 12. Thus, even if the premise is accepted that process schizophrenics are learning disability children grown up, the question arises whether or not it is too late for remediation.

Experience at Arizona State Hospital suggests that some adults, even those with histories of long hospitalization, can benefit to a greater or lesser degree from treatment aimed at development of sensorimotor integration. The fact that improved levels of functioning seem to hold after treatment has been discontinued points to the achievement of a higher level of neurological integration. When treatment stopped, it was the absence of regression that distinguished sensory-integrative treatment of chronic patients from other types of therapies. It appears that integration, once achieved, is not lost, barring damage to the central nervous system. Once the integration involved in skipping is achieved in childhood, a person can skip 40 years later even though there has been no utilization of the pattern in the interim.

Patient Selection

Sensory-integrative treatment through gross

motor activities appears to be effective with autistic and schizophrenic children. Sensory-integrative treatment can be expected to be helpful with adolescents and adults who fit the process schizophrenia description. It has worked well with acutely ill reactive schizophrenics who are primarily nonparanoid in their patterns. However, at our present stage of knowledge, we cannot expect results in treating paranoid patients by the use of sensory-integrative methods.

Neurophysiological approaches, such as utilization of the carotid sinus effect, are useful with agitated depressives and with anxiety states. We know how to calm the manic patient through slow rhythmic rocking and other sedating activities, but the manic seldom wishes treatment. Therefore he is not treatable through an approach that relies essentially upon voluntary cooperation, unless the calming activities can be made pleasurable enough to induce his participation.

If therapists are interested in exploring the possibilities or demonstrating the usefulness of sensory-integrative methods in psychiatry, it is essential to select appropriate patients and to make no claims that the method will work with every type of patient. Many good treatment methods have been discarded prematurely because of the overzealousness of their proponents.

Summary of Rationale

The rationale for using certain gross motor activities in the treatment of schizophrenia may be summarized by stating: 1. Sensorimotor deficit appears to play an etiological role in process and perhaps in reactive schizophrenia. 2. Certain gross motor activities seem to facilitate improved sensorimotor integration in children. 3. Empirical studies show chronic process schizophrenics functioning more adequately following gross motor activity treatment. 4. Gains made in sensory integration tend to be relatively permanent and less subject to regression than gains resulting from verbal therapies. 5. Gains in sensory integration seem to have a self-starter effect. The patient finds that success motivates him to further efforts, and every small increase in neurological integration makes the next step easier to achieve.

Selection of Activities

Proper selection of activities is important if maximum effectiveness is to be achieved. In general one may say that all motor activities suitable for the sensory-integrative treatment of schizophrenia must meet two requirements: cortical (cognitive or conscious) attention must not be centered upon the motor process but must instead be focused upon an object or an outcome. The activity must be pleasurable. It should provoke smiles, laughter, a feeling of mastery, achievement, or pure fun.

Desirable Specific Patterns

In addition to the general requirements, specific prerequisites are important. All requirements will not be met by each activity. Incorporate as many aspects of vestibular stimulation as possible, that is, movement of the head through a significant distance in any plane. A major component is bilateral use of the tonic muscles, preferably against resistance. This would include what Rood[31] describes as heavy work patterns, such as tug-of-war. Recommended are activities that integrate (counteract) primitive reflex patterns, labyrinthine and tonic neck, in particular. Pressure touch should be used where possible. Incorporate activities that have proprioceptive feedback from the joints and tendons, such as jumping rope. Include other aspects of sensory input, such as eye pursuits, color, texture, rhythm, and awareness of space and form.

Activities

Suitable kinds of activities can in general be divided into two categories: recreation and games. The variety is almost endless since elements of skill, chance, surprise, incongruity, and suspense can be combined in myriad variations. Almost anything can by fiat become a game. Trial and error will produce a usable repertoire which should be kept as fresh and spontaneous as the therapists' and patients' imaginations will allow. Purposeful or task-oriented activities can include digging and gardening, sweeping, and folding sheets.

Task-oriented activities will usually be effective after a patient's level of functioning has been raised to a certain point. To be considered are the amount and kind of gross motor activity involved and whether or not it meets the patient's needs as well as the degree to which it meets the general criterion that the activity be pleasurable and give a sense of mastery.

Activities can be individual or group organization. Where staff is limited and there are large numbers of chronic patients to be treated, the group approach appeals on a basis of sheer efficiency. However, the group approach also facilitates fun, laughter, and unselfconscious participation. Competition should be avoided in group activities since it is often damaging to an already fragile self-concept. The individual's performance should be compared only with his own past performance. There is a place, of course, for one-to-one treatment, especially with the patient who cannot yet tolerate a group.

Equipment

While gross motor activities require few pieces of equipment, there are some objects which are useful. One is the parachute, which can be used best by groups of 8 to 25 and lends itself to many activities. Balloons, which move slowly enough for easy eye pursuit, do not hurt if they hit someone, have a pleasing color, texture, and softness, and can be rubbed against the body (tactile stimulation) to produce static electricity effects. Beach balls move faster, are colorful, lightweight, and harmless, and come in several sizes. Bean bag chairs are useful for learning to fall and to get proprioceptive input through crawling and rolling over a shifting surface.

Many of the activities developed for use with children also can be used with adults. Kuizenga and Wilbarger[40] suggested games that can be adapted for groups of adults.

Implications for Prevention

If subsequent research validates the hypothesis that developmental deficits in the tactile–vestibular–proprioceptive components of sensory integration are an etiological factor in process–reactive schizophrenia, then there will be important implications for preventive programs. Several research projects are focusing on identifying infants who are high risks for schizophrenia.[41–43] Of these, the work by Fish is perhaps most closely related to the hypothesis discussed in this article. Fish found that the most significantly predictive factor found in high-risk infants is abnormality of postural responses; these responses are closely related to vestibular function and can be identified in the first few weeks of life. Carefully controlled long-term studies of the results of developmental training with high-risk infants should shed more light on the relative importance of sensory-integrative mechanisms in the etiology of schizophrenia.

Conclusion

Activities designed to stimulate the development of the sensory-integrative capabilities of the central nervous system appear to offer promising results in the treatment of process and reactive schizophrenia. Current research suggests avenues for the preventive training of children. Occupational therapists' training in developmental sequences and in the analysis of activity places them in a crucial position for doing further research in this significant area.

REFERENCES

1. Ritvo E, Ornitz EM, Tanguay P, et al: Neurophysiologic and biochemical abnormalities in infantile autism and childhood schizophrenia. Paper presented at the 47th Meeting of the American Orthopsychiatric Association, 1970
2. Cole JO: Psychopharmacology and psychopathology. In Neurobiological Aspects of Psychopathology. Edited by Zubin and Shagass. New York, Grune and Stratton, 1969
3. Hoskins RG: The Biology of Schizophrenia, New York, Norton Co., 1946
4. Kantor RE, Herron WG: Reactive and Process Schizophrenia, Palo Alto, Science and Behavior Books, Inc., 1966
5. Sullivan HS: The Conceptions of Modern Psychiatry, Washington, DC, William Allen White Psychiatric Foundation, 1947
6. Cole JO: Schizophrenia: the therapies—a broad perspective. In Schizophrenia, New York, Medcom–Roerig, 1972
7. Fowles DC, Watt NF, Maher BA, et al: Autonomic arousal in good and poor premorbid schizophrenics. Br J Soc Clin Psychol, 9: 135–47, 1970
8. Bleuler E: Dementia Praecox or the Group of Schizophrenics. Translated by J Zinkin. New York, International Universities Press, 1950
9. King HE: Reaction time as a function of stimulus intensity among normal and psychotic subjects. J Psychol, 54: 299–307, 1962
10. Mednick S: A learning theory approach to research in schizophrenia. Psychol Bull, 55: 316–27, 1958
11. Silverman J: Scanning control mechanisms and cognitive filtering in paranoid and nonparanoid schizophrenia. J Consult Clin Psychol, 28: 5, 385–93, 1964
12. Spohn H, Thetford P, Cancro R: Attention, psychophysiology and scanning in the schizophrenic syndrome. In The Schizophrenic Reactions. Edited by R Cancro. New York, Brunner/Mazel, 1970
13. Raush HL: Perceptual constancy in schizophrenia. J Pers, 21: 176–87, 1952
14. Funkenstein DH, Greenblatt M, Solomon HC: Autonomic changes paralleling psychologic changes in mentally ill patients. J Nerv Ment Dis, 114: 1–18, 1951
15. Venables P, Wing J: Level of arousal and the subclassification of schizophrenia. Arch Gen Psychiatry, 7: 114–19, 1962
16. Lipton MA: A consideration of biological factors in schizophrenia. In Neurobiological Aspects of Psychopathology. Edited by Zubin and Shagass. New York, Grune and Stratton, 1969
17. Ayres AJ: An interpretation of the role of the brainstem in intersensory integration. In The Body Senses and Perceptual Deficit. Edited by H Coryell. Boston, Boston University, 1973
18. Ayres AJ: Sensory Integration and Learning Disorders, Los Angeles, Western Psychological Services, 1972
19. Ayres AJ, Heskett WM: Sensory-integrative dysfunction in a young schizophrenic girl. J Autism Child Schizo, 2: 174–81, 1972
20. Kraepelin E: Lectures in Clinical Psychiatry, Darien, Hafner Publishing Co., 1968
21. Chapman J: The early symptoms of schizophrenia. Br J Psychiatry, 112: 225–51, 1966
22. Sechehaye M: The Autobiography of a Schizophrenic Girl, New York, Grune and Stratton, 1951
23. Schilder P: The vestibular apparatus in neurosis and psychosis. J Nerv Ment Dis, 78: 1–23, 137–164, 1933
24. Angyal A, Blackman N: Vestibular reactivity in schizophrenia. Arch Neurol Psychiatry, 44: 611–20, 1940
25. Angyal A, Sherman N: Postural reactions to vestibular stimulation in schizophrenic and normal subjects. Am J Psychiatry, 98: 857–62, 1942
26. Leach WW: Nystagmus: an integrative neural deficit in schizophrenia. J Abnorm Soc Psychol, 66: 305–09, 1960
27. Mednick S: Birth defects and schizophrenia. Psychol Today, 5: 49, 50, 80, 81, 1971
28. Feldenkrais M: Body and Mature Behavior—Anxiety, Sex, Gravitation, and Learning, New York, International Universities Press, 1966
29. Heath RG: Schizophrenia, an organic concept. In Schizophrenia, New York, Medcom–Roerig, 1972
30. Holtzman P: Perceptual dysfunction in the schizophrenic syndrome. In The Schizophrenic Reactions. Edited by R Cancro. New York, Brunner/Mazel, 1970
31. Rood MS: Personal communication
32. Gellhorn E: Principles of Autonomic Somatic Integrations, Minneapolis, University of Minnesota Press, 1967
33. Gellhorn E: Motion and emotion—the role of proprioception in the physiology and pathology of the emotions. Psychol Rev, 71: 357–72, 1964
34. Petursson E: Electromyographic studies of muscle tension in psychiatric patients. Compr Psychiatry, 3: 29–36, 1962
35. Orthomolecular Psychiatry, Treatment of Schizophrenia. Edited by D Hawkins, L Pauling. San Francisco, W. H. Freeman and Co., 1973
36. Heath RG, Krupp TM: Schizophrenia as a specific biologic disease. Am J Psychiatry, 124: 1019–24, 1968
37. Kety S: Biochemical etiologies—a review. In Schizophrenia, New York, Medcom–Roerig, 1972
38. Selye H: The Stress of Life, New York, McGraw-Hill, 1956
39. Barsch RH: Achieving Perceptual Motor Efficiency. In A Perceptual-Motor Curriculum, Vol 1. Seattle, Special Child Publications, 1967
40. Kuizenga J, Wilbarger P: Activities for the Remediation of Sensorimotor Dysfunction in Primary School Children, Santa Barbara, Goleta Union School District, 1969
41. Fish B, Shapiro T, Halpern F, et al: The prediction of schizophrenia in infancy, III. A ten-year follow-up report of neurological and psychological development. Am J Psychiatry, 121: 768–75, 1965
42. Mednick S, Schulsinger F: Factors related to breakdown in children at high risk for schizophrenia. In Life History Research in Psychopathology. Edited by M Roff, DF Ricks. Minneapolis, University of Minnesota Press, 1970
43. Schulsinger F: The implications of heritability. In Schizophrenia, New York, Medcom–Roerig, 1972

Movement Therapy for

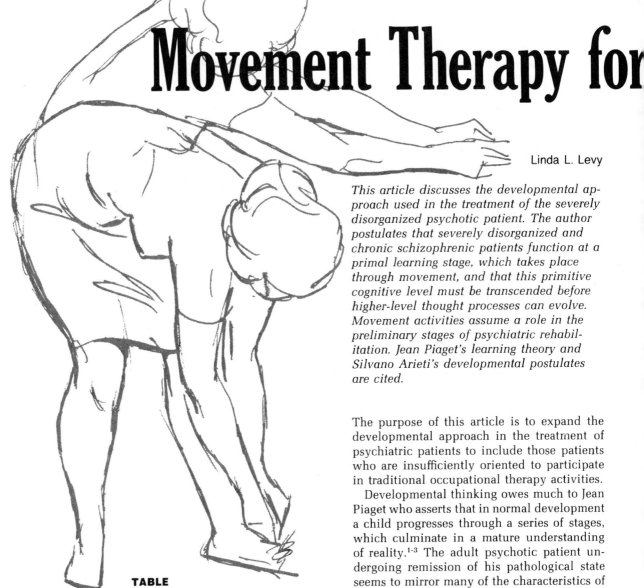

Linda L. Levy

This article discusses the developmental approach used in the treatment of the severely disorganized psychotic patient. The author postulates that severely disorganized and chronic schizophrenic patients function at a primal learning stage, which takes place through movement, and that this primitive cognitive level must be transcended before higher-level thought processes can evolve. Movement activities assume a role in the preliminary stages of psychiatric rehabilitation. Jean Piaget's learning theory and Silvano Arieti's developmental postulates are cited.

The purpose of this article is to expand the developmental approach in the treatment of psychiatric patients to include those patients who are insufficiently oriented to participate in traditional occupational therapy activities.

Developmental thinking owes much to Jean Piaget who asserts that in normal development a child progresses through a series of stages, which culminate in a mature understanding of reality.[1-3] The adult psychotic patient undergoing remission of his pathological state seems to mirror many of the characteristics of these stages. The central thesis of this developmental approach is that psychopathological symptoms are inherently logical if viewed within a developmental framework; therapists should understand the stages of development if they wish to deal effectively with remission of symptoms. When applied to major thought disorders, the developmental approach assumes that thought processes under stress revert to earlier developmental levels of functioning. Remission from a psychotic break thus necessitates rebuilding the steps toward integrated cognition in normal developmental order.

This paper examines the developmental treatment of the severely disorganized psychotic patient under the assumption that severely disorganized psychotics function at a primitive learning stage on the developmental scale, and that new learning in this stage is attained primarily through movement.

Linda Levy, O.T.R., is supervisor of the psychiatric occupational therapy department at the Hospital of the University of Pennsylvania in Philadelphia.

TABLE

Piaget's Stages and Predictable Behaviors in the Adult Psychotic

	Cognition	Behaviors
Stage 1	Functional assimilation	Will perform available schemata
	Generalizing assimilation	Will generalize available schemata to new situations
Stage 2	Able to repeat behavior of models if similar to own behaviors (approximately, at first)	Will imitate if his own body movements are modeled for him
	Beginning to be interested in moderately novel events, actively seeks new stimulation	Will respond to introduction of moderately novel movements
Stage 3	Beginning to perceive effect on environment	Gross-motor activities critical
	Is learning to imitate new behaviors	Is learning direct imitation through progressively more accurate imitation
Stage 4	Is able to imitate directly simple new behaviors	Is able to deal with object-oriented activity

Psychiatric Patients

Piaget's Theory of Sensorimotor Learning and the Remission Process

Developmental theorists, and especially those who are concerned with cognition, support the thesis that movement-oriented exploratory behavior is an essential precursor to thought. This idea is especially applicable to the severely disorganized patient who is undergoing processes of thought reorganization. Piaget expresses the concept most cogently in his writings of the stages of sensorimotor cognitive development[1-3] and demonstrates that, during the sensorimotor period, the infant develops a remarkable set of behaviors which allows him to distinguish among various features of the environment and modify his behavior accordingly. Piaget recognized that the preliminary investigations and early construction of reality in the child are attained through movement. Remission processes, including reorganization of thoughts and reorientation to reality in the adult psychotic patient, are similarly encouraged through movement.

Piaget's Stages of Sensorimotor Development Four of the six hierarchical stages in which Piaget conceptualizes sensorimotor development provide a serviceable framework upon which to base movement-oriented treatment. His stages define primitive levels of thought organization, and may be used to assess the kinds of behaviors presented by the severely disorganized psychotic (table).

In Stage 1 (0–1 month) the newborn depends principally upon his reflexes for interaction with the environment, although, even at this stage, there is evidence that these reflex schemata are modified by experience. Two principles, functional assimilation and generalizing assimilation, get the newborn's behavior started. Piaget emphasizes that, even in the first few days of life, the infant often seeks stimulation. The principle of functional assimilation is that, when an organism has a structure available, there is an inherent tendency to exercise that structure, that is, to make it function. This is particularly true when the structure is new or in need of improvement; behavioral schemata seem to require exercise in order to consolidate. The infant does not indiscriminately suck because he is hungry; rather, he sucks because there is an inherent tendency to make available schemata, such as sucking, function. Piaget's principle of generalizing assimilation asserts that, since schemata need exercise and repeti-

tion, varying objects are required for satisfying this need. Hence the sucking schema tends to extend itself—to generalize to a variety of objects. When the infant is capable of activity, he tends to perform it; when he has a structure available, he tends to generalize it to new situations.

In Stage 2 of sensorimotor development (1–4 months) the infant begins to acquire behavioral patterns that are simple and centered around his body but not directly related to the feeding situation. At this stage, if an infant's chance movements lead to a result that is pleasurable and centered around his body, he immediately tries to repeat the behavior and reinstate the event. The infant at this stage is able to repeat the behavior of models, if such behavior is similar to that already known to the infant. At this age the infant learns in a primitive way to anticipate future events. He begins to associate such kinesthetic cues as feeding position with subsequent behavioral schemata such as sucking. In this primitive awareness of something to come in the future is the beginning of development of time concepts. Finally, in Stage 2 the infant begins to become interested in events that are moderately novel to his established schemata. An experience becomes interesting not for its familiarity, or even for its own characteristics, but for its difference. In this stage the infant actively seeks new stimulation.

In Stage 3 (4–10 months) the infant begins to extend beyond exclusive interest in his own body and to find that his motor actions can affect the external environment. He may discover that by kicking he will make a noise. He tries to isolate the appropriate cause for a chance effect. Through movement the infant is beginning to perceive that his actions are related to an external result: that he is the cause of an effect. Piaget asserts that if this connection is not made no further learning is possible. Another cognitive step in Stage 3 is that imitation of familiar schemata becomes increasingly systematic and precise. Because the infant's schemata have become more extensive and varied, a wider range of new experiences can be matched to that which is known.

Considerable progress in imitation occurs during Stage 4 (9–12 months). The infant begins to imitate the novel behavior of models even if he is not successful. It is in this stage, Piaget found, that an infant can no longer be expected to ignore a new movement because it is new, and will try to imitate it in an approximate manner.

In summary, Piaget's investigations are important for developmental thought because he defines qualitatively distinct stages of mind that precede mature cognition. Further, his investigations assist in revealing that during the sensorimotor period the infant begins to elaborate on basic dimensions of space, time, and causality, and makes his preliminary investigations of those dimensions in terms of movements. Piaget emphasizes that the infant's initial understanding of the world is entirely based on movement, and that only after a progessive development can that movement be translated into thought.

Similarities to Piaget's Sensorimotor Stages in the Psychotic Manifestations of both functional and generalizing assimilation occur in psychotic patients functioning at a low level who seem to have been reached by therapists only on a movement plane. The patient who is functioning at this low level and who repeats only one movement schema, can be motivated to learn new schemata, first by repeating and reinforcing the old schema and then by extending it for him to new situations. For example, the therapist adopts the schema of a patient who rocks in his chair all day and reinforces it for him by sitting down beside him and rocking back and forth with him in different chairs and eventually in varied positions. Gradually, the therapist extends the schema by standing up on the upswing and sitting back to follow through with the backswing. An original schema must be sufficiently consolidated before an extension can be successfully introduced. In this case, the kinesthetic cues associated with pendulum motion are an important part of the original schema and must be maintained. A new addition to the patient's old action must be simple. Any isolated movement that a patient exhibits as part of his movement repertoire can, with a degree of imagination, be extended to promote new learning. Even regressed patients are able to respond to the gradual introduction of extension of walking or running schemata. In fact, most gross motor-behavior patterns can be used as the primary teaching medium for regressed patients who have not yet reached a level where they can learn, and so reconstitute, through objects, the traditional medium for occupational therapy. In all cases, in accordance with the principle of functional assimilation, it appears that when a patient is capable of an activity, he tends to perform it. In accordance with the principle of generalizing assimilation when he has a structure available, he tends to generalize it to new situations.

Manifestations of Stage 2 are observed in patients who are capable of certain behavioral schemata when therapists mimic those schemata for them to follow. Thus, the patient was able to imitate his own rocking schema from a model. This is the initial step that must precede later forms of imitation. Similarly, the learning of time concepts can be structured and reinforced for reconstituting patients, if a consistent sequence of events is maintained during daily therapy sessions. Thus, a patient can learn to expect that rocking will precede walking and running in his therapy session. In this stage the remitting patient, like an infant in Piaget's Stage 2, will actively seek out new stimulation. For this reason, gradual extensions of a reconstituting patient's behavioral patterns with movements that are not too "new," are successful, and are not vehemently resisted. When presented with experiences utilizing schemata that are only moderately novel, the patient seems to want to function.

Severely disorganized patients must go through a stage in their remission process equivalent to that of an infant in Stage 3. It is during this stage of cognitive development that simplified sports such as basketball, volleyball, baseball, badminton, shuffleboard, and basic dance activities are particularly relevant. These activities are especially helpful if the patient's motor responses to them had been habitual and near reflexive before the psychotic break. Here the patient's previously acquired motor behavior is influential in inducing a consistent result. The message that he is indeed causal to an environmental effect is thus conveyed. In games, simplified scoring adds an even more concrete dimension.

When treating psychotic patients, Stage 3 is an important level because it is the immediate precursor to, and lays the basis for, the ability to imitate new skills. Imitative calisthenics are particularly applicable at this point since the reconstituting patient can use previously acquired behavioral schemata—gross motor skill—to match his behavior to that of a model. Through constant exposure to consistent sequences of exercise patterns, he learns to match his behavior more precisely to that of his model. Only after this skill is integrated can he begin to imitate simple behaviors that are not already a part of his repertoire. At this level, a reconstituting patient can, through imitation, begin to learn simple new skills, and therefore work to integrate succeeding levels of cognition through those new skills. The simple new learning opportunities available to him in occupational therapy will probably be the most valuable therapeutic experiences for him from this level on through the balance of cognitive development. The occupational therapist can most easily structure his traditional action-oriented activities to serve the developmental functions of the levels of cognitive development that remain. Movement-oriented activities retain their importance by reinforcing and supporting the old learning, providing much-needed sure-success experiences, and promoting the processes of new learning.

Arieti's Contribution to Development Theory

Piaget's empirical investigations and cognitive theory do not define the place of emotions in the structure of intellect. Silvano Arieti incorporates the affective dimension into his discussion of the structures underlying human development, and asserts that severely disorganized patients are overwhelmed by primitive affect that they cannot control with their primitive cognitive processes.[4] In his works he posits the existence of the "exocept," a concept that has significant implications for this paper.

The Exocept   The exocept is a mental construct or inner representation that is subsequently embodied in movement or overt action. The exocept is important because it reflects a degree of sensory organization that follows immediately from instincts and reflexes. It is the primal thinking that precedes an appropriate response to a specific set of stimuli. By definition, exocepts are immediately translated into motor behavior. They are the motor "concretizations" of primal concepts and appear at a basic developmental level.

Exoceptual activity, as Arieti conceives it, dominates the first two years of life. In Piaget's framework the developmental correlate of the exocept is in Stage 3. Exocepts develop when an infant sees an object that is unfamiliar but similar to a known object and initiates the motor response appropriate for the familiar object. For example, an infant sees a new ball and immediately rolls it as he would his own ball. The infant seems to deal with new stimuli in terms of a primitive memory of his action responses to similar stimuli. In the adult, exoceptual mentation usually does not assume a significant role except in sports, games, or other predominantly motor activities. When a basketball player responds to the stimulus basketball, he usually manages to produce an appropriate response. When an ice skater responds to the stimulus ice conditions, he usually manages to produce appropriate responses. Exoceptual mentation is most often reflected in motor acts that have become near reflexive and automatic in response to a certain set of stimuli.

Exoceptual Activity and Therapy   Psychotic patients who have regressed to low-functioning levels do not seem to lose their exocepts. A patient who was previously a star on the tennis courts can still play an adequate game of tennis during early stages of his remission process, despite frustration and confusion on most other fronts. A basketball player can play an abbreviated game of basketball, while at the same time exhibiting extremely bizarre symptoms on the ward. A patient in the severe agitation of an acute psychotic break can respond appropriately to a short game of catch despite severe disintegration when faced with most other tasks.

Exoceptual activity can, and should, be used to serve valuable therapeutic functions. Indeed, it is probably the most powerful validating tool for reconstituting patients because exocepts are the only thought processes that can be capitalized upon for patients functioning at a low cognitive level.

Conclusion

A significant manifestation of a schizophrenic break is the regression of thought processes to early developmental levels of functioning. Remission from that break hinges on rebuilding the steps toward integrated cognition in developmental order. Movement is the plane on which primal learning must take place, and it is this cognitive level that must be integrated before higher-level thought processes can evolve.

Recreation therapists, dance therapists, and movement-oriented occupational therapists have relevant roles as adjunctive personnel in the psychiatric rehabilitation of severely disorganized patients because they may be the first to reach the patient. They can work with him toward cognitive integration at a primitive level and can help the patient with the tension and confusion surrounding cognitive disintegration. Movement-oriented activity should be involved in psychiatric rehabilitation as the preliminary step toward capacitating the severely disorganized patient for occupational therapy and subsequent sociotherapeutic approaches. ∎

REFERENCES

1. Piaget J: The Construction of Reality in the Child, New York, Basic Books, 1954
2. Flavell JH: The Developmental Psychology of Jean Piaget, Princeton, N.J., Van Nostrand, 1963
3. Ginsburg H, Opper S: Piaget's Theory of Intellectual Development, Englewood Cliffs, N.J., Prentice-Hall Inc., 1969
4. Arieti S: The Intrapsychic Self: Feelings, Cognition and Creativity in Health and Mental Illness, New York, Basic Books, Inc., 1968

The American Journal of Occupational Therapy
1971, Vol. XXV, No. 6, 291–294

Occupational Behavior—A Perspective on Work and Play

Janice Matsutsuyu, M.A., O.T.R.

As trends toward extended health care services in community practice gain momentum, the study and knowledge of the work-play phenomena provide treatment strategies for occupational therapists. Such a strategy represents a shift from the treatment of symptomatology to one of identifying the nature of adaptations or the acquisition of new skills, and examining socialization patterns to support the daily living performance of patients in their life role. Within the frame of reference of occupational behavior three processes are discussed: occupational choice. occupational role, and socialization.

Among the many issues that face occupational therapy today, one is the degree to which members of this profession are able to free themselves from certain generalized assumptions about clinical practice. The professional identity has been based largely on the medical model for guiding practice, curriculum, and theory building. Occupational therapists have become technically competent at identifying deficit and dysfunctional states and their efforts have been directed towards adding to the diagnostic process and reduction of symptoms.

This has not been without rationale as their arena of practice has been firmly posited in hospitals, clinics, and institutions for the ill and disabled. This has required a working knowledge of pathology, of disease entities, of symptoms and course of illness. Occupational therapists, therefore, broadened their knowledge about anatomy, neurophysiology, and psychopathology.

Currently the trend towards extending health care services to community practice is gaining greater momentum.[1] Occupational therapists share with other health professions the goal of returning or keeping patients functioning in their community roles. As yet most of their understanding and knowledge about patient history is based on etiology of disease, on current functions of symptomatology and future planning on stabilization of the disease process. Clinically the reduction or stasis of disease does not necessarily lead to improved function and

Janice Matsutsuyu is chief of the rehabilitation services of the Neuropsychiatric Institute at the University of California Center for Health Sciences in Los Angeles.
This article is based on a paper presented at the symposium, "The Skill Continuum from Play through Work," conducted by the occupational therapy staff of Walter E. Fernald State School and its university-affiliated Eunice Kennedy Shriver Center, October 28–30, 1970, Boston, and sponsored by the Department of HEW Maternal and Child Health Service.

increased engagement in activity. As therapists struggled from various points of view with the meanings to occupational therapy of *functional levels* and *activity* it was found that the perspective based on pathology held few guidelines for working knowledge of healthy function. It is not enough to accept the definition of health as absence of disease.

If occupational therapists value their role as activators of residual functions, as teachers and nurturers of daily living skills, and if they believe in the potentialities of patients striving for independent living, then the therapist's knowledge must be broadened and deepened beyond the medical sciences.

Reilly identified the need for the profession to increase its knowledge about the work-play phenomena as a productive area of study and from which occupational therapy programs for patients could be planned.[2] She reminds therapists of their early beginnings and the Meyerian challenge of 1921[3] and stated that occupational therapy's philosophical and operational base could be found in the understanding of human organization as a balance between work, play, rest, and sleep.[2] More recently she wrote, "Play, in a chronological or a longitudinal sense, we believe, is the antecedent preparation area for work. In a cross-sectional sense we have found it clinically useful to see an adult social-recreation pattern of behavior as a sublatent support to a work pattern. The entire developmental continuum of play and work we designate as occupational behavior."[4]

Occupational Behavior

The frame of reference called occupational behavior is proposed as one approach for adding to the body of knowledge in occupational therapy.[4,6,7,9] It is guided primarily by the sociological concept of role and socialization and by psychological theories of achievement motivation, problem solving, and personality development. Such a behavioral science base, combined with the medical science and knowledge, creates a view of patients not only as diagnostic entities but as individuals occupying life roles with both assets and problems in daily living. Occupational behavior is studied through the play and work phenomena. These phenomena provide the conceptual base and support the premise that adult work and social recreation roles evolve from childhood play, chores, and crafts.

Guided by Reilly's formulations in both the clinical and graduate study areas the early findings were that an almost layman's point of view about work and play existed in occupational therapy. It seemed to be generally assumed that since children's work is play, they know how to play, and since adults work, naturally they know about work. But patients who have been incapacitated or developmentally impoverished in their achievements deserve more from occupational therapists and therefore it becomes critical to seek more informed and systematic ways of looking at maladaptive play and work behavior. The assessment problem for occupational therapy becomes one of acknowledging the present state of dysfunction or disease and also one of examining the quality of socialization patterns in the acquisition of skills for life roles. The treatment strategy becomes one of identifying the nature of adaptations or the renewal or acquisition of new skills needed to maintain, support, or raise the daily living performance of patients in their current life role.

Within the broad frame of reference of occupational behavior three processes became essential for study. These are occupational choice, occupational role, and socialization.

Occupational Choice. Occupational choice is conceptualized as a series of developmental stages culminating in the selection of an occupation.[5] Studies of occupational choice most clearly identify the bridge between childhood play and adult work role. It is a phase when the backlog of experience gained through childhood play and daily living can be seen as adding substantive material from which one can make an occupational choice. The concepts on play proposed by Takata, Florey, and Michelman in this series, identify those elements of childhood that are not only considered important to their growth and development as children but also are relevant to assuming and successfully performing adult roles.

Pezzuti identified certain factors as significant in promoting occupational choice throughout development. Major themes are those of encouraging exploratory and achievement-relevant performance and behavior, and providing objects to play with and manipulate in the environment. Her schema includes the development of a sense of trust in infancy, a sense of competence in one's ability to interact with the

environment through exploratory play, and the development of motility, speed, and control in early childhood. Childhood was characterized by an awareness of sex roles, identification with a worker, learning the rhythm of daily routine, and the mastery of self-help skills. School age was characterized by learning the rudiments of work skills through chores and homework, learning to organize time and energy, and the acquisition of social competence and basic mental skills. Adolescence was marked by the achievement of sex and social role, a sense of competence in role behavior and work tasks, independence from parents, and the selection of an occupation. She further concluded that conscious choice requires experience and opportunity in which to develop skills and the making of choice and decisions. It required cognitive development, and awareness of one's values, interests and abilities, and motivation.[6]

The consensus is that occupational choice is not a single event occurring when an individual reaches a certain age. It is a developmental process extending over many years. It can be seen in the adaptational sense as a series of choices and the elimination of choices, leading to narrowing of choice, and eventually to reconciliation of decision as changes occur in the individual and the environment. It can be seen in the achievement sense through gaining mastery and competence, through striving for excellence and understanding of one's personal resources, within the context of one's environment, and opportunities found in the family, community, and economic realities. And it speaks for the cumulative effect of childhood play and chores, through exploration to mastery to practice, of a variety of skills in the performance of everyday behavior.[5, 6, 7, 10]

Occupational Role. Concurrent with the studies on play of children, the phenomenon of work was being investigated through adult roles. The sociological concept that role can be divided into three systems—family roles, personal-sexual roles, and occupational roles—was accepted. Although acknowledging that family and personal-sexual roles are part of the individual role complex, the studies were initially focused on occupational roles as being most relevant. Since occupational role is also identified as much by social position as by the tasks performed, the concept was further expanded to include the housewife, student, retiree, and preschooler as well as worker.[4, 7, 9]

Moorhead made a significant early contribution to our clinical understanding of the derivatives of socialization, role theory, and occupational role in her study and development of an occupational history instrument.[7] It is based on the assumption that adult occupational behavior reflects an attempt to assimilate oneself into some identified group that meets one's own need for productivity, belonging, and life structuring activities. From this she derived three phases in occupational development. The first involves the events and stages in preadult years culminating in occupational choice; second, the mobility within and between jobs during the adult years, and third, at retirement, the reconstruction of life patterns of activity without the supportive structure of occupational institutions. Through Moorhead's assessment, evidence can be gained about an individual's occupational development. The findings include data about the learning and socialization that occurs in childhood roles, the exploration and decision-making process around occupational choice, and the patterns of achievement and failure within the context and the environmental conditions influencing mobility and solidification in an adult occupational role.[7]

Socialization. The learning of relevant occupational role behaviors occurs through the socialization process. Schmaltz summarized this process for occupational therapy as "a learning based on maturation, a learning in the sense of processing social data, a learning of norms and roles, and developing of a personal system in relation to the social system."[8] She proposed a model of socialization in the occupational therapy setting as one of role maintenance, role learning, and role relearning. Role maintenance occurs if there has been a history of adequate occupational role function. It is to assure adequate opportunities for keeping existing skills operational for daily living. Role learning refers to the acquisition of new or additional occupational role skills if the individual is assessed as being in the growth stage. If there has been an interruption by dysfunction role relearning takes place so that adaptive skills congruent with past occupational history and function and relevant to current or expected life roles can be learned.[8]

The occupational therapy setting is seen as a milieu or culture which must be built and functioning in order that learning relevant to life roles can take place.[2] Essentially Reilly's six specifications provide the occupational frame of reference for the occupational therapy program. She states that first there must be an examination of life roles and identification of the various skills that support them; next that the program should reflect the developmental stages present in the acquisition of life skills; and third, the programs should provide natural and legitimate decision-making areas for patients. The fourth specification states that the milieu must acknowledge competencies, arouse curiosity, deepen appreciation, and demand behavior across the full spectrum of human abilities. Fifth, the occupational therapists must take action beyond the single activity and fragment of time in occupational therapy with concerns for work, play, and rest extending throughout the days, evenings, and weekends. Finally, she specified that the program structure must provide opportunities for the practicing of life skills in a balanced pattern of daily living, take into account individual interests and abilities, and tailor events to age, sex, and occupational roles.

Summary

Through focusing both clinical and graduate studies on play and work, and by shifting the initial perspective of patients from diagnostic labels to those of the occupational roles of worker, student, housewife, retiree, preschooler, and even career patient, occupational therapists have begun to identify what is important and what should be included in programs for daily living. The occupational behavior frame of reference has caused therapists to broaden and raise the level of knowledge about the play and work phenomena and the complex sets of variables from which occupational role evolves.[9] It became evident that prerequisite experiences are to be found in childhood play, especially when concepts such as exploration, mastery, decision making, achievement, and competence emerge as recurring themes.[9]

This frame of reference has led us to the conclusion that work behavior does not automatically begin at society's definition of work age, nor does it spontaneously exist once early conflicts are resolved or disease stabilized.[10] Occupational therapists have come to understand that maladaptive play and work need not necessarily be seen as a result of illness only. Further they have learned that occupational development and vocational preparation are not synonymous and that vocational training for a trade or profession is only one component of occupational development.

It has been encouraging to learn that this profession's early common sense and intuitive approach to work and play principles can be systematically investigated. The behavioral sciences offer rich resources for occupational therapy. Many aspects still must be clarified and studied for further elaboration and clinical applicability. This exploratory phase of building and formalizing both the theoretical base and clinical tools continues with every indication that the occupational behavior frame of reference is a sound one. And, as the consumer of health services begins to demand more involvement in his own treatment process this frame of reference guides occupational therapists towards having the consumer become an active partner in the identification of his problem, in acknowledging his strengths, in setting achievable goals, and in planning a course of action.

REFERENCES

1. Bockoven JS: Challenge of the new clinical approaches. Amer J Occup Ther 22: 23-29, 1968.
2. Reilly M: A psychiatric occupational therapy program as a teaching model. Amer J Occup Ther 20(2): 61-67, 1966.
3. Meyers A: The philosophy of occupational therapy. Read by Adolf Meyers at the Fifth Annual Meeting of the National Society for the Promotion of Occupational

Therapy (Now the American Occupational Therapy Association), held in Baltimore, Maryland, Oct. 20-22, 1921. Arch Occup Ther 1: 1-10, 1922.

4. Reilly M: The educational process. Amer J Occup Ther 23: 299-307, 1969.

5. Ginzberg E, et al: Occupational Choice, New York, Columbia University Press, 1951.

6. Pezzuti L: An exploration of adolescent feminine and occupational behavior. Master's thesis, Department of Occupational Therapy, University of Southern California, Los Angeles, California, 1970.

7. Moorhead LC: The occupational history. Amer J Occup Ther 23: 329-338, 1969.

8. Schmaltz H: Occupational therapy as a socialization process. Master's thesis, Occupational Therapy Department, University of Southern California, Los Angeles, California.

9. Shannon PD: Work adjustment and the adolescent soldier. Master's thesis, Occupational Therapy Department, University of Southern California, 1966.

10. Super DE: The Psychology of Careers, New York, Harper, 1957.

AN ALTERNATIVE: THE

BIOPSYCHOSOCIAL MODEL

This paper suggests a biopsychosocial model as an alternative to the use of the medical or health model for occupational therapists. The concept label for the model was selected because it seems to reflect not only the theories basic to the profession but also the present-future orientation of occupational therapy. The paper outlines how the proposed model facilitates ordering of the theoretical base and thinking about the client care process. The proposed model takes into consideration man as a physical being who suffers from the effect of illness and injury; man as an individual with thoughts, emotions, needs and values; and man as a player of many and varied social roles. The biopsychosocial model moves away from the illness-health continuum to an emphasis upon information, abilities, and values necessary for productive community living.

Anne Cronin Mosey, O.T.R., Ph.D., F.A.O.T.A.

One hears much discussion of late about leaving the medical model as the occupational therapy point of orientation and moving toward another model. The health model has probably been the most frequently suggested. The purpose of this paper is to explore the nature of the medical and health models and to propose an alternative: the biopsychosocial model.

Current Models

The term model as used in this paper refers to the typical way in which a profession or discipline studies and organizes data and devises action plans relative to its domain of concern. It usually includes certain assump-

Dr. Mosey is program director of the occupational therapy curriculum, New York University.

The American Journal of Occupational Therapy

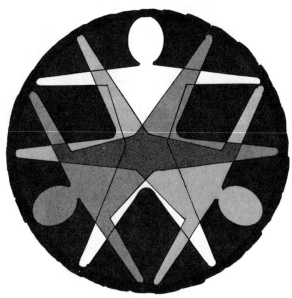

tions, a theoretical base, and a set of operating principles.[1,2,3]

The model used in medicine structures information within the framework of signs and symptoms, cause, pathology, treatment, course and prognoses, and occasionally sequela or abnormal conditions resulting from a disease. The major assumption of the medical model is that man has a right to life. Its theoretical base is derived primarily from the biological sciences. Its set of operating principles is oriented to the diagnosis of disease and the minimization or elimination of a disease process through intervention directed toward causal factors or pathology.

The health model as it has been proposed is vague. There is no specific way to structure a theoretical base. Its major assumption is that man has a right to a fruitful existence despite his disabilities. The theoretical base continues to be derived primarily from the biological sciences with some slight concern for normal growth and development and learning theories. Its set of operating principles is oriented to somewhat more concern for the patient's assets as opposed to his liabilities.[4]

Reasons for Rejecting the Medical Model

The medical model is disease-oriented. But occupational therapists are concerned with sequela and what the patient will be doing after he leaves the treatment center. The medical model is primarily concerned with acute conditions. Occupational therapists are concerned with the sequela of acute conditions, but even more concerned with the long-term consequences of a disease process.

It has become increasingly apparent that the medical model is a poor structure for considering the entire area of psychosocial dysfunction: the cause of psychosocial dysfunction is unknown; there is no agreement about what is symptom, pathology, or sequela; and treatment is often not specific to diagnosis.

The medical model provides no structure for

information regarding alteration of sequela. The considerable information used by a therapist to alter sequela, therefore, remains unsystematized and "homeless."

The medical model emphasizes treatment. Treatment by definition is the process of eliminating or minimizing the cause of a disease process or the resulting pathology. Only by extensive conceptual manipulations can the occupational therapists say their concern is with causal factors or pathology.

Reasons for Rejecting the Health Model

The label "health model" has a euphemistic ring. Many of the patients and clients are chronically ill. It sounds as though occupational therapists might be ignoring the "not being well" aspect of the patient. The patient is interested in utilizing his assets, but he is also concerned about his limitations. He wants help with these limitations.

The health model takes into consideration the occupational therapists' growing work with the socially disadvantaged and clients with learning disabilities. But use of the term health model implies the opposite; lack of health or illness. Questions are bound to be raised by the individual about whether he is sick or well.

The health model as it now stands is not compartmentalized enough to allow occupational therapy to have a systematized theoretical base. It lacks the subdivisions of the medical model. The occupational therapy theoretical base remains amorphous.

The Biopsychosocial Model

The biopsychosocial model directs attention to the body, mind, and environment of the client. It takes these three facets into consideration without any sense of wellness or sickness on the part of the client. The biological aspect of the label focuses attention upon sequela, theories regarding ways of increasing muscle strength, range of motion, coordination, and the anatomy and physiology basic to occupational therapy practice.

The psychological portion of the label emphasizes concern about normal human growth and development and deficits in the maturation process. It provides a place for the various theories used as bases for the teaching-learning process which is so important in most aspects of client care. This portion of the model also includes the need for understanding various theories of psychodynamics, defense mechanisms, and the symbolic process.

The sociological portion of the model points to concern for man as he exists in a group of meaningful others. Here are housed the theories of group dynamics and processes in verbal and activities groups. Here also are the theories of group socialization and the development of various role patterns.

The major assumption of the biopsychosocial model is similar to that of the health model: that man has a right to a meaningful and productive existence. This includes the right not only to be free of disease but to participate in the life of the community. For patients with chronic diseases, the biopsychosocial model emphasizes what can be done to make the chronic illness of the patient more bearable. Man does not have to suffer if there are ways of relieving suffering.

The set of operating principles of the biopsychosocial model are oriented toward the delineation of learning needs and the teaching-learning process.

The therapist is concerned with delineating the overall goals or ultimate orientation of the program. These general aims are then translated into clearly defined and concrete knowledge, skills, and attitudes. Ideally, specific objectives are stated so as to be measurable. General aims and specific objectives are relative to the program in general and not to an individual. These are developed through knowledge of the nature of individuals who will be participating in the program and societal and cultural demands and values of the community.

The assessment and delineation of the individual's learning needs relative to the objectives of the model refer to initial evaluation. However, rather than focus on symptoms, the therapist may speak of behavior indicative of learning and behavior indicative of lack of learning. Knowledge of basic principles of measurement and testing is necessary in order to devise or select appropriate tools for assessment.

The learning sequence or priorities of the model involves specifying what knowledge, skills, and attitudes are to be focused on during various stages of the program. Planning involves consideration of the patient's set of priorities as well as the principles being used to guide the teaching-learning process.

The selection and organization of learning experiences are essentially a statement of the teaching plan. It is derived from knowledge of the nature of what is to be taught and postulates regarding change which are appropriate to the desired learning. The process may be directed toward adding to or deleting from the individual's repertoire.[5,6]

Principles of Teaching-Learning

The teacher begins where the learner is and moves at a rate that is comfortable for the learner. A good teacher takes into consideration the learner's inherent capacities, age, sex, interests, assets, limitations, and cultural group membership. The learner should be an active participant in the learning process. The consequences of an action are important. Opportunity for trial, error, and imitation enhances learning. Frequent repetition and practice facilitate learning. Learning goals set by the learner are more likely to be attained than goals set by someone else. Practice in different situations encourages generalization and discrimination. The learner should understand what is to be learned and the reasons for learning. Planned movement from simplified wholes to more complex wholes enhances learning. Innovative solutions to problems should be encouraged as well as more usual or typical solutions. There are individual differences in the ways anxiety affects learning.[7]

The evaluation of the effectiveness of the learning experience is continued evaluation. As in initial assessment, it requires an understanding of the basic principles of measurement and testing.

Advantages of the Biopsychosocial Model

For several reasons the biopsychosocial model would be useful for the practice of occupational therapy. It provides a means for systemization of our knowledge which is one of the criteria of a profession. It provides a statement of the profession's goals and focuses attention upon theories of change in many aspects of life.

The biopsychosocial model is oriented to the client-in-community. It emphasizes the reality of the client's life outside the treatment center, and the connotation of the proposed model may enhance our relationship within the community. There is less of an orientation toward "medicine" or "treatment" and more of the connotation of working together to solve problems in living.

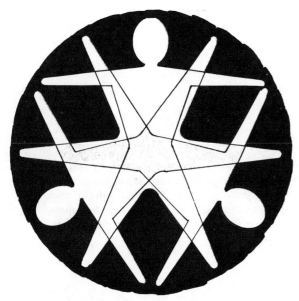

The biopsychosocial model is sufficiently concrete to differentiate it from the medical model, a distinction which the health model does not make clear at this time. The proposed model can help to clarify the roles of occupational therapy relative to medicine and the other health-related professions.

The biopsychosocial model is based upon knowledge necessary for clinical and academic teaching. Thus, transition to these areas of practice may be easier. This is also true in the case of consultation and prevention.

The proposed model seems to be well suited for occupational therapists working without a medical support team immediately available. In these community-based programs, the occupational therapist must be acutely aware of the physical health needs of her clients. The therapist must ensure that these health needs are met. Sociological concepts often serve as the bases for dealing with family, work, and leisure-time problems. Securing financial support and the dynamics of initiating social action for neighborhood groups fall well within the range of the biopsychosocial model.

For occupational therapists working in a psychiatric setting, the biopsychosocial model presents a way out of a chronic difficulty presented by the medical model. There is no concern for what is symptom and what is pathology. If the patient's problems are seen as due to chemical imbalance, the therapist attempts to diminish sequela. Use of the proposed model also allows the therapist to think and act in terms of unconscious conflict or development of skills for fuller participation in the life of the community.

Problems Related to Changing to the Biopsychosocial Model

One of the problems of moving from the medical model to the biopsychosocial model has to do with change itself. Any change is uncomfortable. However, it must be remembered that occupational therapists really did not use the medical model for ordering a theoretical base or practice.

A realistic problem concerns the professional self-concept: a therapist treats. The biopsychosocial model has a much heavier emphasis upon the teaching-learning process. The connotation of *teacher* does not sit well with many occupational therapists because they have worked for many years to eliminate from their public image the idea of being arts and crafts teachers. Thus, any suggestion of teaching is immediately rejected. It is as if such a concept has become a negative archetype in the collective unconscious of occupational therapists. But occupational therapists are teaching skills for living. We may sometimes use arts and crafts as a vehicle for teaching such skills. However, we also teach living skills directly or through the use of activities other than arts and crafts.

One last problem area is again related to the emphasis upon the teaching-learning process. This may immediately bring to mind operant conditioning, "M and M treatment," or a "token economy treatment unit." This is not the intent; the therapist draws upon many different theories of teaching and learning. There was an attempt to emphasize this point in the presentation of common principles of teaching-learning.

Summary

The biopsychosocial model is suggested as an alternative to the medical and health models. Movement away from the medical model is suggested because it does not include a place for organizing our theoretical base nor does it reflect occupational therapy practice. The health model is criticized both for its lack of specificity and for its connotation of the illness-health continuum. The biopsychosocial model is proposed because it focuses upon man as a biological entity, a thinking and feeling person, and a member of a community of others. ∎

REFERENCES
1. Abraham MH: Psychology of Science, Chicago, Henry Regency, 1966
2. Reilly M: The educational process. Am. J Occup Ther 23: 299-307, 1969
3. Stein J: Random House Dictionary of the English Language, New York, Random House, 1966
4. Johnson J: Report of the Task Force on Social Issues. Am J Occup Ther 26: 332-359, 1972
5. Anderson, V: Curriculum Improvement (2nd ed), New York, Ronald Press, 1965
6. Taba W: Curriculum Development, New York, Harcourt Brace & World, 1962
7. Hilgard E, Bower G: Theories of Learning, New York, Appleton-Century-Crofts, 1966

The behavioral model can be a useful tool to occupational therapists in changing specific behaviors of patients. The process of behavior modification is involved in daily patient treatment, but the direct, conscious application of behavioral principles and procedures is not widely used in occupational therapy. When occupational therapy terminology in planning a treatment program is compared to behavioral terminology in applying the behavioral equation, the treatment session becomes the disposition; the activity becomes the discriminative stimulus; the patient's performance becomes the response; the treatment plan the contingency; and the treatment goal the consequence. To systematically apply these behavioral techniques, the therapist must have an understanding of the basic systems of applied behavioral analysis as well as the procedures for designing a behavior modification project that includes: identifying the terminal behavior; timing, counting, recording and charting; selecting the reinforcer; choosing a fixed or interval schedule of reinforcement; and shaping, chaining, and modeling to establish new behaviors. These concepts are presented in the context of their application in occupational therapy.

Applying the Behavioral Model

TO THE OCCUPATIONAL THERAPY MODEL

Kay W. Sieg

Occupational therapists are involved daily in the modification of patient behavior,[1,2] yet there are few reports of systematic application of operant techniques and principles to occupational therapy treatment.[3-11] While several such studies were conducted through the cooperative efforts of occupational therapists and personnel from other disciplines, the high incidence of first authorship by the latter suggests that the occupational therapist played a secondary role in the engineering of the projects.[5-9] In order for the occupational therapist to systematically apply operant techniques, it is necessary to have a basic understanding of the principles and procedures of designing a behavior modification project. This article will acquaint the therapist with the rudiments of designing a behavior modification project and

Kay W. Sieg, O.T.R., M.Ed., is assistant professor in occupational therapy at the University of Florida in Gainesville.

the simplicity of the basic techniques. It is not purported to be an all-inclusive review of the information that is available about behavior modification.

Much of the following information is derived from *The Handbook of Applied Behavior Analysis* by W. D. Wolking.[12] Other suggestions are from the author's experience gained through teaching and supervising students in behavior modification projects for learning-disabled children.

Definitions of Applied Behavioral Analysis

A number of terms are used by disciplines when referring to applied behavioral analysis. *Operant conditioning* is B.F. Skinner's term, which holds that an organism operates on its environment toward some goal and, when this goal is attained, the likelihood that the behavior will recur is increased. *Behavior modification* is used in the clinical application of operant conditioning laboratory methods and is the process by which the frequency of a behavior is modified by the consequences of the behavior. *Learning theory* states that both maladaptive and adaptive behaviors are learned. In *behavior therapy* the emphasis is on designing conditions that will change the behavior and thus alleviate the problem, rather than delving into psychic or mental reasons for the problem.[13,14]

In the past decade, special educators developed procedures for applying Skinner's operant conditioning principles in the classroom.[15,16] *Precision teaching* is a recording and measurement system for identifying the functional control of the environment upon the learning of the child. The aim is to determine which environmental events produce maximum learning for that child. The process consists of designing a unit of instruction for the child, implementing the program, and recording the child's responses. These measures provide direct and continuous feedback for the student and the teacher, and enable the teacher to make "data decisions" based upon the efficacy of the instructional unit.[12]

Four Systems of Applied Behavioral Analysis

The four systems of applied behavioral analysis are determined by whether a pleasing or an aversive stimulus is either withdrawn or presented *contingent* upon the response. When a pleasing stimulus is presented, this is termed *positive reinforcement;* when an aversive stimulus is withdrawn, this is termed *negative reinforcement;* when a pleasing stimulus is withdrawn, this is termed *extinction,* and when an aversive stimulus is presented, this is termed *punishment.* Positive and negative reinforcement increase responding; punishment and extinction decrease responding.[12] These four systems are summarized in the table.

Positive Reinforcement

In positive reinforcement, the aim is to increase the desired response by presenting a pleasing stimulus contingent upon that response. When a child behaves well in order to obtain certain privileges, he is positively reinforced for good behavior. Positive reinforcement is also used indirectly to decrease undesirable behavior by increasing desirable behavior through attractive, positive reinforcers.

Procedures to increase desired responding include the following: *Shaping, chaining, and modeling* are procedures for establishing a new behavior. *Differential reinforcement for high rates* (DRH) maintains high rates of responding once the behavior is established. The reinforcement is available provided the rate has stayed equal to or above a set level during a stated time period, such as reinforcing a patient for weaving at least ten rows in a five-minute interval.[17] *Differential reinforcement for low rates* (DRL) is used to maintain a behavior at a low frequency during a certain interval, such as maintaining verbal interaction at a rate that does not interfere with working behavior.[17]

Procedures to increase desirable responding by decreasing undesirable behavior include the following: *Differential reinforcement for*

TABLE

Four Systems of Applied Behavioral Analysis

	Positive Reinforcement	Negative Reinforcement	Punishment	Extinction
Present	Positive stimulus		Negative stimulus	
Result	Increases responding		Decreases responding	
Withdraw		Negative stimulus		Positive stimulus
Result		Increases responding		Decreases responding

other behaviors (DRO) is used to reinforce any behavior occurring during an interval, except the undesirable behavior. If the undesirable behavior occurs, none of the other behaviors during that interval are reinforced.[17] *Reinforcing incompatible behaviors* strengthens behaviors that cannot coexist with the undesirable behavior, such as increasing working behavior incompatible with nonworking.[17] *Desensitization* has been used to reduce anxiety by conditioning incompatible behaviors in the presence of anxiety-provoking stimulus.[18] For example, while imagining the feared object (anxiety provoking), deep muscle relaxation is practiced (incompatible behavior). *Decreasing the discriminative stimulus for the undesired response* involves removing the discriminative stimulus that sets the occasion for the response.[19] For example, not having sweets (discriminative stimulus) available when trying to diet will decrease the occurrence of eating sweets (undesired behavior). *Group contingency* may be used to initiate group control of behavior of the individuals within the group, in which each member of the group must emit the desired behavior in order for each individual to be reinforced.[12] *Reinforcement satiation* may be used to decrease undesirable behavior by the application of excessive quantities of the pleasing reinforcer. Towel hoarding behavior of a psychiatric patient was decreased by delivering large quantities of towels to her room.[20]

Negative Reinforcement

Negative reinforcement may be used to increase desired behaviors that avoid (postpone) or escape (terminate) an aversive stimulus. The subject can postpone or terminate a negative stimulus by emitting a desired response.[19] Self-feeding (desired behavior) was increased by psychiatric patients in order to avoid the messy feeding by nurses (aversive stimulus).[21] In a toilet training project, severely mentally retarded children escaped the aversiveness of being restrained in a pottie chair by voiding there.[22] The term "negative reinforcement" is often confused with punishment procedures in which aversive stimuli are applied to decreasing responding. In behavior modification terminology, "negative reinforcment" describes the procedure of increasing desired behaviors that avoid or escape an aversive consequence. The term "reinforcer" is used when a stimulus increases responding and is therefore common to negative as well as to positive reinforcement.[17] The difference is that an aversive stimulus is used as a reinforcer in negative reinforcement and a pleasing stimulus is used as a reinforcer in positive reinforcement.

Punishment Punishment may be used to decrease the rate of an undesirable response by delivering an aversive stimulus or withdrawing a positive stimulus contingent upon and following the occurrence of the undesired response. It has been used when other approaches have proved unsuccessful, such as a mild electric shock in the treatment of chronic rumination when counseling and antiemetic medication were ineffective.[23] Punishment has also been used in the treatment of such deviate personal or social behaviors as transvestism and alcoholism.[24] The effectiveness of punishment is increased when alternate methods of responding are provided. Treatment should entail not only control of the undesirable response but also an expansion of the patient's desired behavior repertory.[25,26] The restraint of prison inmates that prevents the occurrence of the undesirable behavior while other behaviors are shaped in rehabilitation programs is one example.[19] The primary criticism of punishment is that it is ethically improper as a form of professional treatment. Other criticisms are: that punishment of one response may depress responding in general; that the subject is driven away from the punishing agent and the relationship is destroyed; and that the subject may become aggressive to nearby persons. Punishment is also said to negatively reinforce the punisher who escapes the aversive stimuli of the undesirable behavior but does not deal with the reasons for the undesirable behavior.[24] A parent who spanks a child for whining is negatively reinforced if the spanking terminates the aversive stimulus (whining).[19]

Extinction In extinction, the therapist identifies and terminates the stimuli reinforcing the undesired response. Extinction is the *removal* of reinforcer in order to decrease the rate of responding, in contrast to punishment in which an aversive stimulus is *delivered* to decrease responding. Time-out and response cost are two extinction procedures commonly used. In the *time-out* method, when a patient is not performing as desired, he may be removed from the situation for a period of time so that he has no opportunity to earn reinforcement. In *response cost,* once an effective reinforcer is found, the reinforcer is reduced a certain amount for undesirable behavior.[27]

Defining the Behavioral Equation in Terms of the Occupational Therapy Program

Lindsley, a special educator, has designed a behavioral equation for developing a precision teaching curriculum unit that, when occupational therapy terminology is used, is similar to the method used by therapists planning a treatment program.

The Operant Behavioral Equation:[12,15]

Disposition→Discriminative Stimulus
   (D)   (SD)
→Response→Contingency→Consequence
  (R)   (K)   (C)

The Occupational Therapy Program:

Treatment session→Activity→Patient performance→Treatment plan→Treatment goal

Disposition/treatment session These are the general, constant environmental features and includes the clinical setting, day of the week, time and length of the session, lighting, sounds, and potentially distracting or facilitating events. *Discriminative stimulus/activity* These are specific environmental stimuli that set the occasion for the desired response. In occupational therapy, it would be the task selected to meet the patient's needs. There are two kinds of discriminative stimuli: dimensional, including the physical aspects such as materials, tools, presence of the therapist, demonstration of instructions; and instructional, including the spoken or written language. *Response/patient performance* This includes the actual patient behavior desired as he engages in the task at hand. This is the behavior being observed, counted, and recorded. *Contingency/treatment plan* This is the rule that states when the consequence of the behavior is made available to or produced by the patient. In occupational therapy, it would include the time required to complete the project, if upon completion of the project the reinforcer were available; or it could be the number of sanding strokes needed to strengthen a muscle without overtiring it. *Consequence/treatment goal* These are contingent upon the occurrence of the specified behavior only if the desired response is made. Referring to the above examples, the project must be completed for the efforts to be rewarding; the board must be sanded for the muscle to be strengthened. Consequences may be natural, such as reading comics or listening to records, or synthetic, such as pennies and M&M candies. Consequences are termed reinforcing when these are used to increase or accelerate a behavior; and punishing when used to decrease or decelerate a behavior. Consequences are aversive if they are noxious to the subject.

The occupational therapy treatment model is comparable to the behavioral model. The primary difference is that while the occupational therapist plans and executes treatment for the patient, he must often rely on clinical observation to know whether the program is meeting the goals. The application of the behavioral model is a means whereby the therapist can have continual and sensitive data to verify the efficacy of specific activities in the treatment process. He has the information to evaluate treatment and to affect change. The behavioral model increases the awareness of what the therapist expects the patient to do, how the therapist's behavior affects the patient, and if the treatment is producing the desired results.

Because the behavioral model concerns specific behaviors, it is helpful in structuring a means of modifying a specific patient problem. The therapist may apply the behavioral model to a precise behavior within more general treatment goals. For example, one goal for the mentally retarded is to increase self-esteem, and a means of achieving this may be through success in the specific task. The behavioral model becomes one systematic tool for some patients, although it is not advocated as the best approach to all patient problems.

Designing the Program

Identifying the Terminal Behavior The initial step in designing a behavioral modification program is to identify the behavior to be increased, decreased, or shaped. The behavior must be observable and countable. One may begin by asking "If I could change one behavior, which would it be?"

There are several guidelines for pinpointing the behavior. The first is to use a positive approach, to select a behavior to accelerate rather than decelerate, since increasing a behavior involves positive stimuli, while decreasing a behavior involves aversive stimuli.[12] In identifying behavioral objectives for chronic mental patients, one occupational therapist specified that the patient be "on time for the session," rather than that he "not be late," and that he "initiate relevant, appropriate conversation," rather than "not engage in inappropriate, bizarre speaking."[5] Retention of the desired behavior is more likely to occur when a behavior that is rewarding personally and socially is increased, rather than only when an undesirable behavior is diminished.

An observable behavior should be described but not an inner emotion.[12] Identify smiles, not happiness, identify the frequency with which the patient complies with requests, not cooperativeness. Action words, such as hammering, sanding, throwing, hopping, are helpful in defining the behavior. The behavior should be described completely and accurately so that it is obvious where it begins and ends.[12] If someone who is unfamiliar with the patient and the procedure can read the description and readily observe and count the behavior, then it is defined accurately and completely. The terminal behavior in one study was "70 units of work in 50 minutes for one cigaret" and the unit of work was further described.[8] One occupational therapy student identified increasing verbalization as the desired terminal behavior defining verbalization as "anything spoken distinctly enough for a listener to understand, regardless of how many words were spoken at a time."

A behavior that occurs with moderate frequency is most manageable.[12] Behaviors that occur frequently are difficult to count, while very low frequency behaviors make the reinforcement less effective. Counting every stitch knitted could be time consuming, while counting every afghan would negate the power of the reinforcement. Counting every ten rows or counting every granny square completed might be a realistic approach.

Counting the Behavior   Counting the occurrence of the behavior provides precise information for identifying the efficacy of the treatment. While standardized tests are used initially to assess the problem areas, or to assess the effect of the treatment, the rates of specific behaviors may be used on a daily basis to assess the treatment. This permits immediate adjustments to be made.

Once the terminal behavior is identified and before making any changes related to this behavior, baseline rates are gathered by counting the behavior as it usually occurs. This provides a basis for comparing the effects of the treatment. Counting the behavior three or four times before introducing changes is usually sufficient.

When the pinpointed behavior occurs infrequently, some system of counting every occurrence of the behavior must be made. It may be a simple matter of counting the units of completed work,[8] noting whether the patient was well groomed,[5] or checking whether the patient could successfully use an orthotic device. For most pinpoints it is not necessary to count every occurrence of the behavior. A behavioral sample may be taken at any appropriate time during the session. Every occurrence of the behavior is counted during a brief period, such as muscle testing, during the last 5 minutes of the session. Rates are derived by counting and timing the pinpointed behavior. Counting is done by the therapist or other personnel by using an inventory counter, golf or knitting tally, marking an index card, or any other means that is effective. A weekly chart may be used when a number of related behaviors are pinpointed such as those involving work habits, including punctuality, working without stopping, and initiating conversation.[5] Timing involves the use of a wristwatch, stopwatch, or timer to measure the amount of time during which the behavior occurred. If the time is less than five minutes, seconds are used. Timing is done by the same person doing the counting. Both the number of occurrences of the behavior (movements) and the number of minutes are recorded on a raw data sheet, with columns for movements, minutes, and rates. The rate is computed by dividing the movements per minute.[12]

Recording the Rates   There are three recording plans: movement-based or ratio, time-based or interval, and first come. In the movement-based method, the number of responses is set and the time will vary depending on how long it takes for the desired number of responses to occur.[12] For example, in increasing verbalizations, the subject earns one point for each responsive verbalization, two points for each voluntary verbalization, and is not reinforced until he accumulates ten points. In this way, the subject must emit the desired response a certain number of times in order to be reinforced.

In using a time-based or interval plan, the time is fixed, while the movement numbers vary.[12] In a student's project to increase verbalization, the number of verbalizations occurring during a five-minute period were recorded. The number of movements varied but the number of minutes remained constant.

This recording method is the plan of choice in the clinical setting where the length of the treatment is fixed. For example, the number of times the patient swallowed prior to verbalizing to decrease drooling was counted during the 25-minute speech therapy session.[28] In one study, a psychiatric patient was reinforced with cigarettes for completed units of work within the 50-minute treatment session.[8]

The use of the interval plan may be applicable to behaviors occurring with high or low frequency. A cerebral-palsied patient was reinforced immediately for every ten-second interval he maintained standing balance.[9] In one case, the treatment session was divided into 360 ten-second intervals and the patient was reinforced every five minutes for each ten-second interval spent working on the task.[7] Psychiatric patients were reinforced after seven- to ten-consecutive daily sessions in which their performance exceeded a minimum criteria.[5]

Shortcuts to rate computation are possible when intervals of 1/10/100/1000 are used and the rate is calculated by moving the decimal to the appropriate place to the left. Interval units of .5/5/50/500 may be used and the rate computed by multiplying the number of responses by 2 and moving the decimal accordingly. When units of 2/20/200 are used, the number of responses must be first divided by 2 and the decimal moved accordingly.

A final plan is the "first come" basis where both the number of responses and the amount of time are fixed. Counting is terminated each time the set number of responses occurs or at the end of a specified time, whichever comes first.[12] In physical therapy, treatment of a cerebral-palsied child was reinforced each time he exceeded a certain number of unassisted and uninterrupted steps within 9 one-minute periods. If the required number of steps had not occurred during a one-minute trial period, counting stopped, he was not reinforced and counting in a new time period started.[29]

Recording should be done consistently regardless of the recording plan selected. The number of movements should be counted during every treatment session, at the same time each session, and by the same person.

Charting the Data Once the behavior has been counted, timed, and the rates computed, the information is charted to provide graphic feedback. The charting may be done privately or publicly but should be done consistently, since the method used may influence the behavior. Public charting is recommended since the expectations of the therapist and the performance of the patient are openly stated. Therapy becomes a shared responsibility, rather than something placed upon or given to the patient by the therapist. Physical therapists found that significantly greater gains in upper extremity strength of spinal cord-injured patients were produced with a planned program of positive reinforcement. Patients in the experimental group were praised and encouraged, the program was explained, progress and charted performance discussed, while the control group received the usual verbal interaction and the typical process of private program planning and charting of performance.[30]

Charting should provide clear information about the rate over a period of time. Tally cards have been found useful when the patient can assume some responsibility for charting, or when he retains the card and contacts the therapist who marks it when the work is completed.[5,31] Six-cycle log paper may be used that provides space for 20 weeks of charting.[32] Graph paper may be substituted to plot rates over a long period. A solid, vertical line is drawn to separate the phases of the project: the baseline period, the introduction of the reinforcer, and changes in the treatment. Specified changes should be introduced singly to identify the influence of each.

Selecting a Reinforcer After pinpointing and counting the baseline occurrence of the behavior, the reinforcement is introduced. When selecting the reinforcement, first analyze what is supporting the behavior. Attending to the patient only when he is having difficulty performing may reinforce his nonperforming behavior. This was the case with one quadriplegic patient who was left alone to practice typing. When the therapist's attention was made contingent upon typing, the typing increased from 5 to 30 minutes in two sessions.[6]

A second guideline is to individualize the reinforcement.[12] Although there are many extrinsic reinforcers, social reinforcement is often effective with rehabilitation patients who, because of their disability, are deprived of positive social reinforcement.[6] When pa-

tients are similar in their functioning level, the individual differences must be considered, as was demonstrated in one study of toilet training of five severely mentally retarded boys. The effective reinforcers discovered included baby food, a ride in a wheel chair, a shower, a ball, and allowing a subject to return to his bed. Stimuli that served as a positive reinforcer for one subject were neutral or aversive to another; the shower used as positive reinforcement for one patient was found to be an effective aversive consequence for another.[22]

Reinforcement should be presented immediately after the occurrence of the desired behavior so that a direct consequence of the behavior is obvious to the subject.[12] Reinforcers that are immediately consumed or engaged in may be used, such as a spoonful of ice cream,[33] thirty seconds of music,[29] or five minutes of talking with the therapist.[6] To give immediate recognition of the behavior but to postpone the consumption of the reinforcer, tokens may be used. Tokens are realistic in terms of society's expectation that one learn to delay gratification. Tokens may be exchanged for a variety of reinforcements that the child selects from a reinforcement menu. Tangible tokens such as metal washers or buttons, or transmittable tokens such as clicks from a grocery tally may be used. It is advisable for the therapist to retain the tokens, although these may be distributed in full view of the subject, such as dropping a plastic counter into a cup with the subject's name on it. This prevents the subject from counterfeiting, selling, stealing, losing them, or being distracted during the session.[27] The subject should be able to understand the system of reinforcement. A mentally retarded child reinforced by points may not make the connection between work performed and a potato chip at the end of the hour.

The reinforcer should be given only if the desired behavior occurs. If the desired behavior is not occurring, then the pinpointed behavior is probably too high for the patient's functioning level and should be refined, or a review of the program may be in order.

To make use of reinforcers in the environment the Premack principle may be used. This principle states that a behavior that occurs at a low rate will be increased when followed by a behavior occurring at a high rate.[34] A preferred activity may be used as a reinforcer for a nonpreferred activity. For example, the psychiatric patient who was reinforced with points for working in occupational therapy (nonpreferred activity), with which he could purchase cigarettes, coffee, or television (preferred activity).[7] The preferred activities are identified by observing the patient, by asking him or other staff or family members.[27]

When a strong but artificial reinforcer is used, a weak but more socially acceptable reinforcer may be paired with it, such as pairing a smile and positive comments (weak reinforcer) with candy (strong reinforcer).[12]

Depriving the patient of a reinforcer can increase its subsequent effectiveness. A 47-pound female patient with anorexia nervosa was deprived of visitors, television, music, flowers, a pleasantly decorated room, and coaxing to eat. When these stimuli were made contingent upon her eating, she responded, stabilizing at 80 pounds after three months and maintained this weight in a five-year follow up.[19,35]

A reinforcer should be successful and fair. The objective in a modification project is to program success; it is imperative to proceed at a rate at which the patient can succeed. The reinforcer should be in keeping with the demands for performance and not so scant that it discourages trying, or so abundant that it encourages only minimal effort. Fairness is stating the contingencies clearly, in positive terms, and by involving the patient in the decision-making when possible.[36]

Selecting the Schedule   Once the reinforcer is selected, the rule for when it is to be given is selected. The *continuous schedule* is used initially to acquire a behavior or strengthen a weak behavior. Every occurrence of the behavior is reinforced, such as one token given for each figure-ground picture identified. This produces high, steady rates of responding.[19,37] When the behavior is occurring with frequency on the continuous schedule, *intermittent schedules* may be selected depending upon the type of responding desired. The fixed ratio may be chosen to maintain the strength of the reinforcer and prevent reinforcement saturation. Every *n*th response is reinforced, such as one token for every three pictures identified. This produces high rates of responding.[19,37]

The fixed interval schedule may be used to reinforce various related behaviors during a given period. Reinforcement is available after a certain period for behaviors occurring during that period, such as reinforcement for three minutes of identifying pictures or shapes. This produces low rates of responding, since the reinforcement is available if the behavior occurs, regardless of the number of times it occurs.[19,37]

Once the behavior is occurring on the fixed ratio or fixed interval schedule, a variable schedule may be used. In this, the reinforcer is available after an average number of responses or length of time, rather than a fixed number or length of time. In the case of the variable ratio schedule, the number of responses varies for each reinforcement yet averages a predetermined number. For example, in a fixed ratio, every fifth response would be reinforced (FR5) during the session, while in a variable ratio schedule, an average of every fifth response would be reinforced (VR5). In the latter case, the reinforcer would be available after every third, then every seventh, then fifth, then sixth, then fourth response or any combination of numbers for an average of five (VR5). Variable ratio schedules produce high sustained rates of responding, since the reinforcer may come at any time.[19,37]

To increase the reinforcer's effectiveness between reinforcement, the variable interval schedule may be used. Reinforcement is available after a certain time period that varies around a mean such as a VI_4 schedule in which the reinforcer is available after the third, sixth, fifth, fourth, and second minutes of responding. This produces low, sustained rates of responding. Because the reinforcement is available at unpredictable times, there is incentive for the behavior to occur continuously but not necessarily rapidly.[19,37]

Rate schedules may be used in which the reinforcer is available after a certain rate of responses within a certain time period. These include the differential reinforcement for high rates of responding (DRH) and differential reinforcement for low rates of responding (DRL), mentioned earlier in this paper.[37]

The effects of extinction vary with the schedule on which the undesirable behavior is reinforced. After a continuous schedule, extinction of the reinforcer will decrease responding fairly rapidly. Following a ratio schedule, behaviors decrease at a moderate rate; after an interval schedule, the decrease is slow.[19]

Shaping, Chaining, and Modeling   When the desired behavior is not in the patient's repertoire, shaping, chaining, or modeling may be used to establish the new behavior. Shaping, or the technique of successive approximations, involves reinforcing closer and closer approximations to the desired behavior.[19] A physical therapist used successive approximations to shape the purposeful reaching of a six-year-old spastic cerebral-palsied child who was functioning at a three-month level in motor skills. The patient had some spontaneous arm motion and was reinforced with a spoonful of ice cream when he moved in the direction of a red hoop suspended over the crib. Later, he was reinforced when he touched the hoop, and finally every 15th time he touched it until he reached it voluntarily.[33]

Once the specific behavior is shaped, a related behavior may be added to this through chaining a series of specific behaviors, thereby producing complex behaviors. In chaining, each response becomes the discriminative stimulus. For example, it gives the signal for the next response.[37] This procedure has been used in teaching dressing skills to the mentally retarded. In one program, dressing was broken down into eleven skills: attention, coming to the technician, sitting down, remaining seated, standing up, removing the shirt or dress, putting on pants, and putting on socks. Each of these skills was first shaped by using successive approximation. For example, in learning undressing, the child was reinforced for removing the pants from the ankles, then from the knees, and finally from the waist.[38]

Modeling or imitation may be used, in which the patient is exposed to another person (or the therapist) who exhibits the desired behavior and that person is reinforced for the behavior in the presence of the patient.[39]

Summary

This paper provides information about behavior modification and the procedures for applying the behavioral model to occupational therapy patient treatment. Included were a brief review of behavioral terminology and a discussion of the four symptoms of applied behavioral analysis: positive reinforcement, negative reinforcement, punishment, and extinction. The behavioral equation was superimposed upon the occupational therapy treatment model. The steps in designing a behavior modification project were discussed including: identifying the terminal behavior, counting the behavior, recording the rates, charting the data, selecting a reinforcer, selecting a schedule, and shaping, chaining, and modeling. ∎

Acknowledgments

The author thanks the following individuals from the University of Florida for their assistance: W.D. Wolking, Ph.D., Peter K. Sieg, J.D., Lela Llorens, M.A., O.T.R., Alice Jantzen, Ph.D., O.T.R., Margaret Morgan, Ph.D., and Donna Schiebel.

REFERENCES

1. Diasio K: Psychiatric occupational therapy: search for a conceptual framework in light of psychoanalytic ego psychology and learning theory. Am J Occup Ther 22: 400–407, 1968
2. Ethridge DA: Behavioral modification techniques in occupational therapy. In Occupational Therapy Today–Tomorrow, Proc. 5th Int, Congress, WFOT, Zurich, 1970, pp 215–219
3. Ellsworth PD, Coleman AD: The application of operant conditioning principles to work group experience. Am J Occup Ther 23: 495–501,1969
4. Ellsworth PD, Colman AD: The application of operant conditioning principles–reinforcement systems to support work behavior. Am J Occup Ther 24: 562–568, 1970
5. Kaye JH, Mackie V, Hitzing EW: Contingency management in a workshop setting innovation in occupational therapy. Am J Occup Ther 24: 413–417, 1970
6. Myerson J, Kerr N, Michael J: Behavior modification in rehabilitation. In Child Development: Readings in Experimental Analysis. Edited by S.W. Bijou, D.L. Baer. New York, Appleton Century Crofts, 1967, pp 214–239
7. Ogburn KD, Fast D, Tiffany D: The effects of reinforcing working behavior. Am J Occup Ther 26: 32–35, 1972.
8. Overbaugh TE, Bucher B: Use of operant conditioning to improve behavior of a severely deteriorated psychotic. Am J Occup Ther 24: 423–427, 1970
9. Rugel RP, Mallingly J, Eichinger M, et al: The use of operant conditioning with a physically disabled child. Am J Occup Ther 25: 247–249, 1971
10. Smith AR, Tempone VJ: Psychiatric occupational therapy within a learning theory context. Am J Occup Ther 22: 415–420, 1968
11. Trombly CA: Principles of operant conditioning; related to orthotic training of quadriplegic patients. Am J Occup Ther 20: 217–220, 1966
12. Wolking WD: Handbook of Applied Behavior Analysis. Unpublished student manual. U. of Fla., Gainesville, 1972
13. Grassberg JM: Behavior Therapy: A Review. In Behavior Modification in the Classroom. Edited by G.A. Fargo, C. Behrens, P. Nolen. Belmont, Wadsworth Pub. Co., 1970, pp 52–71
14. Ullman JP, Krasner J: Case Studies in Behavior Modification, New York, Holt, Rinehart & Winston Inc., 1965
15. Lindsley OR: Direct measurement and prosthesis of retarded behavior. In New Directions in Education. Edited by R.T. Jones. Boston, Allyn and Bacon, 1970, pp 206–234
16. Lindsley OR: Mentally retarded children are not retarded. In Behavior Modification in the Classroom. Edited by G.A. Fargo, C. Behrens, P. Nolen. Belmont, Worth Pub. Co., 1970, pp 182–192
17. Sulzer B, Mayer GR: Behavior Modification for School Personnel. Hinsdale, Dryden Press, 1972
18. Wolpe J: Advances in behavior therapy. Curr Psychiatr Ther 12: 27–37, 1972
19. Riese EP: The Analysis of Human Operant Behavior, Dubuque, Wm. C. Brown, 1966
20. Ayllon T, Azrin NH: The Token Economy, a Motivational System for Therapy and Rehabilitation, New York, Appleton Century Crofts, 1968
21. Ayllon T, Michael J: The psychiatric nurse as a behavioral engineer, J Exp Anal Behav 2: 323–334, 1959
22. Giles DK, Wolf MM: Toilet training institutionalized severe retardates: an application of operant behavior modification techniques. Am J Ment Defic 70: 766–780, 1966
23. White JC, Taylor DJ: Noxious conditioning as a treatment for rumination. Ment Retard 5: 30–33, 1967
24. Azrin NH, Holz WC: Punishment. In Operant Behavior: Areas of Research and Application. Edited by W.K. Honig. New York, Appleton Century Crofts, 1966
25. Hamilton J, Stephens T, Allen P: Controlling aggressive and destructive behavior in severely retarded institutionalized residents. Am J Ment Defic 71: 852–856, 1967
26. Birnbrauer JS: Generalization of punishment effects–a case study. J Appl Behav Anal 1: 201–211, 1968
27. Neisworth JT, Dino SL, Jenkins JR: Student Motivation and Classroom Management—a Behavioristic Approach. Newark, Behavior Techniques, Inc., 1969
28. Garber NB: Operant procedures to eliminate drooling behavior in a cerebral-palsied adolescent. Devel Med Child Neurol 13: 641–644, 1971
29. Chandler TS, Adams MA: Multiply handicapped child motivated for ambulation through behavior modification. Phys Ther 52: 399–401, 1972
30. Troller AB, Inman DA: The use of positive reinforcement in physical therapy. Phys Ther 48: 347–352, 1968
31. Hewett FM: Educational engineering with emotionally disturbed children. Except Child 33: 459–467, 1967
32. Martin MB, Koorland P: Elementary Principles and Procedures of the Standard Behavior Chart, Gainesville, Precision Teaching of Fla., 1973
33. Rice HK, McDaniel MW, Denny SL: Operant conditioning techniques for use in the physical rehabilitation of the multiply handicapped retarded patient. Phys Ther 48: 342–346, 1968
34. Premack D: Toward empirical behavior laws: 1. Positive reinforcement. Psych Rev 66: 319–333, 1959
35. Bachrach AJ, Erwin WJ, Mohr JP: The control of eating behavior in an anorexic by operant conditioning techniques. In Case Studies in Behavior Modification. Edited by T. Ullman, T.P. Krasner. New York, Holt, Rinehart and Winston, 1965, pp 153–163
36. Homme T: How to Use Contingency Contracting in the Classroom, Champaign, Research Press, 1969
37. Reynolds GS: A Primer of Operant Conditioning, Glenview, Scott, Foresman and Co., 1968
38. Minge RM, Ball TS: Teaching of self-help skills to profoundly retarded patients. Am J Ment Defic 73: 74–78, 1967
39. Bandura A: Behavioral modifications through modeling procedures. In Research in Behavior Modification. Edited by T. Krasner, J.P. Ullman. New York, Holt, Rinehart and Winston, 1965, pp 255–263

The Consumer of Therapy in Mental Health

Judith S. Bloomer

The current emphasis on consumer advocacy and accountability in health care has implications for the practice of occupational therapy in mental health. The consumer movement that gained national attention during the 1960s was marked by the passage in 1962 of a congressional bill that affirmed the consumer's right to safety, the right to be informed, the right to choose, and the right to be heard. These four rights, as well as the concept of client self-determination (seen as an additional right of the client to determine his or her own participation in the evaluation and treatment process), can be applied to occupational therapy practice. Occupational therapists must begin to address the aspects of accountability to the consumer by understanding both the concept and the principles of consumerism and the consequences of focusing on the patient or client as consumer. Therapists must then attempt to apply these principles to practice. Principles of consumerism can be incorporated into practice in clinical, administrative, and educational settings.

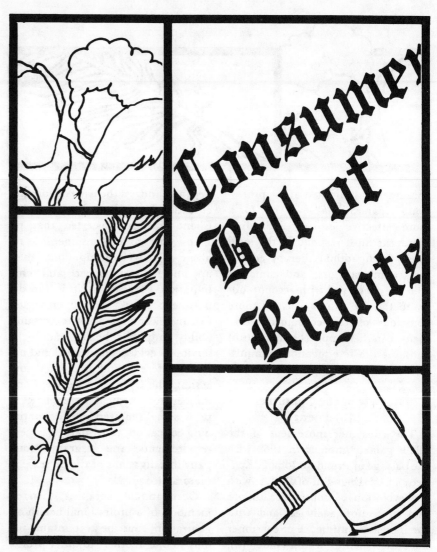

Judith S. Bloomer, M.S.W., OTR, is an occupational therapist, Inpatient Treatment and Research Service, Langley Porter Neuropsychiatric Institute, University of California, San Francisco; and a part-time faculty member, Occupational Therapy Department, San Jose State University.

O ccupational therapists are beginning to address the issue of accountability by establishing peer review standards as a section of Professional Standards Review Organizations (PSROs). However, they have not been systematically accountable to the populations they serve. One attempt to be more accountable to the consumer was initiated by the Office of Advocacy of the American Occupational Therapy Association (AOTA), which proposed a resolution to develop a "Consumer's Guide to Occupational Therapy." The resolution was passed by the Representative Assembly in October 1977 (1). This response to the

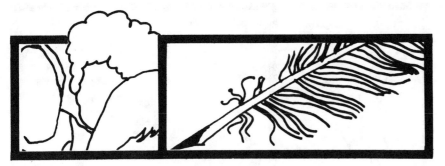

consumer was initiated at the profession's organizational level, but for a more effective impact, individual therapists must respond at the local level. Occupational therapy educators, administrators, and clinicians who are concerned with accountability to the client and who are more conscious of the consumer movement, can then apply the concepts of consumerism to education, administration, and clinical practice.

Review of the Consumer Movement

The consumer movement of the 1960s gained impetus in 1962 with the passage of President John F. Kennedy's Consumer Bill of Rights, with the evolution of consumer's unions and protection agencies, and with the increasing influence of consumer advocates such as Ralph Nader (2). This movement was initiated by and felt most strongly in business and industry where consumer satisfaction has long been a concern. Market research surveys indicated that feedback from the target group was necessary for success in consumer-oriented products or service. As a result, the more useful techniques for involving consumers in decision making have come from the field of business. Consumer advisory boards, suggestion boxes, and brainstorming sessions have been implemented by companies responsive to consumer concerns and demands.

Following the trend of consumerism in the business world, health service organizations and professions

began to address the issue of consumer satisfaction in the early 1970s. Client advocates asserted that responsiveness to the consumer is as realistic a goal for occupational therapy and for social service and rehabilitation agencies as it is for department stores and supermarkets (3). Increasing attention to accountability in public health and social services is evidenced by local and national interests and mandates concerning the Utilization Review Committees for medical care, PSROs, professional requirements for continuing education, third-party payment requirements, and insurance company investigations of the increase in malpractice suits.

Occupational therapists, then, as members of a professional health organization, must be accountable not only to one another, to other professional groups, and to governmental organizations, but also to their consumers directly. Before considering how this objective might be accomplished, some basic tenets of consumer rights are reviewed and these are generalized to the services offered in mental health. The therapist's subjective position as a consumer is explored in order to identify with the client as consumer.

Client/Consumer Bill of Rights

In his Consumer message to Congress in March 1962, President Kennedy outlined a Consumer Bill of Rights that declared the consumer to have: the right to safety, the right to

be informed, the right to choose, and the right to be heard. These rights are applicable to a client's right to ask for and receive psychosocial and occupational therapy services.

The right to safety is determined by laws in every state that require the individual, particularly the psychiatric client, to be protected from harm by others or by self. Thus, involuntary psychiatric hospitalization provides a setting where the therapist is responsible for protecting the patient from harm to self or others. The right to safety also extends to the protection of the confidential aspects and records of the client's involvement in occupational therapy services.

The right to be informed should include the mutual sharing of information about expectations and roles by client and therapist. It should also include the provision of any pertinent information that will enable the client to make decisions about the treatment process and problem-solving aspects of the occupational therapy program.

The right to choose includes the choice involved in seeking help initially, in participating in a contractual agreement with the therapist, and in choosing to discontinue services or involvement with a certain therapist at any time, as long as the client is aware and informed of the consequences of such a decision.

Finally, the right to be heard assures that the interests of the client, individually and as part of a consumer group, will be considered in the treatment process, program evaluation, and policy setting. This right should also include the establishment of a mechanism through which other rights can be asserted.

These basic rights seem theoretically sound, but can they be implemented? Two examples—the consumer seeking automotive repair and the consumer seeking mental health service—may help the reader to assess subjective reactions to the implementation of consumer rights in occupational therapy.

The often desperate plight of the typical car owner trying to find a reputable automobile mechanic is well known. Recent consumer demand has resulted in the establishment of various advocacy agencies as well as consumer complaints and protection coordinators to deal with questionable practices in automotive repair shops. The public seems more aware of the avenues of recourse on negligence in auto repair than in other areas of services. Consider whether or not similar methods of recourse should be available in the area of mental health care. Consider a consumer who seeks mechanical service for an automobile. The person must determine where to go for the service, the reputation and qualifications of the mechanic, what type of diagnostic screening the car should go through, and what information is needed from the mechanic. The person would then ask what is wrong with the car, what is the specific problem, what parts are needed, and what are the labor, time factor, costs, and guarantees of the service.

Now consider consumers seeking outpatient or private counseling services for anxiety or depression over a divorce, death of a relative, job pressures, or family crisis. Would the consumer go through the same process to determine where to go for the service, to ask for the qualifications and orientation of the therapist, or to ask the therapist what the diagnosis is, how he or she conceptualizes the consumer's presenting problems, and how long the treatment will last? This process usually is not expected in a medical model. The "patient" (rather than "client") traditionally has been in a dependent role in men-

tal health treatment settings and has been encouraged to trust the therapist to do whatever the therapist deems best. In the business world, such unquestioning trust and dependency has not been beneficial to the consumer. To foster it in clinical practice certainly seems antithetical to the concept of consumerism in health care.

Occupational therapists can incorporate the concepts of consumerism and client rights into their practice. To a certain extent, therapists already include the use of the client's abilities and skills in their working philosophy. How this practice can be emphasized is discussed next.

The Concept of Client Self-Determination

A major premise of our profession is that occupational therapy helps clients to mobilize their resources and capacities so that they can function optimally in their environment. This premise is similar to a concept often invoked in the social work literature, "client self-determination," a phrase used to define the process whereby the client determines the course of treatment by using his or her own resources. A major theorist in the field of social work, Helen Perlman, stated that:

The essence of self-determination is precisely this: that the individual should take cognizance of what he thinks and feels, wants and does not want, and of the possible results of both, and that, then, he should decide upon or mobilize himself to a choice of action or circumstance . . . . (his) *decision to go forward . . . should be self-determined and chosen as freely and understandingly as is possible for him.* (4, p 56)

Incorporating the concept of client self-determination in occupational therapy would mean encouraging clients to assume responsibility for

choosing among alternatives and for using their own skills and resources to deal with their agreed-upon tasks.

There are various practice situations in which client self-determination has certain limitations. One is that the therapist must recognize the client's ambivalence and difficulty in deciding upon or determining goals. Often, self-determination has to be modified because of the reality of certain situations, or legal, social, or economic constraints. There may be a conflict between the client's decisions and the therapist's responsibility for meeting client needs, which may be determined by agency function and the therapist's assessment of the situation (5, 6).

Still, facilitating client self-determination, even with the constraints imposed in practice, is believed by many clinicians to enhance the client's sense of motivation, investment in the treatment process, and sense of self-esteem. For these reasons, it should be an integral part of practice—in establishing treatment goals and expectations of service in occupational therapy.

Expectations of Service

To respond to the client as a consumer responsible for determining goals, it is important to explore the client's perception and expectations of the services offered. Success in treatment can be impeded by the client's misperception of what "help" is when seeking services from a mental health center (7). Clarification of services offered, mutual contractual agreements, expectations, and performance standards are important aspects of accountability to the client.

To help clients decide what is best for them, the therapist must provide them with adequate information concerning resources. Part of the necessary information is a clear definition of the therapist's areas of responsibility to the client. Although little has been published on this topic in the literature of occupational therapy, studies (7, 8) in the social work literature have shown that conflicts in worker-client decision making result from misperceptions of the social worker's responsibility (7). Blumberg and coworkers (8) studied clients' expectations of social workers in medical settings by assessing four factors: the client's perception of his problems and needs to be met by the worker; the client's initial expectations of the worker; the services the client thought he received; the client's degree of satisfaction with the help he received. These investigators found that clients rarely are asked what kind of help they want or what type of intervention they think they have been given. They discovered that almost half of the clients did not know what to expect from the worker and that more than one third said they believed that the worker would give them concrete help, such as financial assistance. Only 18 percent said they had expected emotional support, which was the role function the social worker was primarily prepared to fulfill.

Barton and Scheer (9) measured attitudes about a psychiatric activity program and compared similarities and differences between staff and patient perceptions of the program. There was a significant discrepancy in perception or expectation of certain aspects of the activity program. The authors suggested that the discrepancy might be the result of inadequate client orientation to activity program concepts.

Relationship of Expectations to Practice

In addition to being an important aspect of client orientation, clarification of expectations regarding the therapeutic process is also an essential element of practice because it affects the client's attitude, motivation, and involvement in the therapeutic alliance. Studies that explored incongruities in client-therapist expectations indicated that the client's perception of his or her problem is more important than the therapist's view of the situation (7-9). Emphasis therefore must be placed on the client's perceived need, and an important task for the initial interview is to engage the client as a mutual partner in decision making in both the evaluation and the treatment process. The importance of client involvement in evaluating and participating in therapy is supported by the significant amount of evidence indicating a relationship between involvement and the achievement of therapeutic goals. Shared responsibility for mutual goal setting and decision making, and for the actual treatment, has been shown to enhance the potential progress of the client (3).

Mutual Goal Setting. The concept of mutuality requires mutually agreed-upon goals that are accepted by both the therapist and the client, based on objectives that are realistic, diagnostically sound, and ego-syntonic for the client (10). The goals are to be refined, revised, or continuously modified by both the client and the therapist until the treatment contract is terminated. The contract is a working agreement of mutual promise and duty between two contracting parties. The explicit agreement should include the target problems, the goals, the strategies of intervention, and the roles and tasks of the participants (11). The advantage of using a formal treatment contract, in addition to clarifying objectives and treatment goals and thus preventing "double agendas" of the client and therapist, is that it en-

hances commitment and facilitates maximum participation. Both explicitness and reciprocal accountability are integral parts of contract setting.

Client Evaluation of Service. When goal planning is implemented and treatment is terminated, evaluation of the program and services rendered is initiated as part of a systematic review. Involving the client in evaluating the effectiveness of services received is an essential aspect of consumerism in mental health. Client appraisal is rarely solicited but it should be an important determinant of the kinds of services offered (12, 13). Sachs, Bradley, and Beck addressed this issue convincingly:

Actually there is a great deal of logic in using clients directly rather than workers or research interviewers as the chief judges of outcome. They are the consumers of service. It is they who define their problems and choose where to go for help. It is they who directly experience the helping process and live daily with the results of that help. Only they can really say whether as a result they are or are not better able to cope with their particular problems .... Clients can also report what went wrong, if anything, and why they terminated. They can likewise report what they needed and did not receive. (14, p 103)

Various methods can be used to solicit client reactions to occupational therapy services. Surveys, discharge interviews, and planning sessions for program evaluation can be implemented in most treatment settings. An example of involvement of clients in program evaluation is a program planning session introduced by the author as part of an activity group on an inpatient psychiatric treatment service. Patients were asked to review a range of 15 activities and treatment modalities often scheduled within the program. The schedule might include activities such as art therapy, outings, cooking group, basic living skills, discharge planning, role playing, and a work program. To establish priorities for inclusion in the program schedule, the planning group rank-ordered the activities. In establishing their priorities, the patients considered which activities they perceived to be important in helping them to realize their therapy goals, which activities they enjoyed, which combined both therapeutic and enjoyable aspects, and which activities, if any, they perceived to be detrimental to their rehabilitation process. The results of this evaluation proved to be valuable for revising and refining the overall occupational therapy program. However, soliciting client feedback is not always so pleasant. The appraisal process may produce an evaluation that the provider is not prepared to hear. The reluctance to hear criticism is but one of the obstacles to engaging client/consumer input.

Roadblocks to Professional Acceptance

The four major obstacles to accepting clients as consumers and evaluators of service are:

1. The concept of professionalism in the patient-therapist relationship, with the implied issues of power and control.

2. The status needs of occupational therapy as a profession.

3. The organization and structure of the service delivery system.

4. The gaps in client-oriented research (15, pp 1-17).

Some consumer advocates believe that the concept of professionalism in mental health is antithetical to the philosophy of client self-determination. Thursz (3), for example, sees professionalism as implying expertise, control, and monopoly of decision making. He reviewed sociological evidence indicating that professional groups still striving for "professional" status have difficulty in accepting the notion that an untrained individual can render worthwhile service or that a recipient of service can participate in decision making.

This concept· of professionalism may also contribute to the lack of research drawn upon the client's experiential field. It has been postulated that a major reason for the lack of such research is that psychiatric practice has been heavily influenced by psychoanalytic concepts (3, 15). Practitioners influenced by psychoanalytic theory tend to discount views expressed directly by the client in order to expose alternate or indirect expressions that may have more therapeutic significance. For example, cognitive expressions are often interpreted as representing underlying unconscious material of which the client is not aware, or not aware until the practitioner helps the client bring it to conscious awareness and assimilation. Although many therapists are highly skilled in making such clinical judgments and interpretations, and these often are beneficial to the client who has little insight, an assumption of professional infallibility carries potential danger.

Occupational therapy is a relatively new discipline, still forming an identity and striving for status in the health care field.· One characteristic of a profession is that it has a specialized body of knowledge, and this tends to reinforce the professional's conviction that he or she knows what is best for the client. This might be contrasted with prevailing attitudes in the business world, as reflected in the adage "the customer is always right." A customer knows his or her own needs and will comparison shop in an effort to satisfy them. The customer also feels relatively confident about judging the value of the service or merchandise offered. The client who goes to a professional, on the other hand, finds the professional is dictating what is right for him and has no choice but to accede to the professional's judgment or to seek service elsewhere. Further, the client is not considered able to evaluate the caliber of professional service he or she receives. Finally, the client's perception of the outcome of service may be threatening to the professional, and therefore is not sought out.

The structure of many agencies also hampers the collection of client-oriented studies or opportunities for client-group participation in self-determination. The typical structure often isolates clients from one another; for example, the client coming in for individual therapy rarely communicates with other clients. In contrast, clients in school, prison, or in inpatient units, do interact and can organize into groups to protest poor or inadequate services. These organizational protests often pressure the service providers to be more accountable, to modify services, or to grant concessions to the protesting group.

A final factor contributing to the relative lack of client-oriented research is that new disciplines, in their effort to be more "scientific" or "professional," often discount exploratory studies in favor of those producing hard empirical data. Experimental design and operational research tend to draw away from studies of clients that involve surveys, self-ratings, and exploratory research.

Potential Avenues for Action

There are several possibilities for expanding consumer advocacy in occupational therapy. The occupational therapist who desires to meet the challenge of reaching out to the con-

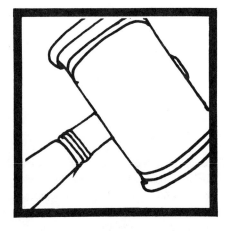

sumer is urged to assume a complementary role, such as researcher, consumer educator, or community organizer.

The role of researcher is an important one, both to the profession of occupational therapy and to the consumers it serves. It has been stated repeatedly in the occupational therapy literature and communications network that further research is crucial to the development of the profession (16). Occupational therapists must address this need for an increase in research activity within the field. As they develop their interests and knowledge in research design and methodology, they can apply these skills to clinical practice and foster client-oriented studies. Developing a project to study the effects of client/consumer participation in evaluation and treatment planning is one example for expanding consumer advocacy through research.

A potential role for occupational therapists could be as consumer advocates. As advocates, therapists could become more active in community organization to develop additional community-based service programs to meet the needs of clients. Expanded program development is possible by engaging the support of such community service clubs as the Rotary, the Lion's Club, and the Shriners. As members of community planning groups, consumer advisory boards, or Health System Organizations (HSOs), therapists can be effective in mobilizing political interest and action in an advocacy project. Therapists assuming the role of community organizer can use the strategies or *locality* development,

social action, and social planning to promote ventures in the interest of their clients at the community level (17).

In *locality* development, the therapist acts as a consultant or catalyst in coordinating the problem-solving attempts of the local citizens of a community. An example of this technique of community organization is the therapist who spearheads an effort to solicit funding for the development of a program for autistic or learning-disabled children. The therapist might consult with groups of interested parents and representatives of various community agencies, such as mental health clinics, special education programs, public school systems, and regional centers for developmentally disabled or crippled children. She or he might coordinate the efforts of active members of the groups toward the accomplishment of various tasks that might include writing and submitting a program proposal, and involving members of power structures (local government and school boards) as collaborators in a common venture.

Using the strategy of social action in community organizations, the therapist assumes an activist approach, often acting as a negotiator or partisan. This technique, applied to the example used above, might have the therapist applying pressure on political groups such as state or county governments and local school boards to provide more programs for the disadvantaged group of learning-disabled or autistic children. In this role, the therapist might speak out in favor of certain bills at legislative hearings or even organize the collection of signatures for a consumer-initiated petition.

The occupational therapist, acting as a consumer advocate and using the social planning approach, can emphasize the planning aspects of

community organization. Using this strategy, the therapist might gather facts about the perceived community problem, analyze the data, and propose a solution. Again, using the example cited above, the therapist, who might be employed within an agency, might begin by documenting the unmet needs of the autistic or learning-disabled child, then systematically exploring the available resources, suggesting a plan to supplement them with additional services, and developing a procedure to implement the desired service program.

Occupational therapists who wish to stay in the clinic, rather than extend their activities into the community, can assume a consumer advocate role within their clinical practice and as staff members of their agency. They can emphasize mutual goal setting in treatment, encourage client self-determination, and reflect their consumer-oriented attitude in their working relationships. Occupational therapy administrators can stress client involvement in program evaluation and can promote organizational change embracing consumerism within their department. Also, by analyzing whether their agency is a closed or an open system (one that incorporates change through either internal or external sources), they can encourage an administrative structure that is receptive to innovation at whatever level that is appropriate to the situation.

The role of consumer educator is also appropriate for occupational therapists. Therapists can take part in the move toward expanded systematic education of the client/consumer group. Many are well prepared to teach community-based adult education classes and offer university extension courses in their specialty areas. The regional education committees of many state occupational therapy associations have developed lists of speakers in their resource files, for speakers at workshops and in the community, to educate the consumer group. More occupational therapists could volunteer for speaking assignments, both to engage consumers in their area of interest and to develop the therapist's own public speaking skills.

Occupational therapy educators, whether in academic settings or as clinicians accustomed to providing inservice education and student practicum training, can incorporate the concepts of consumerism in their teaching. The application of consumerism to education is especially important, since education perpetuates attitudes and knowledge and since occupational therapists educate clients, students and colleagues in all areas of practice. Students, for example, can be encouraged to role-play client-therapist interactions by assuming a consumer and service provider orientation. They might practice mutual goal setting by using a "Goal Attainment Scaling" model that directly engages the client and student in both planning and evaluating the outcome of goals (18). An audiotape/slide program entitled *Consumer-Provider,* which discusses the issue of client accountability, is available commercially and can be used in academic and clinical education settings (19). Occupational therapy educators can raise consumer consciousness in their students by encouraging them to participate in student government bodies and curriculum planning, and by pointing out how this correlates with practice.

Conclusion

The consumer movement has extended into the realm of health care, and occupational therapists have begun to address accountability to their clients. Therapists not only can be held accountable but can incorporate basic client rights into their clinical practice and can encourage client self-determination. Occupational therapy traditionally has believed in helping clients to use their innate capabilities and resources in adapting to their environments and mastering tasks of living. A natural extension of this premise for practitioners is to aid clients "to help us help them" through active participation in mutual goal setting and treatment planning. Therapists can involve clients in evaluation of the services they provide to their clients and can also anticipate and surmount possible personal and professional resistances to this engagement of clients as consumers. There are many opportunities for therapists who wish to assume the role of consumer advocate. They can develop their skills as researchers, consumer-oriented administrators, community organizers, consumer and occupational therapy educators. At the very least, therapists can serve as role models for their colleagues by upholding the philosophy of consumerism in their practice and employment settings.

Acknowledgments

This article is based on a presentation given at the First Annual Symposium of Occupational Therapy in Mental Health, September 16, 1977, Los Angeles, California. The symposium was organized by the Valley Chapter of the Occupational Therapy Association of California.

REFERENCES

1. American Occupational Therapy Association Annual Conference, October 1977, Puerto Rico. Minutes of the Representative Assembly. *Am J Occup Ther* 32: 242-264, 1978 (Resolution #519-77, p 254)
2. Aaker DA, Day GS: *Consumerism—Search for the Consumer Interest,* New York: Macmillan, 1971
3. Thursz D: *Consumer Involvement in Rehabilitation,* Washington, DC: U.S. Department of Health, Education and Welfare, 1970
4. Perlman H: *The Roots of Social Work,* S.C. Kohs, Editor. New York: Associated Press, 1966
5. Travis G, Neely D: Grappling with the concept of client self-determination. *Social Casework* 48: 503-508, 1967
6. Bernstein S: Self-determination: King or citizen in the realm of values? *Social Work* 5: 3-8, 1960
7. Silverman PR: A reexamination of the intake procedure. *Social Casework* 51: 625-634, 1970
8. Blumberg D, Ely AR, Kerbeshian A: Client's evaluation of medical social services. *Social Work* 20: 45-47, 1975
9. Barton GM, Scheer N: A measurement of attitudes about an activity program. *Am J Occup Ther* 29: 284-287, 1975
10. Gottlieb S: Mutual goals and goal setting in casework. *Social Casework* 48: 471-481, 1967
11. Maluccio N, Marlow WD: The case for the contract. *Social Work* 19: 29-35, 1974
12. Fidler JW: The patient's view of occupational therapy. *Am J Occup Ther* 3: 170, 1949
13. Jantzen AC: Patient evaluation: Of occupational therapy programs. *Am J Occup Ther* 19: 19, 1965
14. Sacks JG, Bradley PM, Beck DF: *Clients Progress Within Five Interviews,* New York: Family Service Association of America, 1970
15. Mayer J, Timms N: *The Client Speaks: Working Class Impressions of Casework,* New York: Atherton Press, 1970
16. Yerxa EJ, Gilfoyle E: Research seminar. *Am J Occup Ther* 30: 509-514, 1976
17. Cox FM, Erlich JL, Rothman J, Tropman JE: *Strategies of Community Organization,* Itasca, IL: F.E. Peacock, 1974, 2nd Edition
18. Kiresuk T, Sherman R: Goal attainment scaling: A general method of evaluating comprehensive community mental health program. *Comm Ment Health* 4: 443-453, 1968; and Bloomer JS: The use of goal attainment scaling in occupational therapy. Presented at the American Occupational Therapy Association Conference, San Diego, May 8, 1978, handouts are available from the author upon request.
19. Tigges K, Herold J, Gross D: *Consumer-Provider,* Audio Tape/Slide Program, Catalog #257501. Communications in Learning, Inc., 2929 Main Street, Buffalo, New York 14214

THE THERAPEUTIC USE OF SELF

JEROME D. FRANK, M.D.

First of all, I should like to express my appreciation for this opportunity to address you today. As a psychiatrist I have become increasingly aware that our central task is rehabilitation—that is, helping individuals who are chronically maimed or stunted to use their assets more effectively and minimize their liabilities. In this we are similar to all those who treat chronic illness, and most psychiatric illness is chronic. Occupational therapy obviously plays a crucial part in all rehabilitation efforts, and I have come increasingly to appreciate the role of occupational therapy in our work at Phipps. So I welcome this opportunity to test a few ideas with you.

Although I was happy to receive the invitation to speak to you, I must confess that the topic, "The Therapeutic Use of the Self," somewhat stunned me. "The self" is a term which covers just about all aspects of personality development and functioning, and the adjective "therapeutic" has come to refer to all personal influences which facilitate helpful change. In the hope of carving out an area from this vast field which is particularly relevant to our work and which will keep our discussion within manageable limits, I have decided to focus on the interrelationships of certain perceptual and behavioral aspects of the patient's self, and their implications for the therapeutic use of the therapist's self.

Since the self is an aspect of human nature, we must pause for a brief moment to consider the nature of human existence. Like all living creatures, man is a fragile and transitory organism at the mercy of huge forces which seem indifferent to his fate and which inevitably and eventually destroy him, but he differs from the rest of creation in being aware of his destiny. The poet A. E. Housman has well expressed the human predicament:

> "I a stranger and afraid
> In a world I never made."[1]

Man is always faced with the threat of nothingness, of obliteration, and this is probably the root of the anxiety that all humans feel. In order to combat this anxiety and to gain the positive values of life, man must construct a meaningful world out of his environment. To do this, he learns to make *predictions* as to what the effects of his behavior will be, based on his past experiences. He learns that if he drops a stone it will fall, that if he sticks his hand into a flame, it will hurt him, and so on. These predictions are based on what are called *perceptual constancies;* that is,

after he has learned what a stone is, he will perceive anything that looks like a stone as having a stone's attributes, such as heaviness and hardness. After he has seen several different kinds of flame, when he sees a new kind of flame, he will assimilate it to the other kinds and will perceive it as hot. Thus we build up a universe of perceptual constancies, and this is a basic human function.

An important aspect of these perceptual constancies is that they are "time-binding." They are based on past experience, are guided by our present purposes, and imply a prediction or expectancy as to the future. The past experiences may be unique to the individual, or they may be those of the groups to which the individual belongs. The child does not actually have to burn himself to expect that fire will burn him—his mother's alarm when he reached for a live coal may have been sufficient to establish this expectancy.

Let me give some examples to illustrate these points. The perception of a stone involves a set of expectancies based on past experience. This was vividly demonstrated to me when I first met something called pebble candy. This candy looks exactly like little rocks. All my past experience told me that these things were stones; therefore I automatically expected them to be hard and have no taste and probably break my teeth. Even though I knew they were candy, this expectancy was so strong that it was all I could do to taste one. A universal experience is that nearer objects are larger than distant ones; hence, if two similar objects are shown to us, we inevitably perceive the larger one as nearer.

Space perception and pebble candy are examples of perceptual constancies and their accompanying expectancies based on widely shared experiences. Here is an example of how perceptual constancies are influenced by the groups to which we belong. In an experiment subjects were presented with ambiguous stimuli by means of a stereopticon, an apparatus which presents a different image to each eye in such a way that they are superimposed. Thus the observer has three choices; he can see only the left hand image, or only the right hand image, or fuse both of them into a new image. The choice he makes is, of course, not deliberate but automatic, depending on his past experiences and present purposes. To illustrate the role of group influences in determining these choices, some Mexican and American school teachers were shown through the stereopticon superimposed photos of a baseball player and a bullfighter. An overwhelming proportion of the Americans "saw" the baseball play; an overwhelming proportion of Mexicans "saw" the bullfighter.[2]

Finally, perceptual constancies can be determined by strictly personal experiences, as the following amusing example shows. Dr. Hadley Cantril presented to various persons through a stereopticon superimposed pictures of a statue of a Madonna and a statue of a young nude from the Louvre. Among his subjects were two college professor friends of his. As he describes it, one of them first saw a Madonna and Child. "A few seconds later he exclaimed, 'My God, she is undressing!' What had happened so far was that somehow she had lost the baby she was holding and her robe had slipped down from her shoulders and stopped just about the breast line. Then in a few more seconds she lost her robe completely and became the young nude. For this particular professor, the nude never did get dressed again. Then my second friend took his turn. For a few seconds he could see nothing but the nude and then he exclaimed, 'But now a robe is wrapping itself around her.' And very soon he ended up with the Madonna with Child and as far as I know still remains with that vision. Some people will never see the nude; others will never see the Madonna."[3] In this case individual life experiences and purposes seemed to determine what the two professors saw.

I hope these examples make clear that perception is not a passive process by which outside stimuli register upon us as upon a photographic plate, but an active transaction between the person and his environment. The world we live in—the world we perceive—is, in a sense, created by us from a welter of experiences. It consists of a set of *expectancies or predictions,* based on past experiences, selected in accordance with our purposes.

From the fact that each of us constructs a world based on his expectancies, it follows that to the extent that we can influence another person's expectancies, we can affect how he feels, thinks and behaves.

A very striking example of this is to be found in the phenomenon of faith cures. The evidence for these cures is as great as that for anything else we accept as fact. There seems little reason to doubt that faith cures can heal damaged tissues very rapidly under certain circumstances which we still do not understand. The least common denominator of all faith cure situations seems to be an environment in which the atmosphere creates an expectancy that healing will occur. This is true of shrines of miraculous healing which have existed throughout recorded time and in all religions. It also exists in the doctor's office where, because of the doctor's role, the patient expects him to be able to heal him. It has been demonstrated repeatedly through what has been called the placebo effect—the astonishing influence on bodily functioning of an innocuous medication which is offered to the patient as a means of helping him. For example, many dermatologists have shown that painting warts with an inert dye is just as effective a way of healing them as X-ray or surgery. Warts are physical manifestations due to a definite virus. They are obviously not imaginary. Yet the power of the expectancy conveyed by painting the wart blue will in many people be sufficient to produce a change in the skin so that the virus can no longer take hold.

It would take us too far afield to discuss the ramifications of the placebo effect for medicine and psychotherapy.[4] I use it merely to illustrate the tremendous importance of expectancies in influencing our feelings, behavior and bodily states.

So far I have not distinguished between the world of things and the world of people in describing how we carve a meaningful world out of the chaos of stimuli impinging on us by constructing perceptual constancies and expectancies. In order to get on with the topic of the therapeutic use of the self, for the rest of this talk I shall focus exclusively on the personal world. Here the major division we make is between a group of phenomena labelled "myself" and another group labelled "other persons." The importance of a person's notion of his "self" in influencing his feeling, thinking and behavior has long been recognized. Unfortunately, each of us possesses not one self but several. The essayist and novelist, Oliver Wendell Holmes, just ninety-nine years ago in "The Autocrat of the Breakfast Table" expressed this point charmingly:

"It is not easy, at the best, for two persons talking together to make the most of each other's thoughts, there are so many of them . . . When John and Thomas, for instance, are talking together, it is natural enough that among the six there should be more or less confusion and misapprehension . . . I think . . . that there are at least six personalities distinctly to be recognized as taking part in that dialogue between John and Thomas.

THREE JOHNS

1. The real John; known only to his Maker.
2. John's ideal John; never the real one, and often very unlike him.
3. Thomas's ideal John; never the real John, nor John's John, but often very unlike either.

THREE THOMASES

1. The real Thomas.
2. Thomas's ideal Thomas.
3. John's ideal Thomas.

"Only one of the three Johns is taxed; only one can be weighed on a platform-balance; but the other two are just as important in the conversation. Let us suppose the real John to be old, dull, and ill-looking. But as the Higher Powers have not conferred on men the gift of seeing themselves in the true light, John very possibly conceives himself to be youthful, witty, and fascinating, and talks from the point of view of this ideal. Thomas, again, believes him to be an artful rogue, we will say; therefore he is, so far as Thomas's attitude in the conversation is concerned, an artful rogue, though really simple and stupid. The same conditions apply to the three Thomases. It follows, that, until a man can be found who knows himself as his Maker knows him, or who sees himself as others see him, there must be at least six persons engaged in every dialogue between two . . . No wonder two disputants often get angry, when there are six of them talking and listening all at the same time."[5]

For our purposes it will be sufficient to distinguish between three "selves": the acting self, the perceived self, and the ideal self. Since there must be something which perceives and acts, we have to postulate another self—the "real" self "known only to his Maker," to use Oliver Wendell Holmes' phrase. But he is beyond my reach, so I shall say no more about him.

We are, of course, not born with a full set of selves but develop them through our transactions with other people and the successes and failures to which these lead. The infant at first is simply a bundle of more or less unrelated interactions with his environment, and his behavior is met by a corresponding variety of responses from others. He cries and is fed. He moves his bowels and is diapered. He smiles and people smile back. Gradually there emerges out of this welter of behaviors and responses a set of *roles*—that is, consistent and enduring ways of behaving which are elicited by certain situations having something in common. Each of us has many roles, each consisting of a different set of actions. A man who plays the role of the autocratic boss in the office may play that of a henpecked husband in the home. A child who is a terror on the playground may be a docile mama's boy at the supper-table. The sum total of the roles with which we respond in different situations may be termed the *acting self*, the self we present to others. Ideally this self is both flexible and self-consistent; that is, we are able to modify our roles to fit the demands of the different situations in which we find ourselves. But also underneath them all we remain recognizably ourselves. They all have a common core. Furthermore, ideally the roles which make up the acting self are appropriate to the different situations. The person is a good boss in the office and a good father at home. That is, he carries out his roles in such a way as to yield the maximum satisfaction for himself and for those with whom he is interacting.

Each of an individual's roles implicitly demands a *reciprocal role* from other persons which tends to reinforce it. The henpecked husband is reciprocal to the domineering wife; the autocratic boss to the submissive employee. Of course, others do not always respond in the way the role calls for, but they do respond in some fashion.

In using terms such as role and acting self, I am trying to emphasize that our behavior always has an audience, which responds actively to it. The terms should not be taken to mean that the person puts on an act deliberately. Roles are assumed automatically and unconsciously.

A person cannot directly perceive his own acting self. What he does perceive is the responses of others to the roles he plays. Other persons are, as it were, a set of mirrors reflecting back our acting selves, with more or less distortion. These images gradually fuse to form a *perceived self* and an *ideal self*—what I am and what I would like to be or should be.

The child, for example, whose parents regard him as basically good and well-meaning will usually grow up to perceive himself as this sort of person. The child who feels unwanted and is made to feel wicked and evil may grow up overburdened with a sense of guilt. That is, he perceives himself as evil.

The perceived self emerges somewhere in childhood. Richard Hughes in that remarkably perceptive book about children, *A High Wind in Jamaica*, describes how his heroine, Emily, at the age of 11 suddenly becomes aware of herself:

"And then an event did occur, to Emily, of considerable importance. She suddenly realized who she was . . . She had been playing houses in a nook right in the bows . . . (Emily is on a ship) and tiring of it was walking rather aimlessly aft, thinking vaguely about some bees and a fairy queen, when it suddenly flashed into her mind she was *she*.

"She stopped dead, and began looking over all of her person which came within the range of her eyes. She could not see much, except a fore-shortened view of the front of her frock, and her hands when she lifted them for inspection; but it was enough for her to form a rough idea of the little body she suddenly realized to be hers.

"She began to laugh, rather mockingly. 'Well!' she thought, in effect: 'Fancy *you*, of all people, going and getting caught like this!—You can't get out of it now, not for a very long time: you'll have to go through with being a child, and growing up, and getting old, before you'll be quit of this mad prank!'

. . . .

"Well, then, granted she was Emily, what were the consequences, besides enclosure in that particular little body . . . and lodgement behind a particular pair of eyes?

"It implied a whole series of circumstances. In the first place, there was her family, a number of brothers and sisters from whom, before, she had never entirely dissociated herself; but now she got such a sudden feeling of being a discrete person that they seemed as separate from her as the ship itself. However, willy-nilly she

94

was almost as tied to them as she was to her body. And then there was this voyage, this ship, this mast round which she had wound her legs. She began to examine it with almost as vivid an illumination as she had studied the skin of her hands. And when she came down from the mast, what would she find at the bottom? There would be . . . the whole fabric of a daily life which up to now she had accepted as it came, but which now seemed vaguely disquieting. What was going to happen? Were there disasters running about loose, disasters which her rash marriage to the body of Emily Thornton made her vulnerable to?"[6]

In this passage the emphasis is on the discovery of the perceived bodily self. The author singles out two implications of the discovery of one's self which it is well for us to keep in mind. One is that when I become a person, other people become persons, too, and I am aware that they exist and function to some extent independently of me. The other is that as soon as "I" exist as an entity, I can become a target, I can be hurt. The integrity of myself can be threatened. As a result, a great deal of our activity seems to be devoted to preserving the constancy of the perceived self, for the same reason that we try so hard to preserve the constancy of our perceptual environment. The perceived self is our base of operations. It is the concept on which we base predictions as to how our behavior will effect others, so we try hard to hold it steady.

Dr. Cantril has shown experimentally that one's perceived bodily self has much greater constancy than the perceived bodies of other persons. He put glasses on people which distort the human form so that the upper part of the body seems to lean forward with the upper and lower half of his body distorted in length. He found that if a person wearing these glasses looks at himself in a mirror, he sees only minor and detailed distortions; for example, the hands or feet may be slightly misshapen. But when he looks at a stranger, he sees more general bodily distortion plus the appearance of leaning one way or another.[7]

Our perceived self includes various aspects such as physical and intellectual abilities, tastes, emotions, and values and standards. The caretaker of these latter is the *ideal self*—the person I would like to be or feel I ought to be. Against this ideal self I continually measure my perceived self. In the normal person there is enough discrepancy between the perceived and ideal selves to stimulate him to try to better himself. Such a person is self-confident or self-respecting. If a person's ideal self is identical with his perceived self, he sees no room for improvement; he is smug. If his ideal self is too far removed from his perceived self, it no longer acts as an incentive for improvement but instead becomes a source of discouragement. Such a person is self-derogatory; he lacks self-confidence.

We try even harder to maintain the constancy of our ideal selves than of our perceived selves. Morality is based to a large extent on the need to maintain intact one's image of his ideal self. Most of us do not respond to the temptation to steal, however great, because to steal would violate our pictures of ourselves as honest persons. In fact, the need to maintain our ideal self intact may be stronger than the drive for self-preservation. Many millionaires have committed suicide after losing a lot of money although they still have more than enough to live on, because they cannot bear to see themselves as failures. The hero marches off to certain death because he cannot stand the thought of being a coward.

Like the perceptual constancies described earlier, the perceived and ideal selves are based on past experiences and imply expectancies about the future. These expectancies are important determinants of feelings and behavior. Psychiatrists have found that a particularly useful question to evaluate a suicidal risk is "How does the future look to you?" It is the prospect of a hopeless future, more than an unbearable present, which makes life insupportable.

If the process of self-development runs smoothly, the person ends with a self-system which has certain properties. First of all, it shows a balance between flexibility and firmness. His acting self, perceived self and ideal self are all clear and definite, but not so rigid that he cannot adapt to different situations. With respect to his acting self, though he can easily assume the roles demanded by different situations, they are all consistent with each other. Secondly, the perceived self and the acting self are in harmony. The person can reasonably accurately predict how he will respond in different situations and how he will look to others. As a result, his acting selves, his roles, are well tailored to the different environments in which he finds himself. Thirdly, the perceived and ideal selves are optimally close together. The person likes himself pretty much as he is, though granting room for improvement. Finally, since the self-image includes the future, a person with a healthy self-system predicts implicitly that he will be at least as successful in the future as he has been in the past. In short, such a person is self-confident and self-respecting.

So far I have described the healthy organization of the self. It is obvious that many of our patients have pathological self-structures. They lack self-confidence. They cannot predict the effects of their own behavior on others. Their expectancies of the future are often much too pessimistic which leads them to give up in the present. I should like now to discuss briefly how these miscarriages of development of the self come about and then return to a brief description of some of the major ones as an introduction to a discussion of how the occupational therapist can use his or her self to correct some of these difficulties.

Some of the miscarriages in the development of the human self undoubtedly depend on constitutional factors which we only dimly understand at present and which are of little relevance to our current work. I therefore will pass over them with this mere mention and focus entirely on the role of life experience in leading to pathological self-information. I have suggested that each of us develops his self-picture out of the responses of others to him, especially those who mean the most to him such as members of his immediate family. If a person's parents handle him inconsistently, mistreat him, or derogate him constantly, he cannot develop a consistent and workable self-image. The most damaged persons psychiatrists see, from the standpoint of their self-image, are schizophrenics and the so-called sociopathic personalities. The families of these patients are almost always severely disturbed. As Dr. Theodore Lidz and his colleagues are finding, the parents of schizophrenics were often in a state of constant warfare and the child was the battlefield.* Often the dominant parents is of the opposite sex from the child and continually derogates and humiliates the same-sex parent. The mother, let us say, holds the father up to scorn, so the boy, who tends to identify himself with his father, comes to see himself as unworthy and inadequate. The parents of sociopaths are often disorganized, without consistent standards, and treat the child unpredictably. They may be neglectful, over-indulgent, or brutal—not in response to anything the child does, but because of their own emotional state at the time. The child has great difficulty developing any kind of consistent self-image from this welter of unpredictable parental responses to him. Let me hasten to add that this is not the whole story of the etiology of schizophrenia or sociopathy by any means, but it may serve to illustrate how early experiences may lead to maldevelopment of the self.

An important determinant of a pathological self-image which deserves the particular attention of occupational therapists is a physical handicap. The actual nature and extent of the disability is important in determining the person's self-image, of course. But probably more important is how the person perceives his disability. This, in turn, largely depends on how it has been perceived by others important to him—what kind of image they have reflected back to him. Thus a visible handicap, especially a disfiguring one, is apt to be more disturbing to a person's self-image than an invisible one such as a damaged heart. A handicap which a person regards as shameful is much more damaging to the self-image than one that is not. Recently I have been working with a patient faced with eventual blindness because of familial eye disease. Several members of his family are already severely afflicted. Though distressed by the threatened disability, he is much more disturbed by his feeling, which he picked up from his family, that it is a disgrace which must be concealed from others at all costs. He sees himself as marked by ancestral sin, as it were, and this is the major problem. For example, it implies that if others knew of his affliction they would scorn him, and it prevents him from even thinking about rehabilitation, because to do so would require a public admission of his handicap.

Inconsistent or derogatory parental attitudes are bound to arouse much anxiety, because they create a situation which is not only threatening but, what is worse, is unpredictable. There is nothing that creates more anxiety than not knowing what to expect. Mild anxiety is a great stimulus to experimentation and change, but excessive anxiety is paralyzing. The more anxious the person is, the more he clings to his habitual ways of perceiving and behaving. At least they have enabled him to survive, however inadequate they may be, and he cannot risk the danger that might result from changing them. The child's anxiety, therefore, make it very difficult for him to change his pathological picture of himself. Thus, most of our patients are saddled with a self, usually the reflection of attitudes of persons to them in their past, which is not very useful in the present. Because this self is not appropriate to their present condition, they experience failures and frustrations instead of successes in their dealings with others which heighten their anxiety and rivet them even more strongly to their past selves. The poet Robert Burns long ago pled for the power to see ourselves as others see us. Our patients cannot see themselves as others see them, because they see themselves as others *saw* them, and they are unable to shake themselves loose from this image.

The best-known example in psychopathology of not being able to free oneself from the past is the so-called *transference reaction*, with which I am sure most of you are familiar. This simply means that an individual reacts to someone in the present as if he were a significant person in his past. He reacts to a boss as if he were a father; to a fellow group member, as if he were a sibling, and so on.

Three ways in which we maintain the constancy of our pictures of ourselves in spite of experiences which might tend to cause changes are: *avoidance, selective inattention*, and *the self-fulfilling prophecy*.

We tend to *avoid* experiences which would cause us to change our pictures of ourselves. Recently I saw a person who expressed this very bluntly. Whenever things do not go to his liking, he states, he just walks off. But one doesn't have to go to psychopathology to find examples of avoidance. I wonder during the last presidential election how many supporters of Ike listened to Stevenson's speeches. How many of us, who listen to say Fulton Lewis, Jr., also listen to Eric Severeid, or vice versa? Most of us avoid reading or listening to persons whose views disagree with ours.

A somewhat more subtle way of protecting the constancies which we have built up is through what H. S. Sullivan has termed *selective inattention*. We simply do not attend to those aspects of situations which are at variance with our established constancies. To hark back to the example of the nude and the Madonna, both stimuli were present. One man attended to the Madonna and "inattended" to the nude; the other attended to the nude and not the Madonna. In all our personal relationships we tend to single out from the behavior of other persons those aspects which fit our preconception and to ignore those which do not. This, in conjunction with the point I am about to mention, I think is chiefly responsible for the fixity of our self-perceptions.

Not only do we selectively inattend to responses of others which might be inconsistent with our pictures of ourselves, but we tend to act in such a way as to elicit behavior from others which confirms our self-picture. This has been termed the *self-fulfilling prophecy*.

The patient with congenital eye disease clearly illustrates this phenomenon. He cannot see in the dark, so he stumbles at night unless somebody helps him. He does not tell people of his difficulty, so when he stumbles they snicker or laugh or think he is drunk, which confirms his opinion that his disease is shameful and disgraceful. Recently in the group he was able to confess in detail his feelings about his night blindness and became quite moved in so doing. As can be well imagined, nobody snickered; nobody thought it was the least disgraceful; and the group was very supportive. At this moment his self-fulfilling prophecy was not met. On the basis of this experience, in a vacation which subsequently ensued he immediately told a couple whom he and his wife had met about his affliction. Then when he stumbled at night, they understood what the trouble was and did not laugh, and he began to get evidence that people did not regard his blindness as a joke. His behavior up to that moment had been such as to reinforce his prophecy that people would have contempt for him if they knew of his difficulty.

What makes these self-fulfilling prophecies hard to modify is that most of the behavior which elicits them is automatic and goes on outside of awareness. I think of a patient in group therapy who wore a habitual frown and wondered why people seemed to react unfavorably to her. She was quite astonished when the group pointed out that she presented a sulky face to the world. We do not know that we are doing things which cause people to react to us in the way that we expect; therefore, it is hard to change.

Many of our patients have disturbed self-structures. I have suggested that the disturbance starts because parents reflect back to the child an inconsistent or derogatory picture of himself. From this he molds a defective or disorganized self-image and then, because he is anxious, he cannot readily change it. Instead, by such devices as avoidance, selective inattention, and the self-fulfilling prophecy he prevents new experiences from correcting his self-image.

I should now like to turn to three common types of disturbance of the self that our patients present: first, difficulties in the acting self; secondly, difficulties with the perceived self; and, thirdly, discrepancies between the perceived, acting, and ideal selves.

The acting self can go awry in two diametrically opposed ways. Frequently it is too rigid; the patient's repertory of roles for different situations is too limited. Now, the narrower the range of our roles, the more compelling they are in influencing the behavior of other persons. It is practically impossible to deal for long with a person who responds suspiciously no matter what you do, for example, without becoming irritated at him. When he finally succeeds in angering you, this confirms his suspiciousness. This pattern is nowhere better seen than in the paranoid patient, whose chronic hostility inevitably engenders like reactions in others which he then uses to justify his feeling that people are against him. Since the more limited a patient's role repertory is the more likely he is to evoke confirming behavior from other persons, the person with a rigid and limited acting self is apt to become more and more committed to the few roles available to him. Thus he meets increasing failures and frustrations, heightening his anxiety and making it even more difficult for him to change his patterns.

At the other extreme the acting self remains diffuse. The patient remains like the infant in responding too directly to the demands of the different situations in which he is placed. His repertory is so wide that no stable acting self becomes organized. He is like a chameleon.

This difficulty with the acting self leads directly into a very important type of self pathology—the failure of a perceived self, and therefore of an ideal self, to jell. The patient is confused about who he really is. Patients often express this by saying, "All my life is an act." This difficulty is particularly common in our society for two reasons. The first is that it is such a complex and changing one that we are exposed to many different groups with inconsistent expectancies and value systems. Furthermore, these expectancies may change rapidly in time. For example, the modern male is expected to behave quite differently at work, in his home, in church, and when out with the "boys." The modern woman often finds it very hard to reconcile the roles of housewife and career woman, to name just two. Thus the lack of unity in our culture becomes reflected in our multitudinous acting selves and in a confusion in our perceived selves. To use E. H. Erikson's term, we suffer from *role diffusion.*

The situation is aggravated because our culture places such a high value on pleasing other persons. Fromm has described this aspect of our life brilliantly in his discussion of what he calls the marketing character, by which he means that we have adopted the values of the market place in which saleability, not use, is the main criterion of worth:

"The market concept of value, the emphasis on exchange value rather than on use value, has led to a similar concept of value with regard to people and particularly to oneself. The character orientation which is rooted in the experience of oneself as a commodity and of one's value as exchange value I call the marketing orientation . . . Like the handbag, one has to be in fashion on the personality market, and in order to be in fashion one has to know what kind of personality is most in demand . . . Since modern man experiences himself both as the seller and as the commodity to be sold on the market, his self-esteem depends on conditions beyond his control. If he is 'successful,' he is valuable; if he is not, he is worthless.

"In the marketing orientation man encounters his own powers as commodities alienated from him . . . Both his powers and what they create become estranged, something different from himself, something for others to judge and to use; thus his feeling of identity becomes as shaky as his self-esteem; it is constituted by the sum total of roles one can play: *'I am as you desire me.'* "[9]

This diffusion of the perceived self and failure to form an ideal self is seen in many patients called sociopathic and in some alcoholic patients, who in a single interview can box the compass in their descriptions of themselves. They will, for example, first say that alcohol is not a problem for them, that they can conquer it easily if they only make an effort; and a few minutes later they will point out how impossible it is to overcome their drinking since they have to associate with people who drink. Or they will brag about how independent they are and how able they are to do without other people, and a little later explain how lonely they are and how much

they need people. The fact that they can make these statements without any awareness that they are contradicting themselves strongly suggests that they do not have a perceived or ideal self against which they can measure their statements.

Finally, there are various *discrepancies between the different selves* which plague people. Patients often misperceive the physical attributes of their acting selves. I think of a person who always saw himself as much smaller than his teachers in college. When he returned for a reunion he discovered to his astonishment that he was taller than many of them.

The perceived self may deviate from the acting self in two opposite ways, either of which leads to failures and frustrations. The person may over-estimate his acting self, as in the fictitious example given by Oliver Wendell Holmes of the man who was a bore and thought he was brilliant. More commonly, especially among our patients, he is apt grossly to under-estimate his acting self. He does not appreciate his assets and abilities. The man I mentioned who is threatened with blindness, for example, sees himself when blind as utterly helpless and dependent; though perfectly aware that blind people lead useful, productive lives, this simply does not register with him emotionally. One source of this in our society is related to the prevalence of the marketing character with its emphasis on competition to be liked. This leads each of us to develop quite a skillful acting self; we take each other in quite readily. We accept the other person's acting self at its face value, while at the same time being aware of how much we do not live up to our own acting selves. As a result, we tend to under-estimate ourselves in relation to other people. This becomes clearly evident in group therapy or in any type of group where the emphasis is on free and honest interchange of feelings and ideas. The most common single benefit reported by members of these groups, whether mental patients or captains of industry, is the discovery that other people also have problems, that other people are no better adjusted than they are, that behind their acting selves each has doubts and hesitations.

The tendency to underestimate one's own acting self is related to the final type of discrepancy I want to mention—the discrepancy between the ideal self and the perceived self. This discrepancy is perhaps the most potent source of misery that I have mentioned. It seems as if the more doubts we have about our perceived selves, the more rigid and more lofty we make our ideal selves in a vain effort to compensate for this. For example, a hysterical patient who presents to the world a picture of almost superhuman poise, charm and forbearance feels herself to be full of hate, and is wretched because of this. Her ideal self demands that she should be full of Christian charity and forgiveness at all times and always in complete control of her emotions. Another patient, a man who is very competent in his work, a good husband and father, is frequently depressed and panicky because he is not living up to his ideal of being utterly independent, a complete he-man who is able to tackle anything that comes along without hesitation and without asking anyone else for advice. The man with the failing sight, although he has many successes in business and in social life, can never accept them as real. From the standpoint of his ideal image, you may recollect, his eye disease is evidence of his moral unworthiness, so he cannot admit his successes. He immediately decides each one was a fluke and goes on underestimating himself. In all these cases the excessive height and rigidity of the idealized image blinds the person to his actual successes, because in comparison with what he would like to be they fall far short. Thus, he is unable to gain self-confidence from his actual achievements. Moreover, the situation is a self-aggravating one. The higher the ideal self, the worse the perceived self seems by contrast, causing the person to raise his ideal self still higher, so that neurotic patients characteristically show what might be called a split self-esteem. On the one hand they feel lower than the low and on the other, secretly and in brief moments, they feel far superior to most other people—a truly miserable state of affairs.

One can sum up these different forms of failure of the self to develop with the word "disintegration." They are all aspects of failure to form an integrated self, expressed either by too great a rigidity of the acting self, inadequate structuring of the perceived self, and discrepancies between the three different selves.

To recapitulate, much of the distress of our patients can be viewed as springing from disorders of their self-systems. As a result of misperceptions of themselves in relation to others, they guide their behavior by incorrect expectancies and predictions, leading to experiences of failure and frustration which increase their emotional difficulties. Their disordered self-systems have grown up through damaging experiences with others and have been maintained and strengthened by a variety of mechanisms such as avoidance, selective inattention and self-fulfilling prophecies.

All forms of psychotherapy, including the psychotherapeutic aspect of occupational therapy, try to reinforce the healthy aspects of the patient's self and help him to modify its flaws. They do this by trying to engage him in new and different interpersonal transactions which will confirm his healthy expectancies and disappoint his pathological ones.

The main therapeutic tool for this purpose is the self of the therapist, and here, at last, I shall address myself briefly to the title of this presentation—the therapeutic use of the self.

The first questions is, how much of the therapist's self is relevant to therapy? I do not know what occupational therapists are taught about this, but in psychiatry there is a tendency to assume that the psychotherapist's total self must be involved if treatment is to succeed. Much has been written about the qualifications of the psychotherapist which leaves the impression that he must be a paragon of warmth, maturity, altruism, able to give freely of himself, acutely sensitive to the feelings of others and so on. Some writers on therapy go so far as to maintain that genuine therapy only occurs when the therapist becomes deeply and personally involved in the process. It seems to me that this is unsound theoretically but, more important, that it is decisively refuted by everyday experience. We all know that the therapeutic skill of our colleagues bears little relationship, within wide limits, to their own maturity, idealism, nobility of soul or sensitivity.

There is no question but that some persons have greater healing powers than others, and that this depends on attributes of their personalities which are ill-defined and probably cannot be taught. Moreover, obviously one cannot play one's therapeutic role successfully unless this aspect of oneself is supported by a reasonably sound self-structure in other respects. A therapist may have personal problems which are so severe as to interfere with his role as a healer, in which case he should certainly seek to straighten himself out by himself submitting to psychotherapy.

But if successful therapy were solely a matter of the therapist's innate gifts or qualities he has achieved through his own psychotherapy, there would be nothing to teach or learn, and a meeting such as this one, for example, would have no purpose.

My own belief is that most of us have enough innate healing potentialities, and are well enough organized to be able to present an acting self to the patient which enables him to achieve a better integration of himself.

If we do not keep our therapeutic role distinct from the rest of ourselves, we run the risk of impeding our therapeutic efficacy in several ways. One is that we may try too hard to help—we may expect too much of ourselves, forgetting that like all skills, those of the occupational therapist have only a certain range of usefulness. This may play right into the exaggerated and unrealistic demands of certain patients, briefly arousing in them false expectations of a miracle. So they end up more disappointed and embittered. Or it may feed their already excessive dependency and impede the development of a more independent outlook.

More importantly, to the extent that we do not keep our therapeutic role clearly separated from the rest of ourselves, we are at the mercy of the patient who fails to improve. Occupational therapists like psychiatrists are practitioners of a healing art who perceive themselves as help-givers; that is, persons able to relieve suffering and improve the effectiveness of others. If we invest too much of ourselves in this role and cannot carry it out successfully, we become frustracted and react with anger or depression. We are exposed to exactly the same type of damaging failure experiences from which many of our patients suffer, and thereby in the long run become less effective because of our own exhaustion or irritation. Certain types of patients make it very difficult for the occupational therapist to offer help successfully. Patients who fail to improve despite our best efforts and return always with renewed complaints or accusations that we are making them worse are a great trial, because they do not display the behavior which would be reciprocal to our role. Sometimes one cannot maintain the proper role with such patients, and then it may be well to refer them to another person. But the best protection against such patients is to remind ourselves of the limitations of the therapeutic role. Through this we may be able to maintain the objective attitude which represents the best possibility of thwarting their self-fulfilling prophecies that all those from whom they seek help are angry at them and will eventually reject them. In this way we may be able to help them after all.

The therapeutic role of the occupational therapist is confined to trying to bring about modifications in the acting self of the patient. He tries to help the patient modify his expectancies in a limited area of his functioning—the task he is doing—in the hope that the self-confidence thus gained will generalize to other areas of the patient's life. This will lead to modifications of his behavior which will, in turn, elicit different behavior from others. This further strengthens his favorable expectancies, leading to progressive improvement. The point to emphasize is that whatever the occupational therapist's hopes as to the final outcome of this train of events, he is responsible for aiding only in one of its initial steps.

Within these limits, the therapeutic goal of the occupational therapist is the same as that of any psychotherapist; namely, to strengthen healthy aspects of the patient's self-picture and weaken

the unhealthy one. The latter is accomplished by acting in such a way as to disappoint his pathological expectancies. The real art of therapy is to do this under such conditions that it will lead to a modification of his expectancies in a healthy direction. For the patient has many ways of maintaining his habitual expectancies despite contradictory experiences. Therefore, special conditions have to be met if the therapist's behavior is to be effective.

First of all, the therapist must act in such a way that the patient perceives him as someone who wants to help and is able to do so. As already mentioned, the expectancy that something helpful is going to happen may in itself be a powerful healing force, as faith cures bear witness. In addition, the patient's faith in the therapist may give him the initial courage to experiment with changes in his behavior, to become more spontaneous and flexible and thereby mobilize his assets more effectively. In any case, it is only if the patient perceives the therapist as an actual or potential help-giver that he will be influenced by the therapist's behavior.

The therapist gets across to the patient that he can be helpful by demonstrating his belief in himself, and in the patient. He demonstrates his belief in himself by showing competence in his role—by doing his job in a self-assured manner. Let me emphasize again, this does not require that the occupational therapist be self-confident with respect to all aspects of himself, but simply that he know his job and show it.

Demonstrating one's belief in the patient's capacity to be helped is a more complex business. How one does this depends on how one sizes up the patient's reactions to praise and blame. Direct reassurance may be the right approach to many—perhaps most—patients, but for some it has the opposite of the desired effect. Schizophrenic patients, for example, are suspicious of praise. They are apt to experience it as an attempt to seduce them into a state of emotional dependency so they can be manipulated and exploited in the service of the therapist's nefarious plans. All of us may experience praise which is given too easily as at best a dubious compliment, because it implies that the praising person does not expect very much of us. So, many patients get more of a feeling of your belief in them if you offer reassurance sparingly, thus implicitly reinforcing their self-confidence. Under special and rare circumstances the best way to convey one's faith in a patient may even be to get angry at him. If it is clear that the anger is directed, not at his total self, but at his acting self of the moment and that it is based on the therapist's conviction that the patient can easily do much better, then it can be supportive.

In addition to conveying his ability and desire to be helpful, the therapist increases his chances of disappointing the patient's pathological expectancies by striking the proper balance between *clarity* and *ambiguity* in his behavior. Let us consider each of these aspects in turn. The therapist must act clearly and consistently because it usually takes a long while for behavior which contradicts a patient's expectancies to break through into the patient's awareness. Moreover, consistent behavior in itself may disappoint a major expectancy of many patients who display a variety of inconsistent—or even conflicting—behaviors. They may express utter discouragement one moment, over-optimism the next; alternate between resentment and gratitude; demand a great deal of help or insist on doing it themselves. And they implicitly expect from the therapist the reciprocal responses to these behaviors. Once the therapist has decided what his most effective role should be with the patient, he should maintain it consistently. This not only disappoints a lot of the patient's expectations, but gives the patient a model of steadiness which may help him to settle down.

Consistency, however, does not mean rigidity, but rather *predictable flexibility*. The occupational therapist must be flexible in the sense of changing his behavior to fit the needs of different patients and will want to modify his behavior in keeping with a particular patient's progress. The essential points are that all of the therapist's behavior be such that the patient can perceive it as consistent with the goal of offering help, and that it be predictable. However wide the range of responses that a therapist offers a patient, the patient should have the feeling that if he acts in a certain way, the therapist will respond in a certain way. In this way the patient has a chance to build up new expectancies as to the effects of his behavior which will tend to counteract his habitual faulty ones.

The ideal of consistency, finally, must leave room for *spontaneity*. The therapist obviously should not function like a machine, and an important aspect of demonstrating confidence in one's role is being able to be spontaneous at times. The person who obviously calculates every move inevitably conveys the impression of being unsure of himself. Moreover, we hope our patients will develop more spontaneity, and can help them to achieve this by presenting ourselves as a model in this respect.

I have stressed the importance of presenting a clear and consistent picture of oneself to the patient. It now remains to round out the story by adding that a certain degree of *ambiguity* may also be appropriate. To the extent that everyone fears the unknown, an ambiguous situation is anxiety-provoking. If the patient cannot figure out what is expected of him, he may become so anxious that he is even less capable of learning than usual. On the other hand, with certain patients ambiguity has a diagnostic value in that it helps us to determine how the patient copes with stress. From the therapeutic standpoint it tends to increase the patient's involvement in the situation. He is forced to engage himself in order to cope with the uncertainties and deal with them. Finally, it can help his self-confidence if he copes successfully with the ambiguity and manages to create out of it an adequately structured situation. Thus the optimal balance between clarity and ambiguity depends on how well-organized the patient's self-system is. Schizophrenics and sociopaths, whose selves are chaotic, usually benefit only from crystal clear, definite behavior on the therapist's part; mild neurotics may profit more from being left to their own devices.

It should be apparent from this discussion that all generalities about the therapeutic use of the self should be regarded with suspicion. In the last analysis, the therapist's success in acting so as to usefully disappoint the patient's expectancies depends on his diagnostic acumen with respect to the patient concerned, and the repertory of behavior at his command. His aim, always, is to respond differently enough from the patient's expectancies to force the patient to take another look as it were, but not so differently that the patient perceives it as totally irrelevant to his behavior. Furthermore, it must be different enough to arouse an optimal amount of anxiety in the patient, since this is a powerful stimulus to learning, but not so different as to arouse excessive anxiety, which is paralyzing and serves merely to reinforce the patient's original behavior.

Let me, in conclusion, try to pull this rather complicated presentation together. Many of our patients have faulty self-structures, which contribute significantly to their difficulties. I have tried to describe some of these faulty selves and how they may arise, stressing particularly the role of expectancies, based on past experience in determining how we see the world and how we behave. One of the tasks of the occupational therapist is to use himself to help the patient develop a more workable self of his own. This requires, first of all, that the therapist make a correct diagnosis, that he understand what is going on, and one aim of this presentation has been to offer a framework for thinking about problems of the self. To use himself effectively the therapist must also have a clear realization of his own abilities and limitation. He must have confidence in his methods, but should not expect them to work miracles, and he must set limits to his own self-involvement in his therapeutic efforts.

In trying to use himself therapeutically, the occupational therapist has two general goals. The first is to get the patient to make an emotional investment in the therapeutic situation—to perceive it as important to his welfare—since if he does not, nothing the therapist does will make any difference. The second goal is to reduce the patient's anxiety, or raise his self-confidence, to the point that he can dare to take a fresh look at himself, and begin again to profit from new interpersonal experiences. Aspects of the therapist's behavior which can help to achieve these goals are his use of reassurance, the clarity or ambiguity of the treatment situation he creates, and the consistency, flexibility, and spontaneity of his actions.

REFERENCES

1. *Collected Edition of the Last Poems of A. E. Housman.* New York: Scribners, 1937.
2. Cantril, Hadley. "Perception and Interpersonal Relations," *American Journal of Psychiatry*, 114:119-126, 1957.
3. *Ibid.*
4. Rosenthal, David and Jerome D. Frank. "Psychotherapy and the Placebo Effect," *Psychological Bulletin*, 53:294-302, 1956.
5. Holmes, Oliver Wendell. *The Autocrat of the Breakfast-Table.* New York: The Heritage Press, p. 46-48, 1955.
6. Hughes, Richard. *A High Wind in Jamaica.* New York: Modern Library, p. 188-195, 1932.
7. Cantril, Hadley, *op. cit.*
8. Lidz, Theodore, Alice R. Cornelison, Stephen Fleck, and Dorothy Terry. "The Intrafamilial Environment of Schizophrenic Patients: II. Marital Schism and Marital Skew," *American Journal of Psychiatry*, 114: 241-248, 1957.
9. Fromm, Erich. *Man for Himself.* New York: Rinehart and Co., Inc., pp. 68-73, 1947.

Termination: That Difficult Farewell

LEONARD T. MAHOLICK, M.D.*
DON W. TURNER, M.D.* | *Atlanta, Ga.*

Termination is usually a difficult and painful, yet powerfully significant life experience. It is experienced in multiple contexts beginning with birth and ending with death. This article addresses itself to these issues and the when and how of goodbyes.

At the Church Gate

The play is done; the curtain drops,
　　slow falling to the prompter's bell;

A moment yet the actor stops,
　　and looks around, to say farewell.

It is an irksome word and task;
　　and when he's laughted and said his say,

He shows as he removes the mask,
　　a face that's anything but gay - - -

Thackeray

Termination, be it in individual or group psychotherapy, can present a powerful analogy to how we deal with the farewells of our lives. We view termination as one of those natural pausing points which present us with the opportunity to say goodbye. The critical issues we shall deal with include the when and how of goodbyes. The following remarks refer to the natural, voluntary, or spontaneous terminations mutually agreed upon by the patient and therapist as well as other types of terminations, which shall be acknowledged.

We have noted how little has been written in the professional literature on the nature and the clinical management of group termination. A few clinicians have attempted to deal with these issues in the context of group psychotherapy and we acknowledge their efforts, including Kitchen, McGee et al., Kadis et al.[1-3] Some pioneers, Ferenczi, Freud, Alexander, Frieda Fromm-Reichmann, and Rickman[4-8] among them, wrote about termination matters related to individual psychoanalysis and psychotherapy.

PHILOSOPHICAL ROOTS

Increasingly during the past four or five years we have come to view the whole spectrum of human experience as a continuing series of hellos and goodbyes.

The journey begins with the first hello between the egg and the sperm and their introduction to the mother's womb. Some nine months later begins the first goodbye. At that time the newborn separates from an almost ideal home carefully constructed so as to stimulate growth and development and is introduced to an unknown external world.

This is followed with life journey's inevitable seasonal terminations, such as: leaving the parental nest and family-setting to begin school; graduation from high school; leave-taking from the family; later leaving the college-

*Psychotherapists and Supervisors, Atlanta Psychiatric Clinic on Peachtree. *Mailing address*: 2905 Peachtree Rd., N.E., Atlanta, Georgia 30305.

AMERICAN JOURNAL OF PSYCHOTHERAPY, Vol. XXXIII, No. 4, October 1979 setting. Then there is the ending of the single life; the termination of the dyaditic couple when the first baby arrives. Still later there are the goodbyes to each of the children and then all of the children. There are the succession of job changes usually ending with retirement. There are the numerous sayings of goodbye to various family residences. As age advances there is the inevitable farewell to the various functional organ systems and, often, the goodbye to physical health. This is followed quickly by parting with the spouse, family members, close friends and relatives by way of death. And finally there is the ending of one's own life with which to deal.

From this view there is the recurrent cyclical phenomenon of goodbyes encompassing the entire life journey of man from birth to death.

Termination of therapy can be thought of as a recapitulation of the multiple preceding goodbyes of living. At the same time it is a preparation for being able to deal more adequately and openly with future goodbyes.

CLINICAL ROOTS

Through the years in our personal as well as professional experiences we have become increasingly aware of the power in endings. A choice exists between avoiding farewells with the potential for destruction and continuing unhappiness or for the potential of new creative experiences, once goodbyes are accomplished.

Some recent studies indicate that among the most difficult stresses the human has to contend with, in the context of his social role, is to deal with the loss or separation from a parent, particularly in childhood, the death of a spouse, a family member, a friend or relative, or significant other and separation and/or loss through divorce, relocation, or changing jobs.

In our own experiences, we repeatedly have been struck with the lingering power and persistence of pain related to never having dealt with or talked about early life losses and deaths of significant persons. Quite frequently we have been impressed with the continuing evidences of personal suffering often clearly related to the unfinished goodbyes of the past. When these sensitive roots are touched there is an intense, deep-felt, emotional re- sponse and a freeing up of repressed energy which had been bound by the ungrieved grief and nonacceptance of the loss or separation. It is regrettable that as of yet our culture has not fully recognized the need to talk and deal with the pain of loss, separation, or death when it occurs. So often it will have to be dealt with in a psychotherapist's office ten, twenty, or more years later. These critical issues have such great power in defining the future of individuals in their life journeys that we do not hesitate to stop anywhere during the therapy process to return to them repeatedly. We insist upon dealing with those collective unfinished businesses of the past. Our persis- tent efforts with people's termination struggles have consistently yielded rich rewards.

We psychotherapists are therefore strategically positioned to address these termination issues in intimate private dialogue where we talk straight about the untalkables, assuming we are not avoiding goodbyes in our own past.

TIMES FOR TERMINATION

We think of termination as an issue both patient and therapist are hesitant to consider. Goodbyes are indicated at these points:

1. When the contractual ending of the therapy arrangement occurs. At this time it is appropriate to consider termination with or without maximum progress.

2. When the patient in the group has progressed as far as he wants in gaining awareness and changing behavioral patterns. We feel this is a natural and desirable time to terminate but insist, doggedly if necessary, that the person leave with a respectful and genuine goodbye; not a mechanical, cold, "see-you-around-the-campus" farewell. This allows us to close out the experience with the remaining members of the group and with the patient so that neither the patient nor group carries the others "piggy back" into the future.

3. When terminations are precipitated by unexpected developments such as job changes, shifts in working hours, and financial reversals. It is our suggestion that these farewells be as genuine and persistently dealt with as in the above instances, since these are usually out of the patient's power to manipulate. We want to make sure that a firm goodbye is instituted where the individual will leave the therapy experience with closure even though they may not have achieved the originally defined goals. This is one of the times when people are most hesitant and resistant to saying goodbye because they are not through with each other.

4. When presenting problems have been clarified with some significant resolution and there are indications that old patterns of adapting are not returning to the same degree as before. It is often very tempting to let the patient continue therapy at this point because he is becoming increasingly enjoyable and effective and contributes a great deal to the group. However, there is wisdom in asking what additionally the person wants to "work on." If new goals are defined and mutually agreed upon it may well be advisable to permit the individual to stay and work further if, and this is a major consideration, the person is not using the group as a substitute for real living. Let's face it, there are just lots of things in the living process which are not practical for us to do in a therapy group setting. These are better performed in the field of living rather than in the arena of a therapy group. At this juncture there is the danger that the group becomes an obstacle to effective living, an escape as it were, rather than a facility to enhance the person's coping power in life struggles.

5. When in the therapist's judgment, there is wisdom in either the person's or the group's terminating without mutual consent. If at a point where either the group or any patient in the group is consistently destructive to the welfare of the group or any other patient, we think it is mandatory and the therapist's responsibility to consider termination. This obviously should not be done by impulsive, countertransference acting out but rather with consideration and thoughtfulness. One of our colleagues suggested three reasons for the therapist to instigate termination:

(A) Flagrant and recurrent abusive attacking of others;
(B) Flagrant sexual aggressiveness with no regard to the consequences;
(C) Refusal to pay the bill.

These are difficult times when tension in the therapy process usually is at a peak. We think it takes a solid therapist with a good internal support system in order to deal with these explosive issues.

6. When a patient refuses to go on, refuses to deal with therapy issues, and refuses to say goodbye. These are often the least successful termination experiences for the group. They are difficult for all therapists. While the "bolting" patient may not say goodbye, it is still worthwhile for the group to say goodbye to him even if it has to be done in absentia. This reveals the unconscious connections and relationships that were established and lets the whole group's awareness expand greatly.

7. When the patient becomes psychotic or regresses to the point he no longer functions in the group and either has to be hospitalized or has to be

taken out of the group on a permanent or temporary basis. This experience is most difficult to explore. Sometimes the patient who has so decompensated in front of the group will return giving the whole group an opportunity to explore the many meanings of the experience. However, some are lost forever. Unfortunately this is another situation where we are forced to say goodbye before we are ready or have any desire to do so. This is in some way similar to an unexpected death.

8. When the therapist and/or patient experiences no progress in therapy, no change in symptoms, no easing of tensions, or even worse an acceleration of maladapted behavior. This is a most troublesome termination on which few comments can be found. We view this as an unsuccessful hello in the sense that we never had a committed therapeutic beginning or contract. Perhaps a successful goodbye would be the most therapeutic thing for the person at that particular nodal point in his living.

Some of these issues are dealt with in the literature by Zimmerman, Grotjahn, Koran, and McGee.[9-12]

INDICATIONS FOR TERMINATION

We have an increasing awareness that particular areas of therapy are worth exploring as termination is being started or considered. Some strategies we have found valuable include the following:

1. Examination of the initial symptoms, problems, and areas of conflict to see if they have been ameliorated, eradicated, or otherwise resolved. This means a going back to the original hello to check out the readiness for goodbye and its implementation. The initiation of the therapeutic process not only sets the framework for the therapeutic endeavor, but also predestines the termination as a part of the experience. In this sense, initiation and termination are polar opposites of the therapeutic process. Dr. Maholick includes the use of a set of written materials given to the patient during the initial evaluative phases of therapy which document the patient's problems and pains. These can be used as checkpoints to let patient and therapist together decide if goodbye is really appropriate.

2. Exploration of the extent to which resolution of the precipitating stress has been achieved since the initial hello. This is particularly helpful when no structured symptoms were part of the presenting complaints.

3. Search for indications of improved coping ability. Has there been some modification of the presenting defenses or simply a flight into health.

4. Determination of degree of increased awareness, appreciation, and acceptance of the self and others. Has there been demonstrated a willingness to accept responsibility for one's own actions. Also, to what extent has a growing appreciation of humanness, individually as well as collectively, been demonstrated.

5. Exploring to what degree the capacity to love and be loved has been evidenced: that is, to love thyself, to love thy neighbor, and to love thy God. We realize this capacity is never fully accomplished but represents in some ways the "impossible dream" for which we continue reaching.

6. Reflection on the ability of the person to plan differently and work more effectively.

7. Judging whether the ability to cooperate and play rather then merely to obsess about the heaviness of life has been demonstrated.

These are checkpoints. Just that—checkpoints clarifying indications and reflecting appropriateness to terminate. It would be a most remarkable achievement if we could uniformly state we covered all phases in every termination. We unashamedly are simply not that good, wise, nor effective. Rather we are inviting you to consider these as inner guides among others or reference points to be considered in the process of evaluating when and if the person is ready to consider termination, that is, a goodbye to the therapeutic effort.

We view psychotherapy as a transitional process within itself. Initially some of the responsibility for therapeutic movement is relinquished by the patient. Later he will reclaim it as he goes forward with less tension and anxiety and greater ability to define and fulfill himself authentically. Thus if therapy is successful, termination can be implemented with the full knowledge that the person is now ready, as best anyone can know, to take on responsibilities for his own therapy and to live it in life.

We do not see a foreverness in termination. It does not preclude further contact with the therapist. Rather we view it ás the closure of a unique interpersonal endeavor and remain open to future hellos. These include the following: periodic reviews, brief consultations regarding specific problems and/or additional therapy for new life stresses and personal pain.

Nor does termination necessarily preclude a real-life, social relationship. In a few instances this might be of considerable significance to each person. An example of this is a professional in therapy who later becomes involved in joint clinical activity or becomes a working associate and the like.

TECHNIQUES OF TERMINATION

Termination is a most difficult area about which to find data. Literature seems abundant for the "recipes" on beginning therapy, dealing with resistance, and clarifying transference and countertransference issues. Considerations on the issues of meaningful group terminations are scant. In supervision of psychiatric residents, graduate clinical psychology students, and pastoral counselors a routine question is posed, "Where can I read something on the termination process?" We have been repeatedly struck with how little there is to offer.

Not only for the neophyte, but also for the more experienced group therapist there is a need for a style or a mind-set to help start the termination process whether hearts are in it or not. We find it is usual for the patient and therapist alike to resist dealing with termination. To have a successful ending experience is hard work for both but the therapist is certainly better equipped to bring it about than the patient. The therapist has to become active to assure the beginning and ending of the termination process. If left to the patient exclusively we have noted that many terminations are not implemented adequately.

Ideally we should like to do all of the following over a period of at least two sessions prior to termination. We have a contractual agreement with our group members giving us two weeks notice before termination. Recently we have considered four weeks notice to be more appropriate. This period is not meant to be used to convince the patient to stay or to explore further current dynamic issues, but rather to help clarify his disappointments with the group, what he has achieved and to push on with the saying of goodbye to others. The group as a whole is equally resistant to terminating with the individual's leaving. Some of the steps we have found helpful in the process include:

1. Return to the original case record and check each item presented as the problem or symptom to see where the person is in relation to those presenting issues.

2. Asking the patient to repeat certain items in his personal inventory kit of written materials he was given at the entrance into therapy, using them as comparison and preferably sharing this with the group.

3. Requiring the patient to write and/or present orally a final progress report of what the person has or has not achieved in the group. This can provide an obvious opportunity for inviting each member of the group to respond.

4. Request the patient to report dreams and fantasies during the termination process. He is urged to be particularly alert to how those dreams are related to the group and termination process. We asked this directly, repeatedly, and even dogmatically. The individual is asked to be alert and aware of past events and experiences related to separation, loss, or other goodbyes that invariably surface.

5. Encouraging the patient to explore inner feelings and fantasies of a sense of loss, emptiness, aloneness, grief or depression without side-stepping these feelings or assuming that they will go away. The patient is urged rather to dramatize them and get them clearly into the open.

6. Encouraging any and all group members who wish to make a statement concerning the happenings of termination experience to do so.

7. Asking the terminating individual to make a goodbye to each member of the group and in turn invite whatever response each member might have toward him.

8. Later, after the terminating group member has left, motivating the remaining members to share their own feelings, thoughts, fantasies and dreams, paying particular attention to the sense of loss, emptiness and left-behindness. This may have to be done repeatedly for the following two or three group sessions because of uncomfortable feelings and the continuing natural resistance to deal with termination matters after the fact.

THERAPIST ROLE IN TERMINATION

It needs to be emphasized that the therapist should be free, willing and able to actively address himself to all of the central issues involved in the process of termination if the individual or group, after having been given opportunity to take up some issues, fail to do so. Our clinical experiences point to the simple fact that most people will distance themselves from and deny the inner goings-on related to termination. If the therapist carries within himself his own particular mind-set he can direct the energies of the therapeutic effort with good effect. He may have to return to the central issues repeatedly. Otherwise, too often, a public or a "persona" goodbye might be effected reflecting the social graces of the individual and his particular culture. We make it clear we are not dealing with a polite, socially correct, mechanical goodbye, but rather we are making every effort to get into the inner private feelings, fantasies, and dreams of the individual and group members as they proceed to termination. This way it is quite possible to help the individual and group to take care of current unfinished businesses. We also hope to free thereby the individual to use his own full energies to deal with issues confronting him as he journeys out into life and the real world. If the person can deal with the "death" of the relationship in the therapy group with an effective goodbye, he is much freer to go on to the next hello.

CONCLUSION

> Loss and Possession, Death and Life are one.
> There falls no shadow where there shines no sun . . .
> Hilaire Belloc

We believe life has a quiet, deep, to-and-fro, inner regulating rhythm. The hellos and goodbyes are but one of the significant outer symbols. The termination of each day with the sunset, and the beginning of each day with the sunrise determine the rhythm of our lives. At sea, there are the high tides and the low tides. In the sky, there are the building up of the clouds and then their dissipation, some bringing the waters and the wind of life and others giving clear and dry spells. With the beginning of night we say hello to the stars. With night's end the stars recede out of visual awareness and we say goodbye. Then there are the seasons of each year and the seasons of each particular life journey.

Learning to become increasingly aware and open to the symbols of hello and goodbye during the process of therapy allows us the opportunity to touch, get in tune with this inner rhythm and energy permitting us to move on to the next experience in a more creative and freer manner.

It is of great significance to take the time to deal with as many issues related to farewell as is possible. When this is done adequately we help prepare the person to confront other terminations of his life, yet unknown. More to the point, if accomplished reasonably well, the individual ultimately becomes better prepared to deal with the final termination of life—death.

SUMMARY

Termination in therapy as in life is difficult and painful for both parties. If left to chance it will be avoided or glossed over. Under different conditions suggested dynamics and techniques are presented so to assure a successful ending of the therapy experience. The philosophy and importance of termination is shared along with definitive recommendations, with particular emphasis on a group-therapy setting.

REFERENCES

1. Kitchen, R. On Leaving Group Psychotherapy. *Psychol. Newsletter,* New York University, 1957.
2. McGee, T. F., Schuman, B. N., and Racusen, F. Termination in Group Psychotherapy. *Am. J. Psychother.,* 26:521, 1972.
3. Kadis, A. L., Krasner, J. D., Weiner, M. F., et al. *Practicum of Group Psychotherapy,* 2nd ed. Harper and Row, New York, 1974.
4. Ferenczi, S. The Problem of Termination in Analysis (1927). In *Final Contributions to the Problems and Methods of Psychoanalysis.* Basic Books, N.Y., 1955, pp. 77–86.
5. Freud, S. *Analysis Terminable and Interminable* (1937). In *Standard Edition,* vol. 23. Hogarth Press, London, 1956, pp. 216–53.
6. Alexander, F. *Psychoanalytic Therapy: Principles and Application.* Ronald Press, New York, 1946.
7. Fromm-Reichmann, F. *Principles of Intensive Psycho-Therapy.* The University of Chicago Press, Chicago, Ill., 1950
8. Rickman, J. *Selected Contribution to Psychoanalysis.* Basic Books, N.Y., 1957.
9. Zimmerman, D. Notes on the Reaction of a Therapeutic Group to Termination of Treatment by One of Its Members. *Int. J. Group Psychother.,* 18:86, 1968.
10. Grotjahn, M. Learning from Dropout Patients: A Clinical Review of Patients who Discontinued Group Psychotherapy. *Int. J. Group Psychother.,* 22:306, 1972.
11. Koran, L. M. and Costell, R. M. Early Termination from Group Psychotherapy. *Int. J. Group Psychother.,* 23:346, 1973
12. McGee, T. F. Therapist Termination in Group Psychotherapy. *Int. J. Group Psychother.,* 24:3, 1974.

Characteristics of Staff Burnout in Mental Health Settings

AYALA PINES, PH.D.
Research Associate
CHRISTINA MASLACH, PH.D.
Assistant Professor
Department of Psychology
University of California at Berkeley

To determine the characteristics of staff burnout and ways of coping with it, the authors gathered data on institution-related and personal variables for 76 staff members in various mental health facilities in the San Francisco area. A correlational analysis revealed a large number of statistically significant findings. For instance, the longer staff had worked in the mental health field, the less they liked working with patients, the less successful they felt with them, and the less humanistic were their attitudes toward mental illness. The authors present recommendations for reducing staff stress and subsequent burnout, including allowing more chances for temporary withdrawal from direct patient care and changing the function of staff meetings.

■Many health and social service professions require that the practitioner work intensely and intimately with other people over extended periods of time. Such professional interactions often arouse strong emotional feelings and thus are extremely stressful for the staff member. Yet most human-service professions have traditionally been client- or patient-centered, with little attention given in the literature or in training to the many stresses experienced by the professional. When the stresses are not acknowledged and adequately dealt with, they may result in staff burnout. Burnout can be defined as a syndrome of physical and emotional exhaustion, involving the development of negative self-concept, negative job attitudes, and loss of concern and feeling for clients.

In a series of preliminary studies in 1973-75, we tried to define the social and psychological dimensions of burnout. Our initial samples consisted of more than 200 social welfare workers, psychiatric nurses, poverty lawyers, prison personnel, and child-care workers. Besides making field observations, we conducted extensive questionnaire studies and in-depth interviews. Our data showed that the majority of the subjects had experienced similar changes in themselves, in their perceptions of their clients, and in their feelings toward them. They also used a comparable set of techniques to try to combat burnout, including the following:

Detached concern. To defend against their disruptive emotions and try to perform efficiently in stressful situations, professionals who were more successful in coping with burnout maintained a strong sense of caring and concern for their clients but also used various techniques of detachment, such as intellectualization or physical or psychological withdrawal. Within some of the human-service professions the balance between the handling of clients in a more objective, detached way and yet maintaining a real human concern for them is called detached concern, a term that conveys the difficult and almost paradoxical position of having to distance oneself from people in order to help or cure them.

Intellectualization. Professionals tried to experience stressful situations more objectively by recasting them in more intellectual and consequently less personal terms.

Compartmentalization. Professionals often made a sharp distinction between their jobs and their personal lives by in effect leaving their work and their entire occupational role at the office and not bringing it home with them. Thus they were able to confine the emotional stress to a smaller part of their lives.

Withdrawal. Professionals tried to minimize their involvement in stressful interactions by several kinds of withdrawal, such as spending less time with clients, communicating more impersonally with them, and interacting with other staff rather than with clients.

Reliance on staff. Those experiencing stress often turned to other professionals for advice, comfort, tension reduction, help in achieving distance from the situation or intellectualizing it, and a diffusion of responsibility.

Our preliminary studies indicated that the incidence of burnout is often very high in health and social service

Dr. Pines' address is department of psychology, University of California, Berkeley, California 94720. A fuller account of the study, including statistical data, is available from Dr. Pines. The research was funded by a biomedical sciences support grant from the National Institutes of Health.

To combat burnout from intense work with clients, staff in the human services use such techniques as detached concern, intellectualization, withdrawal from clients, and sharp separation of work from home life.

professions and is a major factor in low worker morale, absenteeism, high job turnover, and other indexes of job stress.[1,2] In addition, it may be a factor in the poor quality of health and welfare services.

To obtain further information on burnout and ways of coping with it, in 1975 we conducted a more extensive study with 76 staff members of various mental health institutions in the San Francisco Bay Area. The subjects included psychiatrists, psychologists, nurses, social workers, attendants, and volunteers. They were based in a large state hospital, an Army hospital, a county hospital where the maximum inpatient stay is two weeks, a treatment house patterned after R. D. Laing's Kingsley Hall, and three halfway houses.

Data were collected through interviews based on a specially designed questionnaire. The questionnaire included both open-ended and scale items and was divided into four major areas. The first area concerned background information and included questions about staff members' age, sex, marital status, formal education, training for mental health work, and other professional experience.

The second area dealt with the characteristics of the job. They included patient population (relative percentage of schizophrenics), staff-patient ratio, working hours and schedules, breaks and time-outs (temporary withdrawals from direct patient contact), vacations, working relationships with other staff, work-sharing, staff meetings, staff-patient relationships, and after-hours involvement with the institution.

The third part focused on staff members' attitudes and feelings about mental health work. Included in this section were several sets of questions. One dealt with the present job—how much the staff members liked various aspects of it, what were the best and worst things about it, how separate it was from their private lives, how much freedom of expression and personal control they felt they had, and how successful they felt they were in achieving their goals. A second set of questions concerned attitudes toward patients, changes in attitudes since the staff member began working in

the mental health field, attitudes about mental illness (as assessed by the Custodial Mental Illness Ideology Scale[3]), judgments of patients' problem behavior, and preferred responses to such problems. Additional questions focused on staff members' assessment of the mental health profession in general and of their ideal career if it was different from mental health.

The fourth section of the questionnaire dealt with staff members' perceptions of themselves, as assessed by a 23-item semantic differential checklist of such bipolar sets of adjectives as warm-cold, valuable-worthless, friendly-unfriendly, and intimate-distant. Staff were asked to rate themselves on a 5-point scale on each set of adjectives, with 1 indicating one extreme and 5 the other. They were also asked to rate the average schizophrenic patient on the same checklist.

A correlational analysis was performed on the data. All the correlations presented here are statistically significant at the level of $p < .05$ or higher.

INSTITUTIONAL VARIABLES

In different work settings staff members expressed different attitudes toward their jobs, toward patients, and toward mental health in general.

Over-all staff-patient ratio. The larger the ratio of patients to staff, the less staff members liked their jobs, and the more they tried to separate them from their personal lives. In settings with larger patient-to-staff ratios, staff said they would change their jobs if given a chance. They did not seek self-fulfillment or social interaction in their jobs; to them the best thing about their work was the job conditions—for example, salary. They limited their after-hours involvement with the institution or the patients to handling emergency cases.

Schizophrenic population. The higher the percentage of schizophrenics in the patient population, the less job satisfaction staff members expressed. Staff in settings with more schizophrenics liked their work less, were less likely to view their job situation as the ideal one, and were less consciously aware of what their goals were in their everyday work. They also spent more time in administrative duties and recommended pharmacological rather than psychological intervention for such problems as suicide attempts.

Work relationships. Work relationships were affected by certain working conditions and were also related to staff members' attitudes toward their work, toward the institution, and toward patients. The less seriously ill the patient population and the fewer the work hours, the better were the work relationships. When work relationships were good, staff members were more likely to confer with each other when they were having a problem with a patient, express more positive attitudes about the institution as a whole, enjoy their work, and feel successful in it. They also were more likely to

[1] C. Maslach, "Burned-out," *Human Behavior*, Vol. 5, September 1976, pp. 16-22.

[2] C. Maslach and A. Pines, "The Burn-out Syndrome in the Day Care Setting," *Child Care Quarterly*, Vol. 6, Summer 1977, pp. 100-113.

[3] D. C. Gilbert and D. J. Levinson, "Ideology, Personality, and Institutional Policy in the Mental Hospital," *Journal of Abnormal and Social Psychology*, Vol. 53, November 1956, pp. 263-271.

rate the institution more highly and to list their primary reason for being in the mental health field as self-fulfillment.

When work relationships were good, staff also reported many "good days" and few "bad days." They felt free to express themselves on the job and spent less time with other staff members or in administrative work. But most important, they described the average schizophrenic patient in more positive terms than did staff with poor work relationships.

Staff-patient relationships. The quality of interaction between staff and patients was related to staff members' perceptions of the institution, of other staff members, of the work, and of the patients. When staff-patient interaction was good, staff members liked their work, felt successful at it, and found self-fulfillment in it. They appreciated the other staff members and conferred with them more often when having a problem with a patient. They also rated the institution more highly, described patients very positively, and stayed involved with the institution and the patients after working hours.

Frequency of staff meetings. High frequency of staff meetings was correlated with very negative and dehumanizing attitudes toward the patients. It also correlated strongly with higher average age, higher rank, avoidance of direct contact with patients, and a view of the average schizophrenic patient as tending to be bizarre, cruel, cold, insane, uncaring, and not understanding.

Staff members who participated in more meetings also gave more weight to information about the patient that came from the patient's family or the psychiatric interview than they did to information coming directly from the patient. They saw less chance of curing schizophrenics and tended to have job-oriented goals rather than work-oriented or patient-oriented goals.

Time-outs. Staff who could afford to take time-outs—to withdraw temporarily to other work activities—when they did not feel like working directly with patients showed more favorable attitudes toward patients. They described the average schizophrenic patient as more caring, kind, sane, reliable, and understanding than did staff who did not have opportunities to detach themselves during times of stress. They also saw more chance of curing schizophrenia and expected patients' behavior

High frequency of staff meetings correlated with very negative and dehumanizing attitudes toward patients. It also correlated with avoidance of contact with patients and job-oriented rather than patient-oriented goals.

toward outsiders to be normal most of the time.

Work schedule. Longer work hours were correlated with more staff stress and negative feelings. The more hours a day staff members worked, the less they liked their jobs, the less responsible they felt for the patients, and the less control they felt they had over the patients' lives in the institution. Staff working longer hours also rated themselves higher on the adjectives of bizarre and intolerant.

Time spent in direct contact with patients. Lower-ranking personnel such as attendants and volunteers spent more time in direct contact with patients than did higher-ranking staff such as psychiatrists and psychologists. In addition, the more time staff members had spent working with schizophrenic patients in the past, the less direct contact they currently had with patients. As might be expected, staff who had less direct contact with patients were more likely to spend their time in administrative work and in staff meetings.

Time spent with other staff members. Staff members who spent more time with other staff ranked themselves higher on the adjectives of apathetic, irresponsible, and tense. They were more likely to feel a sense of failure on the job, with patients, and in achieving their goals.

Time spent in administrative duties. Higher-ranking staff members spent more time in administrative work, as noted, as did staff working with a higher percentage of schizophrenic patients. Staff who spent a great deal of time in administrative work liked their jobs less and liked working with patients less. Over time, they developed negative attitudes toward patients and spent less time in direct contact with them. Their original reason for going into mental health work was the job conditions rather than self-fulfillment or interaction with patients, and their attitudes toward patients and toward mental health staff in general had become more negative. They also described themselves as less tolerant.

Work-sharing. Work was perceived as less stressful if the general workload was shared. Sharing of work was also related to an increase in freedom of expression, to a feeling of having a voice in the institution's policies, and to a feeling of personal power.

PERSONAL VARIABLES

Various personal characteristics of staff members were highly correlated with their perception of their jobs, of the patients, and of the mental health field.

Formal education. For staff members with a higher education—that is, some kind of graduate degree—their original reason for going into mental health work tended to be self-fulfillment rather than job conditions. They had entered the mental health professions with higher expectations of patients, but over time they began to view them as more apathetic, weak, and powerless. They were more pessimistic about the possible effects of their work, seeing little chance of curing schizophrenia. When asked to describe themselves, they saw themselves as more tense, distant, and introverted.

VOLUME 29 NUMBER 4 APRIL 1978

Staff who liked their work very much had a smaller percentage of schizophrenic patients, worked fewer hours a day, and spent less time in administrative work. They tended to have positive attitudes toward other staff.

Rank. As noted before, higher-ranking staff usually spent less time in direct patient contact and more in administrative work. Their attitudes toward patients and toward the mental health field tended to change negatively with time. They were more likely to see schizophrenia as internally caused, they were more approving of pharmacological intervention, and they saw less chance of curing schizophrenia. Lower-ranking staff had more direct contact with patients, and their attitudes toward them were less dehumanizing.

Time in mental health work. The longer staff had worked in the mental health field, the less they liked working with patients, the less successful they felt with them, and the more custodial rather than humanistic were their attitudes toward mental illness. They stopped looking for self-fulfillment in work, good days became very infrequent, and the only good thing about their work was the job conditions.

Sense of success and control. Staff members who felt they had input into the institution's policies and who felt free to express themselves on the job had a much more positive view of themselves and of the patients. They were self-confident, felt they had a great deal of control and authority, and also felt better about their work and about themselves on the job.

Staff members who felt successful on the job and successful with patients had a very positive perception of themselves. They liked their jobs, liked working with patients, had many good days, and felt successful in achieving their goals. Yet they did not express humanistic attitudes or particularly positive views of patients.[4]

Relationships with patients. Staff who described their relationship with most patients as a close one spent more time in direct contact with patients and less time with other staff members or in administrative work. They liked their jobs, liked working with patients, and felt successful in both. They were optimistic about their effectiveness in their work and saw more of a chance of curing schizophrenia. They also expressed very positive attitudes about themselves and about patients.

Job attitudes. Job attitudes were related to some working conditions and to staff members' attitudes to-

[4] A. Pines and T. Solomon, "Perception of Self as a Mediator in the Dehumanization Process," *Personality and Social Psychology Bulletin*, Vol. 3, Spring 1977, pp. 219-223.

ward other staff members and toward themselves. Staff members who liked their work very much had a smaller percentage of schizophrenic patients, worked fewer hours a day, and spent less time in administrative duties. They liked working with patients, liked themselves very much, found self-fulfillment in their work, considered it the ideal job, and felt successful. They also tended to have positive attitudes toward other staff members, to see a good chance of curing schizophrenia, and to rate their institution more highly. They did not report becoming as tired during work.

Attitudes toward mental illness. Humanistic rather than custodial attitudes toward mental illness were more characteristic of staff members who had not worked long in the mental health field, who saw their work as overlapping with their personal life, and who expected patients' behavior to be normal most of the time. Those staff members gave more weight to information provided by the patient than they did to information coming from the patient's psychiatrist. They strongly disapproved of the use of medication during crises.

COPING WITH STRESS

Our findings showed that mental health workers experience personal stress as a result of working closely and intensively with patients over an extended time. There are several steps, both physical and social, that can be taken either to reduce the amount of stress the staff member feels, and the subsequent burnout, or to help him or her cope successfully with the stress. The following set of recommendations primarily emphasizes institutional changes.

• Reducing the patient-to-staff ratio. As the number of patients for whom the staff member is providing care increases, the staff member may experience cognitive, emotional, and sensory overload; as the ratio decreases, the quality of care improves.

• Shortening the work hours. The shorter the work hours, the less stressful are the jobs, and the more staff members like them. This recommendation can be implemented by arranging shorter work shifts and more breaks and by establishing more part-time positions. The latter step is especially important for women professionals with families.

• Allowing more opportunities for time-outs. Such temporary withdrawals from direct patient care could be used for non-patient-related work, such as preparing medications, cleaning, and doing paperwork and administrative work or simply for rest and relaxation. But in no case should such time-outs come at the expense of the patients; the structure of the institution should be flexible enough to allow other staff to handle the necessary activities of the staff member who is taking a break.

• Sharing the patient load. Staff members working with only the more seriously ill patients seem to burn out more easily. Sharing the load of the more difficult patients by rotation of staff between wards and by work-sharing are two ways of taking some pressure off

More highly educated staff members tend to enter the field with high expectations. They are not prepared to find themselves in what may be a mundane and uneventful job without opportunity for self-expression.

staff members and of making their jobs more varied and stimulating.

• Changing the function of staff meetings. When we studied health and social service professions other than the mental health professions, we found that staff meetings serve several important functions. They enable the staff to socialize informally, to give each other support, to confer about problems, to clarify their goals, and to exert some direct influence on the policies of the institution. In those professions the frequency of staff meetings is negatively correlated with burnout.

However, in mental institutions, taking part in a large number of formal staff meetings seems to be positively correlated with burnout. Based on our interviews, we believe the reason is that most staff meetings center on case presentations in which a staff member describes a patient in terms of his or her mental illness, using psychological jargon. The patient is reduced to an abstract concept such as "schizophrenic," and thus the meetings serve the purpose of distancing and detaching the staff from the patients. They rarely, if at all, center on problems experienced by the staff.

Staff meetings could give the staff real opportunities to express themselves, to have input into some control over their work routines, and to develop a greater sense of involvement and commitment to the institution. Rather than being solely a place to discuss patients in a detached, intellectualized way, they should also become a place where individual staff members receive emotional and social support and have a chance to confer openly with other staff about themselves and about their patients.

• Improving work relationships. One of the interesting and sad results of the study was the finding that staff members seem to get together in order to avoid direct contact with patients rather than to give each other support and to confer about problems with patients. In general, support systems for staff may often be lacking.

One of our strongest recommendations is for institutions to try to create support systems and improve the social milieu by improving work relationships between staff members. This goal can be achieved by changing or modifying the function of staff meetings or by establishing some other institutional mechanism that allows staff members to express their feelings openly and get

feedback, consultation, and support. Regular group meetings could be helpful for some staff, as could peer counseling, a greater emphasis on teamwork, work-sharing, and institution-sponsored social activities.

• Holding retreats for staff members. One of the most consistent findings from this and related research is the high correlation between years in practice and the degree of burnout. One way of combating or slowing down the process is establishing a system of retreats or workshops outside the institution for the more experienced workers; staff thus could get away from their work and could discuss their feelings about themselves, the patients, and the institution. They also could clarify and restate their goals together with other staff members. In such retreats a formal presentation of the theory and research findings about detached concern and burnout could be very useful.

• Taking precautions as an individual. There are also ways, independent of institutional change, in which individual staff members can prevent the emotional and physical exhaustion and the negative attitudes associated with burnout. They include being aware of work stresses and recognizing the signs of impending burnout, acknowledging vulnerabilities, putting reasonable limits on the amount of work that can be done, setting realistic and achievable goals and, most important, being willing to meet one's own needs as well as those of the patient.

For staff members to change some of their focus from the patient to themselves may be foreign to the traditional view of mental health work. However, focusing only on the patient is self-defeating both for staff members and for patients and may contribute to the process of burnout.

• Training students to deal with future stresses. Our results indicated that the more highly educated staff members tend to enter the mental health field to find self-fulfillment. They come with high expectations of themselves, their jobs, and the patients. They are not prepared for finding themselves a small part of a bureaucratic machine, in what may be a mundane and uneventful job that lacks opportunity for self-expression. They develop negative expectations and become very pessimistic about the effectiveness of their work. Thus we think it is crucial that any advanced psychiatric or other clinical training program should include at least one course that will prepare mental health professionals for the tremendous emotional stresses they will encounter in their work.■

From: Selected papers presented at the general session: Twenty-third annual meeting; Alcohol & Drug Problems Association of North America, Atlanta, Georgia, 1972. Reprinted by permission of Sid Wolf, Ph.D., Director, Mission Valley Center for Psychological Services, 1355 Hotel Circle South, San Diego, CA 92108

COUNSELING: FOR BETTER OR FOR WORSE

Sid Wolf, Ph.D.

An extensive body of information indicates that counseling, psychotherapy, and in fact, all human relationships are for better or worse (Carkhuff & Berensen, 1967). Studies have indicated that there are individuals who are effective in human interactions and are especially competent at helping other people in distress. There are those too who are ineffective in interpersonal relationships and are extremely destructive at efforts to help other human beings. Important research on this matter dates back to 1960 when the efficacy of psychotherapy and counseling was questioned because studies contrasting psychotherapy-treated groups with control groups revealed no significant mean differences (Bergen, 1966). It wasn't until it was discovered that the variance of the psychotherapy-treated groups increased that researchers began to examine the data more closely in an effort to discover why more "treated" individuals received extreme scores on criterion measures of improvement than did their control counterparts. The increased variability of the treated groups indicated that some people were getting better and some were getting worse. Further investigations indicated that therapists contributed significantly to this increased variability, that is, therapists were responsible for people getting better or getting worse (Truax & Carkhuff, 1967).

Research designed to contrast effective versus ineffective "helpers" revealed a number of traits which, when present in counselors resulted in patient improvement but when absent led to client deterioration. These traits and characteristics make up a core of qualities which are present in high-functioning individuals regardless of the specific role, discipline or function they are performing (Carkhuff & Berenson, 1969). For example, regardless of whether one is a psychiatrist, psychologist, social worker, nurse, lawyer, supervisor, physician, manager, parent, teacher, etc., if he or she possesses these traits, he or she is effective in interpersonal relationships. Furthermore, whether the counselor's theoretical orientation is Freudian, Rogerian, Existentialist, etc., if he has the characteristics of the effective individual, he will be helpful in his efforts; when he lacks these traits and characteristics, he will be harmful. These counselor traits are correlated with improvement in vastly different populations. Whether one is working with schizophrenics, alcoholics, college counselees, delinquents, or any other definable group, he will be effective if he is high on the therapist variables. These traits and characteristics have also been correlated with a wide variety of criteria of improvement, such as changes in psychological tests, time out of institutions, independent ratings, self ratings, therapist ratings, supervisor ratings, etc.

Moreover, studies indicate that the therapist variables may be measured reliably and validly, usually on 5 point scales (Carkhuff, 1969). These scales are operationally defined and one may evaluate a helper's performance by reading the transcript to his interactions, listening to audio tapes of his performance, or actually viewing his interactions through one-way mirrors or on video tape. Ratings made in this way by individuals who are discriminating and perceptive are highly correlated with outcome criteria (Cannon & Carkhuff, 1969). Using these scales, normative data on the population at large have been obtained. I will enumerate some of the findings.

On these rating scales, level 3 is arbitrarily set as the point of minimal helpfulness, that is, an individual who scores at level 3 or above is helpful and should achieve statistical outcome rates of improvement in his patients, far exceeding those of low-functioning individuals. Sadly, on the average, most people function at level 2 (Carkhuff & Berenson, 1967). Thus, it is rare in life to find anyone who can provide even minimally facilitative conditions and who is helpful. Furthermore, experienced counselors and psychotherapists function, on the average, at about level 2. That is, even when one is desperate enough to pay money to obtain help, one may obtain a low-functioning therapist who is destructive. Graduate clinical psychology students entering their programs, on the average, function at level 2.5, a quite satisfactory beginning level which suggests a potential for growth. However, later in their training these individuals drop to level 2 (Carkhuff & Berenson, 1967).

Thus, it seems that often we train out the best qualities and characteristics of our potentially most helpful students. In a study where people were asked to give a list of individuals to whom they would turn in time of need and a list of people to whom they would not turn when in distress, independent measures of these individuals' helping abilities revealed that people turn to those who have naturally therapeutic personalities and refrain from contacting those who are low-functioning (Carkhuff & Berenson, 1967).

The variables which have been measured, defined and which separate high and low-functioning individuals are the following:

EMPATHY. Empathy (Carkhuff, 1969) is the ability to accurately perceive what another person is experiencing and communicate that perception. At high levels of empathy, an individual adds noticeably or significantly to the communication, while at low levels, the individual detracts noticeably or significantly from the communication.

RESPECT. Respect implies that a helper appreciates the dignity and worth of another human being. It also implies that the helper accepts the fact that each individual has a right to choose, possesses free will, and may make his own decisions. Respect also indicates that each individual has the inherent strength and capacity for making it in life. At low levels, a person functioning without respect may overprotect, be condescending, or even hold another in low esteem or negative regard. He may make decisions, give advice, be falsely reassuring, or be hostile.

GENUINENESS. Genuineness (Carkhuff, 1969) is the ability of an individual to be freely and deeply himself. It is non-phoniness, non-role playing, non-defensiveness. A person who is genuine is congruent; there is no discrepancy between what he is saying and what he is experiencing. At low levels of genuineness a person may say one thing and communicate another non-verbally. He may be stiffly "professional" or be playing a role (rather than fulfilling a role). He may seem very different in the therapy room from what he is normally. People who function low in genuineness hide behind a facade.

CONCRETENESS. Concreteness (Carkhuff, 1969) implies specificity of expression concerning the client's feelings and experiences. The concrete therapist keeps communications specific and gets to the what, why, when, where, and how of something. Notions, thoughts, experiences are explored, in depth. The concrete therapist maintains relevancy in the communication and prevents the client from avoiding or escaping the issues at hand. A low-functioning therapist who is not concrete is abstract or general. He is very permissive and allows the client to explore irrelevancies, to go off on tangents, and to maintain himself at an abstract level.

CONFRONTATION. Confrontations (Berenson; Mitchell & Taney, 1969) occur when there is a discrepancy between what one is saying and what he is experiencing, or between what one is saying at one point and what he has said before, or between what one is saying and what his actions imply. This variable is totally under the control of the therapist and is initiated when the therapist feels it is appropriate. Confronting is risky and can precipitate a crisis, but it is often through such crises that the beginning of true growth occurs both in the therapeutic relationship and in the client's life. There are different kinds of confrontations possible in a counseling situation. For example, an experiential confrontation is a confrontation that occurs in the here and now, usually because what the client is saying and what he is experiencing are not congruent. There may be strength confrontations, when the therapist emphasizes a client's strength in the face of the client's communicated feelings of weakness. Weakness confrontations occur when the client is ostensibly presenting strength, but in fact, there are difficulties to be resolved and the client is avoiding them. There may be action confrontations when the therapist encourages the client to take action, or didactic confrontations when the therapist transmits factual information.

SELF-DISCLOSURE. Self-disclosure (Carkhuff, 1969) is the revealing of personal feelings, attitudes, opinions and experiences on the part of the therapist for the benefit of the client. The therapist, during self-disclosure, exposes himself and shares with the client some meaningful self-disclosing statements which may be pertinent to the issues. At low levels, the therapist never reveals himself, and maintains a screen of neutrality. Self-disclosure must be used with discretion and an accurate sense of timing and appropriateness. In all cases, self-disclosing statements should occur for the client's sake and not for the therapist's own cathaisis.

IMMEDIACY. Immediacy (Collingwood & Renz, 1969) is dealing with the feelings between the client and the counselor in the here and now. A high level of immediacy exists in the open discussion and analysis of the interpersonal relationship occurring between the client and the counselor, within the counseling situation. This is a very important variable because it provides the opportunity to work out problems and difficulties in an ongoing relationship so that the client profits from the experiences. The client can learn to restructure his interpersonal relationships by finding that it is possible to confront, to reveal oneself, and to express negative or positive emotions to another human being quite safely. Thus, the counselor who is immediate feels comfortable engaging in explorations of the present relationship existing between the client and himself.

POTENCY. Potency (Wolf, 1970) is charisma; it is the dynamic force and magnetic quality of the therapist. The potent therapist is one who has a force of presence. He is obviously in command of himself and communicates to others his sense of competence and security. The person who scores low in potency is milque-toastish, flat, a nonentity. He has little dynamism, little inner power. Such a person cannot evoke feelings of security; rather one feels uneasy in the presence of such an individual and would be reluctant to trust or burden him.

SELF-ACTUALIZATION. Studies have indicated that self-actualization is highly correlated with success in counseling (Foulds, 1969). That is, therapists who are themselves self-actualized serve as models of effective people who can live and meet life directly. A self-actualized person is one whose pleasure to pain ratio is in the direction of pleasure. Though self-actualized people feel stress and tension, they are not incapacitated by these negative forces. Self-actualized individuals can live in the present and are primarily inner-directed. They are able to express themselves freely and openly. Their values are flexible for these people are not judgemental or moralistic. Self-actualized people have the capacity for warm, intimate contact and in general, are extremely effective at living.

METHOD AND PROCEDURE

In order to test the hypothesis that counselors, according to their level of functioning, differentially affect client outcome, the following experiment was carried out. At Spring Grove State Hospital, Baltimore, Maryland, controlled studies testing the efficacy of LSD-assisted psychotherapy have been conducted. In these investigations alcoholics were screened, psychologically tested, and then randomly assigned to therapists who worked intensively with the patients for four to six weeks, seeing each patient between 10 to 30 hours.

Alcoholics were defined operationally as patients hospitalized at the alcoholic rehabilitation unit of the hospital because of excessive and pathological drinking with concomitant destructive emotional and social consequences. Psychotic behavior, brain damage and drinking were contra-indications for inclusion in the study. Screening was done by a five member staff composed of psychiatrists and psychologists, using case histories, medical records and psychometrics to decide whether a patient was qualified for the study. The five therapists involved in treating alcoholics included psychiatrists or psychologists who were highly qualified academically and professionally. After screening and psychotherapy the patients were exposed to drug treatment either a 12 hour high or low LSD experience, dosage being randomly determined. Patients thereafter were followed up, retested, and then usually discharged from the hospital. Independent raters evaluated the patients before their treatment and again at six months subsequent to their treatment. These pre-post ratings of global adjustment were used as the dependent variable. Thus, change in global adjustment was used to determine whether or not patients improved.

The patients in this study were all males and ranged in ages from 26 to 59, with the mean age of 42. All were from lower middle-class socio-economic backgrounds as measured by their income and occupational categories. The level of functioning of the therapists was established on the basis of ratings made by judges listening to recorded 75 minute interviews of the therapists with their patients. The two raters who evaluated each interview were highly trained and discriminating and evaluated each tape, rating global level of functioning.

RESULTS. Table 1 presents therapist level of functioning and the percentage of improvement and essential rehabilitation in their alcoholic patients. Improvement indicates that patients received higher post-treatment global adjustment ratings than they had received pre-treatment. Essential rehabilitation is defined as the attainment of a score of 8 or more on a 10 point scale of global adjustment. An inspection of Table 1 reveals that level of functioning was directly related to percentage of improvement in patients. (Refer to Table 1)

CONCLUDING REMARKS

The impact of the therapist on the client is indeed profound. By employing rating scales to measure the core facilitative dimensions defined above, it is possible to evaluate the strengths, weaknesses, and overall level of functioning of treatment personnel who so differentially affect the outcome of their clients. Training programs designed to inculcate these core qualities and which emphasize communication skills have been designed. The author has been developing such techniques, procedures, and materials to be used in clinical skills development. It has been found that in 60 hour programs, trainees can improve their level of functioning by at least one level. The fact that many individuals are functioning as treatment personnel but are less than effective is indeed sobering, but the development procedures for measuring and improving helping skills hold promise for the counseling field.

TABLE 1

Therapist Level of Functioning and %
of Improvement and Rehabilitation in Alcoholic Patients

Therapist	Level of Functioning	N	% of Improvement at 6 Months*	% Essentially Rehabilitated at 12 Months*
1	4.2	32	78	47
2	4.0	12	75	45
3	2.7	12	66	36
4	2.3	28	61	33
5	1.5	28	60	30

* Positive change in global adjustment
**Attainment of rating of 8 or above on 10 point scale of global adjustment.

REFERENCES

Berenson, B.G., Mitchell, K.M., & Laney, R.C. Level of therapist functioning, types of confrontation and type of patient. Journal of Clinical Psychology, 1969, 25, 111-113.

Bergen, A.E. Some implication of psychotherapy research for therapeutic practice. Journal of Abnormal Psychology, 1966, 4, 235-246.

Cannon, J.R. & Carkhuff, R.R. Effects of rater level of functioning and experience upon the discrimination of facilitative conditions. Journal of Consulting & Clinical Psychology, 1969, 32, 189-194.

Carkhuff, R.R. Helping and Human Relations; A Primer for Lay and Professional Helpers, Vol. 1 Selection and Training. New York: Holt, Rinehart & Winston, Inc., 1967.

Collingwood, T.R. & Renz, L. The effects of client confrontations upon levels of immediacy offered by high and low functioning counselors. Journal of Clinical Psychology, 1969, 25, 224-226.

Foulds, M.L. Self-actualization and the communication of facilitative conditions during counseling. Journal of Clinical Psychology, 1969, 16, 132-136.

Truax, C.D. & Carkhuff, R.R. Toward Effective Counseling and Psychotherapy: Training and Practice. Chicago: Aldine Publishing Co., 1967.

Wolf, S. An investigation of counselor type, client type, level of facilitative conditions and client outcome. (Doctoral dissertation, The Catholic University of America) Dissertation Abstracts International, 1970, 31 Order No. 70-22, 093.

A Conceptual Approach
to Deinstitutionalization

LEONA L. BACHRACH, PH.D.
Sociologist
National Institute of Mental Health
Rockville, Maryland

Many serious problems in deinstitutionalization result from conceptual oversights or confusion. Understanding deinstitutionalization as a process and a philosophy, as well as a fact, permits planning that will accommodate the variety of patient populations that are the products of the deinstitutionalization movement. The role and possible contributions of the state hospital in caring for chronic patients must be assessed objectively. Effective program planning for chronic patients during this period of deinstitutionalization depends on a careful and realistic definition of what individuals are to be treated in the community. Such planning must not only attempt to match patients and appropriate treatment settings but must aim at enhancing rehabilitation, where feasible, through a skills training approach.

■Smith and Hart have written a graphic description of the climate within which mental health services were being delivered in the 1950s: "At that time the setting was right for change. State hospitals had become severely overcrowded, and there were no alternatives for public care. Long periods of hospitalization seemed to be doing more harm than good. . . . The deteriorating conditions in state hospitals, accompanied by the introduction of medication that helped control symptoms and, in military psychiatry, the success of crisis intervention under combat conditions, set the scene that gave impetus to the community mental health movement. Theoretically, if persons received vigorous, early treatment . . . close to home and could stay in the community with the help of medication, chronic mental illness would disappear. It was assumed that there would be no need for long-term hospitalization, and large state hospitals could be closed."

Smith and Hart continue: "Unfortunately no one tested the theory."[1]

Indeed, despite some notable successes over the past couple of decades, the deinstitutionalization movement has, from the beginning, been plagued by a variety of problems. Among other things, it has been accused of overlooking chronic patients—the very people it was designed to help. There is a fair degree of consensus now that community mental health planning is de facto geared toward the care of persons who can, for the most part and most of the time, look after themselves. Chronic patients are alleged to have been shortchanged in community mental health planning. The report of the President's Commission on Mental Health indicates that often the only community-based treatment offered the long-term patient is medication.[2]

How did this situation arise? How may we account for the disparity between the ideal expressed in the 1950s and the realities of the 1970s? It is the premise of this paper that difficulties in deinstitutionalization have arisen largely as the result of conceptual oversights. Only by understanding the process of deinstitutionalization and the philosophy that underlies it can we begin to comprehend the dimensions of the problems that surround the movement.

Deinstitutionalization may be defined as a process involving two elements: the eschewal, shunning, or avoidance of traditional institutional settings (particularly state hospitals) for the care of the mentally ill, and the concurrent expansion of community-based facilities for the care of these individuals. This operational definition focuses on physical properties—that is, on the locations where mental health services are provided—and suggests that deinstitutionalization is more than a unilinear phenomenon involving the movement of patients out of the hospital and into the community. Rather, it is a phenomenon concerned with exchange in the locations of patient care.

There are at least three separate, but closely inter-

Dr. Bachrach was staff sociologist for the President's Commission on Mental Health and staff liaison for the commission's task panel on deinstitutionalization, rehabilitation, and long-term care. Her mailing address is 11001 Wickshire Way, Rockville, Maryland 20852.

[1] W. G. Smith and D. W. Hart, "Community Mental Health: A Noble Failure?" *Hospital & Community Psychiatry*, Vol. 26, September 1975, pp. 581-583.
[2] *Report to the President From the President's Commission on Mental Health*, Washington, D.C., 1978.

related, aspects of deinstitutionalization. Deinstitutionalization is a process. It is a fact. And it is also a philosophy.

THE PROCESS

Deinstitutionalization is a dynamic and continuing series of adjustments involving constant accommodation of all the components of the mental health service delivery system. The concept of continuity of care is a reflection of the dynamic nature of deinstitutionalization. Ideally, at least, with deinstitutionalization, the patient is expected to move about freely from facility to facility or even in and out of the service delivery system. The ideas of "a range of treatment alternatives" and "freedom of choice" are critical elements. Conceptually, deinstitutionalization holds that utilization of facilities is to be determined by the patient's current needs in a kind of free-market model: as service needs change, so will patterns of care change.

In fact, the dynamic nature of the deinstitutionalization movement is evidenced in changes that have occurred in the resident patient population of state mental hospitals. The population pool that at one time comprised the totality of persons resident in state hospitals—a relatively static population that changed primarily only as the result of new admissions and deaths—can today be broken down into five separate subgroups, two in the community and three in the hospital. In the community are, first, patients released from the hospital and, second, persons who have never been hospitalized, though at an earlier time they probably would have been.

In a recently published study of chronically mentally ill persons living in San Mateo County, California, for example, the investigators found that only 4 per cent had been hospitalized in state hospitals within the previous two years, and two in five patients had never been in state hospitals at all.[3] Thus there are now living in the community numbers of mentally ill individuals who 30 years ago would probably have been hospitalized in state facilities but who, as a direct consequence of deinstitutionalization, are not receiving hospital care.

Of the three hospital subgroups, one is composed of old long-stay patients—those who were admitted long ago and have remained in the hospital despite deinstitutionalization efforts. A special study of state hospitals in 13 selected states shows that in 1973 a total of 46 per cent of the patients had been in residence for five years or more, 7 per cent for three to five years, and 12 per cent for one to three years. In all, nearly two-thirds (65 per cent) of state hospital residents had lived there for one year or longer.[4]

The second hospital subgroup consists of recent admissions who are short-stay patients—those who will soon be released to the community. Nearly one-quarter of all admissions to the nation's state mental hospitals in 1975 were released within seven days of admission, and nearly 40 per cent were released within 14 days.[5]

The third hospital subgroup is composed of the new long-stay patients—a build-up of long-term residents from among recent admissions who are unlikely to be considered good risks for community care and probably will not be discharged. A study of state hospital admissions in Illinois estimates that 10 to 15 per cent of new admissions will always require "some form of highly structured care," and 2 to 5 per cent will "remain too disturbed even to be discharged from the hospital."[6]

There is some exchange among these patient (or potential patient) subgroups, most particularly between patients released from the hospital and recent hospital admissions who are short-stay patients. This exchange, of course, is responsible for the situation commonly known as the revolving door. In 1975 a total of 69 per cent of all admissions to state mental hospitals had had prior care in psychiatric inpatient facilities.[7]

The importance of conceptualizing deinstitutionalization as a process is that in so doing, we avoid subscribing to a widespread but narrow definition of the phenomenon. Deinstitutionalization is frequently held to refer only to the release of patients from large mental hospitals. But it is much more than that: it is a complex, multifaceted process that continues to alter patterns of patient care. Ideally mental health program planning should accommodate a variety of patient subgroups, each of which represents fallout from the deinstitutionalization movement.

THE FACT

There is a dimension of reality in deinstitutionalization that cannot be overlooked; evidence is provided in nationwide statistics. Throughout the nation there has been a decrease in the state hospital resident population. The resident population peaked in 1955 at more than a half million, but 20 years later, in 1975, there were only about 191,000 residents of state hospitals, a decrease of 66 per cent.[8]

In 1955 about half of all psychiatric patient care episodes occurred in state mental hospitals; in 1975 the corresponding figure was only about 9 per cent. By contrast, in 1955 outpatient services accounted for only 23 per cent of patient care episodes, but in 1975 seven out of ten patient care episodes took place in outpatient

[3] H. R. Lamb and V. Goertzel, "The Long-Term Patient in the Era of Community Treatment," *Archives of General Psychiatry*, Vol. 34, June 1977, pp. 679-682.

[4] Unpublished data, Division of Biometry and Epidemiology, National Institute of Mental Health, Rockville, Maryland.

[5] *Ibid.*

[6] Smith and Hart, *op. cit.*

[7] Division of Biometry and Epidemiology, National Institute of Mental Health, *Readmission to Inpatient Services of State and County Mental Hospitals, United States, 1969, 1972, and 1975*, Memorandum No. 32, Rockville, Maryland, February 10, 1978.

[8] Division of Biometry and Epidemiology, National Institute of Mental Health, *Resident Patient Rate in State Mental Hospitals Reduced to One-Fourth the 1955 Rate*, Memorandum No. 6, Rockville, Maryland, June 27, 1977.

settings. In 1975 federally funded community mental health centers, which did not even exist prior to the passage of the Community Mental Health Centers Act of 1963, provided the locus for 29 per cent of all patient care episodes.[9]

THE PHILOSOPHY

When deinstitutionalization is viewed as a process, its intellectual foundation begins to become apparent. The deinstitutionalization movement is the expression of a philosophy current in American thought. That philosophy places strong civil-libertarian emphasis on the rights of individuals and on modification of the environment as the primary avenue to social change. In deinstitutionalization, this philosophy is extended to include the care of the mentally ill.

The philosophy of deinstitutionalization proceeds from at least three fundamental assumptions concerning mental health care. First, there is an assumption that community mental health is a good thing—that community-based care is preferable to institutional care for most, if not all, mental patients. Community care is perceived as the more therapeutic alternative, and it represents the treatment of choice in most cases of mental illness.

A second underlying assumption is that communities not only can, but also are willing to, assume responsibility and leadership in the care of the mentally ill. And third, deinstitutionalization is based upon an assumption that the functions performed by the mental hospital can be performed equally well—if not better—by community-based facilities. The idea of deinstitutionalization, in short, implies that the community is capable of providing, outside of institutional settings, the full range of patient services that are available inside the hospital.

These three philosophical assumptions taken together permit an understanding of the charge of deinstitutionalization. The operational definition given earlier, which emphasized the locational aspects of patient care, may now be supplemented with a goal definition. The goal of deinstitutionalization is rooted in the philosophy of the movement. Deinstitutionalization has assumed no less a task than that of humanizing mental health care—a task that would reverse the dehumanizing influences that are perceived to be part and parcel of traditional mental health care.

PROBLEMS WITH THE MOVEMENT

Acknowledgment and consideration of these properties of deinstitutionalization—process, fact, and philosophy—permit a framework for better understanding of the problems associated with the deinstitutionalization movement. Were deinstitutionalization merely an event with locational referents, were it concerned only with the exchange of settings for patient care, many of the problems known to exist would not have arisen. The community would simply have replaced the hospital as the locus of care, and resultant problems would have been of a logistical nature, easily negotiated and resolved.

In fact, however, deinstitutionalization has, since its inception, confronted obstacles every step of the way. There are numerous issues associated with deinstitutionalization of the mentally ill, and the experience of the past decade demonstrates that these issues have often been extremely difficult to resolve. These issues have been analyzed at length in the literature.[10]

Perhaps the most serious single issue is the fact that the deinstitutionalization movement, which was originally designed to provide the chronically mentally ill relief from the inhumane conditions of institutions, has let these patients "fall through the cracks." These patients—the very ones who have been dehumanized through oversight and denial in the past—have somehow, in the process of reducing state hospital populations, largely been lost to the service delivery system.[11] Hansell summarizes this consequence of deinstitutionalization as resulting from such errors in service design as "an unwarranted emphasis on the single-episode user of services, a deficiency of interest in people with lifelong disorders, and unwarranted expectations about the effects that programs of general social betterment can have on serious mental illnesses such as schizophrenia."[12]

Clearly it is time to reassess the deinstitutionalization movement in order to attempt to find solutions for the problems it has generated. One approach is through a sociological, or functional, analysis of the state mental hospital's position in American culture. It was noted above that an underlying philosophical assumption of the deinstitutionalization movement is the premise that the functions performed by the mental hospital can be performed equally well, if not better, in community-based facilities. What exactly are these functions?

A review of the literature suggests that the range of functions performed by mental hospitals is surprisingly complex and is far more extensive than might be supposed.[13] While long-term treatment, asylum, and custody are the roles most often associated with institutional care, the literature reveals a whole series of additional functions that are less readily observed or acknowledged—such as rendering relief to the patient's

[9] C. A. Taube and R. W. Redick, *Provisional Data on Patient Care Episodes in Mental Health Facilities, 1975*, Statistical Note 139, National Institute of Mental Health, Rockville, Maryland, August 1977.

[10] L. L. Bachrach, *Deinstitutionalization: An Analytical Review and Sociological Perspective*, National Institute of Mental Health, Rockville, Maryland, 1976.

[11] "Report of the Task Panel on Deinstitutionalization, Rehabilitation, and Long-Term Care," in *Task Panel Reports Submitted to the President's Commission on Mental Health*, Vol. 2, Washington, D. C., 1978, pp. 356-375.

[12] N. Hansell, "Services for Schizophrenics: A Lifelong Approach to Treatment," *Hospital & Community Psychiatry*, Vol. 29, February 1978, pp. 105-109.

[13] Bachrach, *op. cit.*

family, or providing a sort of hiding place outside the community for some of its less attractive members, or providing an economic base for the hospital community. Some of the functions apply exclusively to patients, some to other elements of society. It is safe to say that some of these roles were not originally intended, but have evolved as the nation's system of institutional care has grown.

It has been demonstrated that the issues in deinstitutionalization are directly related to the functions of the state mental hospital.[14,15] Efforts to reduce the stature of, or eliminate, mental hospitals have placed disproportionate emphasis on the function of treatment and have too often overlooked or neglected to stress the necessity for alternatives to the other functions of mental hospitals. It is inevitable that any movement that so ignores the institutional make-up of society will encounter severe opposition.

Moreover, the deinstitutionalization effort in process has often not been viewed by its champions with sufficient detachment to permit program planners to recognize problems and to introduce necessary modifications. The zeal and dedication that have motivated deinstitutionalization have not in themselves sufficed to mitigate the fact that the movement has left in its wake a series of dysfunctional elements resulting directly from rapid, sometimes heedless, implementation of incomplete program plans. Planning for deinstitutionalization has too often taken place in a sort of functional vacuum. It has certainly largely failed in practice to address the needs of all five of the patient population subgroups described earlier.

However, recent literature indicates greater awareness of the complex nature of deinstitutionalization. Recognition of the variety of functions associated with mental hospitals has become more prevalent in journal articles. This recognition is often accompanied by pleas for more realistic and more meaningful planning, so that entire groups of people are not automatically excluded from the planning process.

It is increasingly recognized now that one of the first steps in implementing successful deinstitutionalization programs must be the careful definition of the target population. Who—what patients—are to be treated in the community? A corollary question is, Are there some patients who cannot be regarded as "good risks" or as appropriate candidates for community care? The answers to these questions are complex and depend very much on the specific community involved and the special resources that community has to offer.

The answers also depend on timing. Some communities are at any given time better equipped—in terms of available services, manpower, and attitudes—to handle chronically disturbed individuals than are others. The fact that a community is not currently ready

It may be necessary eventually to conclude that at least some part of the state hospital's role in the spectrum of services is too difficult to replace by alternative settings in all communities.

for deinstitutionalization by no means necessarily indicates a permanent state of affairs. Preparedness does not occur overnight, and it is an error to assume that all communities are equally prepared for deinstitutionalization at any given time. Lack of readiness may be a temporary phenomenon. Or it may be virtually permanent if the community foresees no way of providing functional alternatives for mental hospitals. Isolated rural communities may be particularly hard pressed to supply such alternatives.[16]

The tentative nature of deinstitutionalization must be acknowledged. If a given community is unable to provide quality community-based care for all of its mentally disabled residents, that should not necessarily be construed as failure in the mission of humanizing mental health care. If there is one lesson that should be apparent by now, it is that the answers are rarely simple. *Thanks for the reminder!*

It may be necessary eventually to conclude that at least some part of the state hospital's role in the spectrum of services is too difficult to replace by alternative settings in all communities—and that the hospital's role should in fact be enhanced through new and innovative programming rather than eliminated.[17] It is really too early to make a comprehensive evaluation at the present time. It is not, after all, where the patient is treated that should be of primary concern, but rather how relevant to his needs a specific treatment program is.

This emphasis on patients rather than on programs is important, and it is reflected in recent literature stressing the role of rehabilitation in deinstitutionalization. Webster says that rehabilitation means to put back in good condition, to re-establish on a firm, sound basis.

To re-establish the patient on a firm, sound basis— that is where the focus of deinstitutionalization needs to be. The emphasis must be moved away from programs and places toward the patients themselves. That is the singular contribution of the growing body of rehabilitation literature. A recent article by Test and Stein urges

[14] *Ibid.*
[15] L. L. Bachrach, *Deinstitutionalization: A Conceptual Framework*, National Institute of Mental Health, Rockville, Maryland, May 1977.

[16] L. L. Bachrach, "Deinstitutionalization of Mental Health Services in Rural Areas," *Hospital & Community Psychiatry*, Vol. 28, September 1977, pp. 669-672.
[17] N. E. Stratas, D. B. Bernhardt, and R. N. Elwell, "The Future of the State Mental Hospital: Developing a Unified System of Care," *Hospital & Community Psychiatry*, Vol. 28, August 1977, pp. 598-600.

the adoption of two guidelines for rehabilitation programs. A program should first ensure that the patient's unmet needs—material and personal care needs, as well as psychosocial needs—are being met. But at the same time the program should not overprovide; it should not meet needs that the patient himself is able to fulfill. It should not encourage dependency where patients can fend for themselves.[18] The second guideline is not only consistent with the patient's right to treatment in the least restrictive environment, but it is also the more humane and therapeutic procedure.

Test's and Stein's guidelines are certainly not bold or new. If at first glance they appear to be somewhat simplistic, they are important conceptually. Too many deinstitutionalization efforts have concentrated so hard on locus of care that they have overlooked these simple but basic principles of treatment.

Anthony appears to pick up where Test and Stein leave off in asserting that the goal of rehabilitation "should be to provide the disabled person with the physical, intellectual, and emotional skills needed to live, learn, and work in the community with the *least possible amount of support from agents of the helping professions*" (italics added).[19] Consistent with this, a former mental patient writes simply: "For me, rehabilitation is not having something done to me."[20]

It must be acknowledged that chronically mentally disabled individuals vary in the extent to which they can benefit from a rehabilitation approach. For those who can be so helped, however, Anthony stresses the need for programs that focus on skill development instead of symptom remission. He suggests a skills training approach in which training departs from a separate rehabilitation diagnosis. This diagnosis supplements the traditional psychiatric diagnosis; the two are, of course, not mutually exclusive. Indeed, they are complementary.

The special value of a rehabilitation diagnosis lies in its identification of skill deficits that prevent the patient from functioning in the community. Such a diagnosis leads to an assessment of the "discrepancies between the patient's skill levels and the levels needed to function in a specific community setting." The discrepancy then becomes the "focus of the rehabilitation treatment intervention."[21] Again, the idea may at first glance appear to be simple, but conceptually it is an important step in providing a focus for planning deinstitutionalization programs.

To summarize, deinstitutionalization planning may proceed in a number of ways, some of them more, some less, sensitive to the needs of individual patients. The least sensitive planning—which is not properly described as planning at all—makes little effort to match patients and settings. It is, instead, wholesale placement of patients without consideration for individual needs. This kind of wholesale placement may occur either in an institution or in the community, and it leads to what has been called "dumping."

Effective planning begins to take place when an effort is made to match patients and settings. The simplest form of matching involves studying the patient's level of functioning and attempting to place him in the setting most compatible with that level. Most patient placements in deinstitutionalization are of these two kinds—either dumping or planned placement in a setting deemed to be consistent with an individual patient's level of functioning. But deinstitutionalization can be even more sensitive and humane if it carries the process one step further to enhance the patient's skill development. In a skills training approach, placements are based on the patient's potential rather than on his current level of functioning. The patient's capabilities—and not his disabilities—are emphasized.

SOME GENERAL PRINCIPLES

The various observations made in this paper lead logically to several conclusions. It is difficult to evaluate deinstitutionalization, because we lack historical perspective. At any one time, we are viewing in cross section an entire social process; what we see is bound to be biased. However, certain broad principles can be extracted from a functional analysis of deinstitutionalization.

First, it is frequently forgotten that deinstitutionalization, for all its positive thrust, is basically a protest movement. Deinstitutionalization is best understood as the obverse of institutionalization. It follows, therefore, that comprehension of the sociology of mental institutions is prerequisite to understanding the nature of deinstitutionalization.

Second, many of the most serious problems in deinstitutionalization result from conceptual oversights or confusion. In the zeal of social reform, deinstitutionalization efforts have, in practice, too often confused locus of care and quality of care. Merely changing the location of care does not in itself ensure fulfillment of the goal of humanizing mental health care. It is necessary to couple changed location with carefully designed programs.

Third, the role and possible contributions of the state hospital in providing patient care must be assessed objectively. It must be acknowledged that state hospitals have historically performed certain functions that cannot, in all instances, be readily duplicated in the community, at least not yet. It is, accordingly, sensible to view the state hospital in terms of its potential. If the state hospital can be incorporated into a unified system of care and given a definite place in the range of treat-

[18] M. A. Test and L. I. Stein, "Special Living Arrangements: A Model for Decision-Making," *Hospital & Community Psychiatry*, Vol. 28, August 1977, pp. 608-610.

[19] W. A. Anthony, "Psychological Rehabilitation: A Concept in Need of a Method," *American Psychologist*, Vol. 32, August 1977, pp. 658-662.

[20] R. Peterson, "What Are the Needs of Chronic Mental Patients?" background paper for the American Psychiatric Association Conference on the Chronic Mental Patient, Washington, D.C., January 1978.

[21] Anthony, *op. cit.*

ment settings—at least until such time as the functions it fills can be placed in community facilities—it can become part of the deinstitutionalization process, and not adversary to it.

Fourth, in this trial-and-error period, during which the problems in deinstitutionalization are being sorted out, we are afforded a unique opportunity to improve planning for the care of the chronically mentally ill. A careful and realistic definition of the target population for community-based care is essential.

Fifth, planning for the chronically mentally ill should identify those patients who can benefit from rehabilita-

tion. Where feasible, rehabilitation should be enhanced through a skills training approach.

Finally, the successful deinstitutionalization program is not one conceived and implemented in haste. Instead it is one in which careful assessment has been made of needs and resources. It is one that strives for a staff adequately trained to recognize and assist in meeting the special needs of chronically ill persons living in the community—both the formerly hospitalized and the never-hospitalized. And it is one that provides for continuing evaluation and modification to meet the needs of the dynamic process of deinstitutionalization.■

Adolescent Role Assessment

Maureen M. Black

Adolescence is a complex period when children are expected to shed their dependencies and achieve a level of independence as adults. Frequently, adult independence is achieved through the occupational role where individuals recognize personal assets and liabilities and participate cooperatively in the society. The decision-making process that guides adolescents in the search for an occupational role is occupational choice. This paper traces the development of skills necessary for the occupational choice process.

An instrument is presented that attempts to identify deficiencies in the occupational choice process and to provide content for occupational therapy intervention. Its usefulness in screening deviant adolescents in order to identify those who may be at high risk in the occupational choice process is discussed.

Adolescence:
Adolescence: Ruth Benedict calls it "Sturm und Drang" (stress and strain) (1); Haim Ginott says it is a disorganized period of curative madness (2); and Benjamin Spock associates it with rebellion and rivalry (3). Parents and teenagers have easily recognized the period from puberty to adulthood as stressful, inconsistent, and at times traumatic.

Adolescence is a stage in human development that separates the dependence of childhood from the independence of adulthood. It is stressful in part because the adolescent does not have a clearly defined social niche. Shannon explains that, although the adolescent is often expected to act as an adult, he is treated

The American Journal of Occupational Therapy February 1976, Volume 30, No. 2

as a child (4). Conversely, when he is treated as an adult he sometimes exhibits childish behavior. Without clear, consistent expectations either from society or for himself, the adolescent immigrates into a peer social system. Within this sheltered environment the adolescent develops and practices skills of occupational choice and eventually acquires the competence to enter adulthood and the larger society.

The social position and activity involved in his occupational role occupies the majority of an individual's time (5). A common progression of occupational roles includes preschooler, student, worker, homemaker, and retiree. Each person develops specific behavioral patterns to define his occupational role. These patterns comprise the occupational role performance and are a primary consideration in an assessment of competence.

Ginzberg and others have outlined occupational choice as a decision-making process that results in the selection of an occupational role (6). Classically, the process extends from childhood through young adulthood, but may be reactivated whenever an individual alters his occupational role (7). For example, the prospective retiree moves through the occupational choice process in planning retirement activities. This paper explores the relationship between the occupational choice process and the adolescent role.

Occupational Choice Process
The occupational choice process is conceptualized in three stages, and each stage is characterized by specific evolutionary tasks (6). The first stage in the occupational choice process is fantasy and the exploration of alternatives; it begins in childhood play. Through play activities children learn the expectations or rules of the society and how to

TABLE 1

ADOLESCENT ROLE ASSESSMENT

CHILDHOOD-PLAY

Activities

Kids spend a lot of time playing. When you were a child what was your favorite age and why? What kinds of things did you like to do? Alone or with friends?

Scoring:
+ —Identifies favorite age and names activity.
0 —Hesitant or vague response.
— —Unable to identify a favorite age, pessimistic.

Rules

What games or physical sports did you do as a child? Did you play team games or other games with rules?

Scoring:
+ —Identifies games with rules.
0 —Vague or only games without rules.
— —No games or sports.

Interactions

As a child did you play with kids your own age, other than brothers and sisters?

Scoring:
+ —Able to interact with peers of same age.
0 —Vague or marginal interaction.
— —No interaction or inability to interact without fights.

Fantasy

When you were a kid did you daydream or have make-believe friends or make-believe games?
Did you dream about what you would be when you grew up?

Scoring:
+ —Identifies fantasy.
0 —Vague, not sure.
— —Can identify no fantasy.

Role Models

When you were a kid how did you learn to do things, such as ride a bike, tell time, drive a car?
Did you teach yourself, learn from parents, friends, brothers, sisters?

Scoring:
+ —Identifies role models.
0 —Vague or difficulty remembering.
— —Unable to do skills or unable to identify role models.

Interests

Sometimes, as people grow, their interests change.
What kinds of interests did you have as a kid?
How do those interests compare with current interests?

Scoring:
+ —Identifies childhood interests, able to discriminate from current interests.
0 —Few interests, basically same as now.
— —Lack of childhood interests.

interact with peers (8). Play is self-directed and children have opportunities to organize games, win or lose, and receive direct feedback from peers. Feedback enables children to distinguish acceptable social behavior from unacceptable behavior.

Through role models and experience, children build references for their fantasy. The stick becomes a director's baton or guitar, the car goes to the store or Disneyland, and the hat transforms the child into a nurse or fire fighter. Children daydream and explore make-believe alternatives as they increase the scope of their reality. From their dreams and fantasies they develop interests and hobbies to guide further exploration.

The second or tentative choice stage emerges when the interests built in childhood are related to personal capabilities, values, and goals. The play of childhood is replaced by a balance of adolescent leisure activities. These activities frequently include social interaction or interest development. The adolescent is no longer licensed to actively fantasize by strumming a stick guitar or pretending to be a fire fighter. The exploration of alternatives requires more subtle outlets as the adolescent seeks to define a consistent pattern of behavior including responsibilities, feedback, and personal effectance (influence on the environment) (9).

The adolescent is expected to assume responsibilities within the family, neighborhood, and school. He receives feedback from his performances and becomes increasingly accountable for his actions. The feedback assists the adolescent in judging capabilities and forming values and goals. As values and goals are compared with interests, the search for possible occupational role alternatives continues.

By late adolescence the alternatives narrow and the individual enters the realistic stage or final phase of occupational choice. This stage is characterized by the individual's thoughts crystallizing on one choice and the development of skills and habits within that choice. To achieve satisfaction and competence in an occupational role, the role expectations must be consistent with the individual's values and within his skill level.

Occupational Choice Deficits

The period of adolescence and the evolutionary process of occupational choice are difficult, but most adolescents become competent adults. Some individuals are unable to survive the inconsistent expectations and discontinuities encountered between childhood and adulthood. These adolescents may act out and become identified by families, neighborhoods, schools, or courts as deviants and troublemakers, or they may passively refuse any responsibilities and remain isolated. There are many unanswered questions regarding deviant adolescents and the effects of childhood on their competence as adults (10).

The evolutionary acquisition of skills in the occupational choice process suggests that deficiencies at an early stage may increase vulnerability at later stages. The deviant adolescent may be handicapped not only by inconsistent expectations and current role pressures, but also by a lack of skills prerequisite to decision making, which are characteristically acquired during childhood. These necessary skills might include ability to play, recognition of rules and feedback, peer interactions, fantasy exploration, use of role models, and development of interests.

Assessment

The Adolescent Role Assessment (Tables 1 and 2) was developed from a review of the literature on child and adolescent role behavior (11). By separating the adolescents' primary spheres of influence into family, school, and peers, the Adolescent Role Assessment investigates performance in a variety of roles throughout the occupational choice process. It was designed to be administered as a semistructured interview through casual dialogue. The questions are phrased in the vernacular and the examiner must be familiar with the purpose of the questions and the rating criteria. The questions yield both an objective rating and a content applicable to treatment planning.

The rating criteria are explained on the assessment form and are based on the literature review of normative behavior (11). The scoring system was designed to reduce value judgments and subjectivity as much as possible. For example, a question entitled "Goals" asks about future plans and is rated by the presence of ideas on goals and ideas on preparation, regardless of the actual goals. The scores are summarized on the Adolescent Role Assessment Scoring Sheet: plus (+) indicates appropriate behavior, zero (0) indicates marginal or borderline behavior, and minus (—) indicates inappropriate behavior. A majority of plus and zero scores signifies no obvious role dysfunction. A predominance of zero and minus scores indicates serious doubt concerning appropriate role behavior and intervention should be considered, using the data gathered from the interview as a basis for decision.

Sample Population

The Adolescent Role Assessment was administered to 12 inpatients at the Neuropsychiatric Institute of the University of California at Los Angeles. They ranged in age from 13 to 17 years with diagnoses that included adjustment reaction of adolescence, anorexia nervosa, school phobia, and depression. The Adolescent Role Assessment was part of a battery of assessments including participatory observation (12), Rosenberg's Self-Esteem Scale (13), Bills' Index of Adjustment and

---

TABLE 2

ADOLESCENCE—SOCIALIZATION

FAMILY

Interactions

Teenagers often hassle with their families.
How would you describe your relationship with your family?
Do you do anything to agitate your family?
What are the positive qualities about your family?
Negative qualities?

    Scoring: + —Relatively positive relationship, recognizes strengths and weaknesses.
          0 —Moderate relationship with vague recognition of strengths and weaknesses.
          — —Negative relationship with no recognition of positive qualities.

Responsibilities

What kinds of responsibilities do you have at home?
Are these responsibilities reasonable?
Do you usually do them on time?

    Scoring: + —Age and sex-appropriate responsibilities, usually completed on time.
          0 —Lack of clarity of responsibilities, occasionally completed on time.
          — —No responsibilities, inappropriate responsibilities, or refusal to do appropriate responsibilities.

Economics

How do you obtain spending money?
Are you satisfied with the amount and arrangement for obtaining it?
Who decides how you will spend it?

    Scoring: + —Manages own money.
          0 —Vague plan for obtaining money with few personal decisions on amount or where spent.
          — —No plan for obtaining money or no personal decisions on how it is spent.

TABLE 3

SCHOOL

Consistent Behavior

What grade are you in?
What kinds of grades do you achieve?
Throughout your life as a student have your grades been consistent?

    Scoring: + —Consistent grades of average to high range.
               0 —Average to low range of grades, some drop in consistency.
               — —All low grades or significant drop in consistency.

Responsibilities

Are you usually prepared for class with assignments completed on time?
Do you attend your classes?
Are you often late?
Do you study regularly after school?
Do you study only for tests?

    Scoring: + —Class attendance regular, usually prepared, regular study schedule.
               0 —Occasionally late for class, occasionally unprepared, studies mainly for tests.
               - —Often unprepared, often misses classes, few study habits.

Feedback

Are you satisfied with your school performance?
What could you do to improve your school experience?
Do you ever follow your teachers' suggestions on improvement?

    Scoring: + —Identifies ways to improve, uses feedback.
               0 —Recognizes improvement potential, but has difficulty using feedback or identifying ways to improve.
               — —Denies improvement potential or does not use feedback.

Effectance and Role Models

Are you treated fairly by teachers?
Are you ever removed from class for your conduct?
Do you have any favorite teachers? If so, what qualities make them your favorites?

    Scoring: + —Usually fair treatment, conforms to norms, identifies positive qualities in a teacher.
               0 —Questionable treatment, occasionally removed from class.
               — —Unfair treatment, often removed from class, or no positive qualities in teachers.

Activities

What activities are you involved in at school?
What activities do you do with your friends (include clubs)?
What activities do you do alone?

    Scoring: + —Several activities mentioned, age and sex appropriate.
               0 —Hesitation with few activities or some inappropriate activities.
               — —No activities or many inappropriate activities.

Values (13), Interest Checklist (14), Rotter's Generalized Expectations for Internal versus External Control (15), and Buhler's Life Goals (16). The analysis of results suggested that patterns of dysfunction could be identified that would serve as a guide for specific program planning (11).

Reilly (17) has advocated the use of the case method in occupational therapy as a heuristic treatment tool for the formulation of questions that would identify problem areas of behavior. One of the adolescents in the sample population was selected from a demographic review as a case study.

Case Study

AK is a 14-year-old male with a diagnosis of adjustment reaction of adolescence. Historical data indicate that, before admission to the hospital, he was failing in several of his ninth grade subjects, had been dismissed from school for smoking marijuana, and had been arrested for stealing. AK was administered the Adolescent Role Assessment and the content was summarized.

AK's childhood fantasies were dominated by jungles and wild animals. At age eight he had friends his own age, enjoyed school, received all As and had no difficulty identifying role models. AK did not participate in team games or sports. His older siblings protected him and allowed him to win in competitive situations.

When AK was ten his parents were divorced, his older sister left home, and he moved several times with his mother and younger sister. At that time he says he re-evaluated his priorities in life and his interests changed. The school system interpreted his fading interest as boredom and AK was advanced an extra year. His academic performance was poor and he entered adolescence without his childhood interests and activities.

AK's mother has had psychiatric care and AK says he loves his mother but considers her crazy and prefers not to depend on her for money. AK has been given household responsibilities and assumes them sporadically. He respects his father, but his father has been physically ill and contacts have been few.

AK exhibits his negative attitude toward school by receiving Fs and cutting classes. He recognizes his potential and does not blame his failure on his teachers; however, he considers school a waste of time and does not participate in any school activities.

AK's friends are generally older and AK appears older than his 14 years. He prefers to be called a young adult and his activities involve sex, drugs, drinking, and stealing. AK spends the major part of his time talking with friends. Alone he reads or daydreams about living in Oregon.

Although AK has never been to Oregon, he fantasizes about a future there with easy living, lots of money, and interesting jobs in the woods. AK has had a few odd jobs—he dislikes the regularity of work, but considers it honest. His occupational choice is based upon his childhood interest in animals, but he no longer pursues that interest and has no plans for implementation. When asked to relate his choice to reality, AK responded that he will probably be "pumping gas." He dreams of accumulating enough money to live without working and is not interested in a family or responsibilities.

Case Study Analysis

AK's childhood role appears to be deficient in behavior formed by rules. Although he engaged in symbolic play and began to develop a relationship between fantasy and reality, his feedback was based on a personal interpretation of reality without rules.

The data from the assessment battery supplements the findings from the Adolescent Role Assessment. The author was a participatory observer as AK learned new techniques of cooking, interacted with peers in a cooperative effort, and practiced skills of decision making. He was skilled in the techniques of cooking; he learned from models as well as by individual experimentation. He assumed a leadership role and was able to make decisions related to coordinating the activities necessary to complete the meal. Scores on Rosenberg's Self-Esteem Scale and Bills' Index of Adjustment and Values suggest that AK has confidence in himself, high personal satisfaction, and ability to form his own values.

He responded negatively to the Interest Checklist by rejecting approximately 70 percent of the items. His only areas of interest were in social recreation. On Rotter's Generalized Expectations assessment, which measures feelings of environmental control and provides implications on the use of feedback, AK received an average score. Buhler's Life Goals Inventory revealed AK's emphasis on immediate satisfaction in necessities and pleasure. He rejected the concept of love and family, and the extremes in his profile suggested an unbalanced goal hierarchy.

As AK approached adolescence, the disintegration of his family and the inconsistencies of his school and peer group caused him to lose his normative agents of socialization. He was attracted to a subculture of older peers and adopted their maladaptive values and activities. As an adolescent he was expected to show an increase in responsibility and reality orientation, but he was deficient in separating fantasy from the rules of reality. He abandoned fantasy and operated on an immediate evaluation of reality.

AK responds to his environment with extremely high self-esteem. Although his technical skills are well developed and he possesses the abstract reasoning necessary for value formation, perhaps the high self-esteem is a protection from the feedback of reality. Without appropriate norms AK has

TABLE 4

PEERS

Activities

After school are you usually alone? With one friend? With a group?
Are your friends older? Same age? Younger?
What do you like about your social situation?
What do you dislike?

    Scoring: + —Positive relationship.
              0 —Mixed feelings about relationship or many friends older or younger.
              — —Poor relationship, few friends or all older or younger.

Time

How many hours a **week** do you spend in the following activities?
How do you decide upon your time schedule?
Do you usually complete activities?
Is scheduling a problem for you?

    School work (outside of school)
    Reading for pleasure
    Watching television
    Doing nothing
    Daydreaming
    Working
    Making yourself and your clothes look good
    Dating
    Hanging around talking with friends
    Playing tennis, swimming, etc.
    Other

    Scoring: + —Balanced, completed activities with no scheduling problems.
              0 —Concentrated time spent in a few activities, some incompleted activities, or some scheduling difficulties.
              — —No activities or multiple disjointed activities without completion, serious scheduling difficulties.

Community

What do you know about your neighborhood?
Where is the nearest food store, park, library?
If public transportation is available do you know how to use it?

    Scoring: + —Knowledge of community.
              0 —Vague.
              — —No knowledge of community.

TABLE 5

ADOLESCENCE—OCCUPATIONAL CHOICE

Work Attitudes

Have you ever worked?
What kinds of work have you done?
What did you like about working?
What did you dislike?
From your experience, what are your attitudes toward work in general (i.e., necessary evil, valuable opportunity, etc.)?

  (Score only for those with work experience)

  Scoring: + —Positive attitudes.
         0 —Mixed attitudes.
         — —Negative attitudes.

Stage of Choice

What occupation would you **like** to enter?
How did you make this selection?
What are your plans for further education or training?
Do you know anyone in this occupation?
What occupation do you think you will actually be in ten years from now?

  Scoring: + —Selection based on interests, capacities, or values with some plans for implementation.
         0 —Selection based on fantasy or interests with few implementation plans, may be role model and recognition that actual occupation is more realistic than idealized occupation.
         — —No selection or selection based on fantasy with no role model or no plans for implementation.

TABLE 6

ADULTHOOD—WORK

Goals

When you think about your future what things do you think will be important to you (i.e., money, free time, feeling young, career, family, etc.)?
How can you prepare yourself for those goals?

  Scoring: + —Some ideas on goals with preparation ideas.
         0 —Vague ideas on goals.
         — —Not future-oriented, has no goals or no preparation ideas.

Fantasy

If your future could be whatever you wanted, what would you want?
If you could change anything in the world, what would you change?
When you daydream, what do you dream about?

  Scoring: + —Able to fantasize about the future.
         0 —Some fantasizing, but minimal.
         — —Unable to fantasize, very concrete.

developed a value hierarchy that leads to deviant, impulsive behavior.

AK is able to use feedback and decision making in a concrete situation; however, he has been unable to incorporate them into the tasks of occupational choice. His paucity of interests and reliance on childhood fantasy illustrate his deficits in the occupational choice process.

From the analysis AK's principal liabilities are rule-oriented behavior, the relationship between fantasy and reality, and identification of norms and appropriate socialization agents; his principal assets are use of modeling and experimentation, intellectual ability to form values, and appropriate use of feedback and decision making in concrete situations. AK's immediate plans are to return to live with his mother and sister and return to public school. Using the assets and liabilities revealed through the assessment battery, specific questions can be raised to guide program planning:

1. *Rule-Oriented Behavior:* (a) Will team sports assist AK in learning to operate within rules?

(b) Could AK begin with a short project with rules and progress to a long-term project with rules to encourage delayed gratification?

(c) Are there responsibilities AK would value that would help him identify rules and responsibilities?

2. *Fantasy and Reality:* (a) Could art projects be used to simulate the symbolic play of childhood to permit AK to express fantasies?

(b) By a balanced program of structured and unstructured activities, could AK learn the rules of reality within an environment that accepts exploration of fantasy?

(c) If AK's high self-esteem serves as a protection from the feedback of reality, what activities would enable him to use feedback without destroying his self-esteem? Could occupational therapy assess AK's skills to find an activity in which he is technically competent and then encourage expression of fantasy?

3. *Norms and Socialization:* (a) Through concrete activities, could AK's decision-making skills be increased to enable him to recognize acceptable norms and reject inappropriate socializing agents?

(b) Through peer group activities where AK acts as both a leader and a follower, could he build socialization skills?

(c) By increasing AK's responsibilities and alternatives in activities, could AK learn to recognize consequences and feedback?

Conclusion

Adolescence is recognized as a stressful period where individuals leave the dependency of childhood and move toward the independence of adulthood. The skills that adolescents must acquire are complicated by inconsistent expectations and lack of clear social positions. Within this turmoil adolescents develop the process of occupational choice in learning to relate hopes or dreams to realistic alternatives.

Adolescents who do not perform successfully and are labeled as deviant are a source of puzzlement and concern. One hypothesis is that these individuals did not develop skills in childhood that would enable them to search for alternatives and to make the decisions required in occupational choice. The Adolescent Role Assessment explores past and present performance and yields content useful for intervention in role dysfunction. This assessment serves as an initial step in attempting to identify crucial variables for adaptive adolescent role performance. •

Acknowledgment

This article is based upon material submitted in partial fulfillment of the requirements for the Master of Arts Degree, University of Southern California, Los Angeles.

REFERENCES

1. Benedict R: Continuities and discontinuities in cultural conditioning. *Psychiatry* 1: 161, 1938
2. Ginott HC: *Between Parent and Teenager*, New York, Avon, 1969
3. Spock B: *Raising Children in a Difficult Time*, New York, Norton, 1974
4. Shannon PD: The work-play model: A basis for occupational therapy programming in psychiatry. *Am J Occup Ther* 24: 215, 1970
5. Pavalko RM: *A Sociology of Occupations and Professions*, Itasca, IL, Peacock, 1971
6. Ginzberg E, Ginzberg SW, Axelrad S, Herman JL: *Occupational Choice: An Approach to a General Theory*, New York, Columbia, 1956
7. Ginzberg E: Toward a theory of occupational choice: A restatement. *Vocational Guidance* 20: 169, 1972
8. Reilly M: *Play as Exploratory Learning*, Beverly Hills, Sage, 1974
9. White RW: Competence and the psychological stages of development. In *Nebraska Symposium on Motivation.* Edited by M. Jones. Lincoln, University of Nebraska Press, 1960, pp. 97-138
10. Muuss RE: *Theories of Adolescence*, New York, Random House, 1968
11. Black MM: The evolution of social roles—a perspective on fantasy. Master's thesis. Department of Occupational Therapy, University of Southern California, Los Angeles, California, 1973
12. Denzin NK: *Sociological Methods*, Chicago, Aldine, 1970
13. Robinson J, Shaver P: *Measures of Social Psychological Attitudes*, Ann Arbor, MI, Publications Division, Institute for Social Research, 1969
14. Matsutsuyu JS; An assessment of interests. Master's thesis. Department of Occupational Therapy, University of Southern California, Los Angeles, California, 1968
15. Rotter JP: Generalized expectations for internal and external control. *Psychol Monogr* 80:609, 1966
16. Buhler C: Human life as a whole as a central subject of humanistic psychology. In *Challenges of Humanistic Psychology.* Edited by JFT Bugental. New York, McGraw-Hill, 1967
17. Reilly M: The educational process. *Am J Occup Ther* 23: 299, 1969

R30202

TABLE 7

ADOLESCENT ROLE ASSESSMENT
SCORING

		+	0	—
CHILDHOOD PLAY	Activities			
	Rules,			
	Interactions			
	Fantasy			
	Role Models			
	Interests			
ADOLESCENT SOCIALIZATION FAMILY	Interactions			
	Responsibilities			
	Economics			
ADOLESCENT SOCIALIZATION SCHOOL	Consistency			
	Responsibilities			
	Feedback			
	Role Models			
	Activities			
ADOLESCENT SOCIALIZATION PEERS	Activities			
	Time			
	Community			
ADOLESCENT OCCUPATIONAL CHOICE	Work			
	Choice Stage			
ADULT WORK	Goals			
	Fantasy			

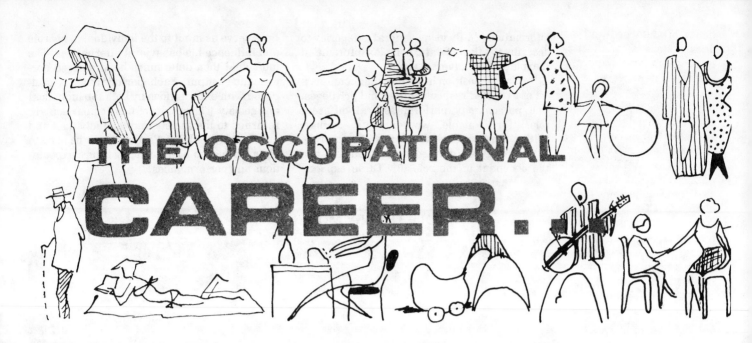

THE OCCUPATIONAL CAREER...

Maureen M. Black

The health care system is responding to the demands for comprehensive services and is extending its services beyond the elimination of pathology to that of providing assistance with problems of daily role adjustment. Occupational therapists are beginning to base their practice on a role theory model, which permits consideration of both pathology and role adjustment. The acquisition of roles throughout an individual's life progresses from infancy through old age and forms a career of roles. Occupational therapists are developing evaluations of role performance to identify strengths and weaknesses of daily role adjustment. By complementing the existing body of occupational therapy expertise with assessments of occupational career, occupational therapists can easily respond to the increasing health care demands.

The public and professional literature is currently emphasizing the increasing demands for health care. These demands reinforce the definitions of health as a state of total well-being, not as a state where disease is absent. Other changes in health are taking place. Instead of "patient," the recipient of health care is called a student or client; institutions are becoming community-centered; families are being incorporated into programs; and the handicapped individual is no longer regarded in sociological terms as a deviant to be isolated by a medical system.

Within occupational therapy literature, Jerry Johnson's 1972 Eleanor Clarke Slagle Lecture proposed a model to focus on health as defined by an individual's ability "to achieve a satisfying interaction with his social system or environment." (1) The 1974 Task Force on Target Populations supported Johnson's proposals with recommendations that occupational therapists move away from pathology-oriented techniques and move toward a consideration of the handicapped individual's role in society (2). By regarding the occupational role as a determinant of health, occupational therapy can then focus on the individual's adaptations to society.

Reilly formulated a frame of reference for occupational therapy entitled occupational behavior, a system that has its origins in the psychosocial concept of role theory (3,4). Occupational behavior is formed on the balanced activities of work, play, rest, and sleep originally proposed by Meyer (5). Through these activities, an individual acquires the skills necessary for role performance and builds the skills into daily habits of behavior. These habits are not behaviors that are repeated in a rotelike manner, but competent steps that enable individual flexibility. Within each role, an individual builds many habits that form a hierarchy of possible behavioral options (6). As competence is gained, the individual selects and uses these habits. The occupational therapist assesses the individual's performance within a role and designs a program that will assist in the formation of skills appropriate to the role that can be practiced and exercised in order to become habits.

Role Theory

Role theory may be explained by using the categories of systems theory. Systems theory is an interdisciplinary method of organizing

Maureen M. Black, M.A., O.T.R. is presently a student in a doctoral program, Department of Psychology, Emory University, Atlanta, Georgia.

information (7). By using general categories to describe the flow of data, complex information is explained in universal terms.

A role is a position in society that contains a set of expected responsibilities and privileges. One person may perform several different roles; for example, worker, wife, mother. Within the boundaries or limits of each role, expectations are formed by both society and the occupant of the role (8). These expecta-tions serve as input to the individual in his role and influence his behavioral alternatives. The individual then determines his preferred per-formance output. Each performance is com-pared with expectations by both the individual and society. The results of this comparison are returned to the society and the individual and are termed feedback. Feedback can be used to alter the system by influencing future expecta-tions and performances.

Internal & External Expectations

ROLE THEORY MODEL

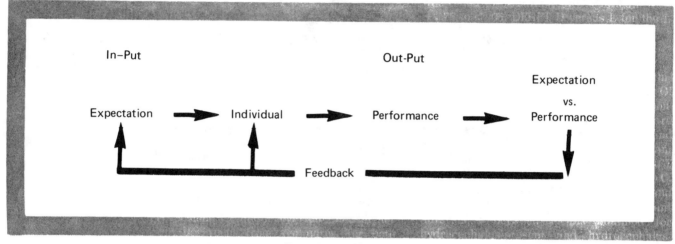

Boundary of Role

Figure 1

OCCUPATIONAL CAREER

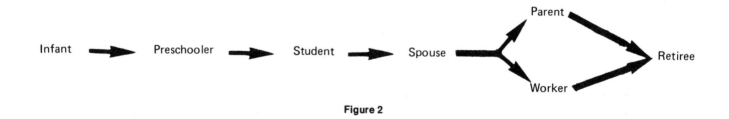

Figure 2

OCCUPATIONAL CAREER

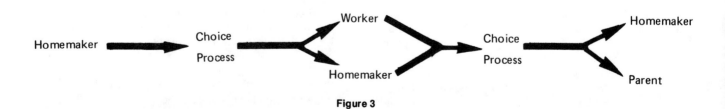

Figure 3

The principal components of role theory may be diagrammed in a systems model (Figure 1).

Role theory offers possible explanations for behavioral differences. The child who misbehaves at home and is complacent at school may be responding to different boundaries and expectations within each setting. In addition to external expectations of society, personal expectations toward behavioral alternatives are important determinants of output. Smith has proposed a theory in which poor personal expectations or negative self-respect initiates a pattern of behavior that results in inappropriate use of feedback and a continuing loss of self-respect (9). Conversely, positive self-respect leads to an ability to profit from feedback both good and bad, and improve future performances.

The construction of adaptive skills and habits within several roles becomes a complex phenomenon. Role theory simplifies the process by identifying the primary variables as boundary, internal and external expectations, feedback, and performance. The evolution of role behavior reveals how skills and habits acquired in one role may be practiced, generalized, and transferred to other roles.

Evolution of Role Behavior

Career has been used in a vocational context to describe movement within a particular job or profession. McCall and Simmons suggest that the concept of **career** can be broadened to study not only movement within one role, but also movement from one role to another (10).

Figure 2 illustrates one possible progression of roles along an occupational career (11).

Roles may be defined by age, sex, family membership, social group, or occupation (12). Thus each individual's occupational career is unique in that it consists of only his particular roles.

The value in conceptualizing lifetime movement during an occupational career is in recognizing that each role is an evolutionary step. Within each role are skills and habits that must be acquired for successful progression to future roles. Conversely, the basis for failure within one role may be explained by failure to build the necessary skills and habits at an earlier stage in the occupational career. For example, the worker who is unable to manage his leisure time may never have learned the play skills inherent in the preschool role.

Occupational Choice

Movement through the worker phase of an occupational career has been described by Ginzberg's decision-making process of occupational choice, which outlines the selection and preparation for a worker role (13). Maurer has outlined the process of vocational development into a series of tasks acquired during childhood, adolescence, and young adulthood

(14). The child progresses from task to task, ranging from a fantasy type of identification with a worker, to the realistic task of applying his own self-concept and skills to a specific occupation.

In a recent publication, Ginzberg expanded the concept of occupational choice beyond the classic adolescent years (15). Throughout an occupational career, each person proceeds through decision-making stages of occupational choice in planning future roles. Therefore, a 45-year-old man, an amputee who is planning his role as a homemaker, fantasizes about future alternatives, explores within these alternatives, evaluates personal attributes, and eventually makes plans to build the skills of a homemaker.

Career

The occupational career emerges as a series of roles bridged by the decision-making inherent in the occupational choice process during a lifetime. Figure 3 illustrates a model of the occupational career that includes the occupational choice process.

Roles are either assigned or acquired (12). Although age and sex roles are assigned, the alternatives and behavior within these roles are influenced by personal attributes and decisions. Family membership, social class, and occupation are initially assigned roles, but as an individual grows, he has opportunities to plan his own family, social status, and occupation. By conceptualizing the progression of roles along the continuum of an occupational career, the occupational choice process emerges as a key variable in personalizing or guiding that career.

Occupational Career Disruptions

The organization of an individual's roles into a career pattern facilitates the recommendation that occupational therapy focus on health rather than pathology. The profession has an established body of knowledge for treating physical and emotional disabilities and the multitude of assessments in those areas identify the target areas of occupational therapy intervention. As Reilly stated, the guidelines of occupational behavior are a "not only, but also" phenomenon (4). While retaining the expertise in treating physical and emotional disabilities, the clinicians recognizing occupational behavior also explore occupational role performance. Using the Role Theory Model shown in Figure 1 as a framework, the homemaking role could be evaluated through the following questions:

A. Expectations

1. What are the societal expectations?
   (i.e., budget, shop)
2. What are the specific expectations and responsibilities?
   (i.e., elderly person in the home on a restricted diet)

B. Boundaries

1. What are the environmental boundaries?
   (i.e., location of laundry facilities, stores)
2. What are the personal boundaries?
   (i.e., must use wheelchair)

C. Individual

1. What are the personal interpretations of expectations and boundaries?
   (i.e., person on restricted diet can cook for himself)
2. What other roles does the individual have?
3. What are the individual's homemaking goals?
   (i.e., vacuum once a week)

D. Performance

1. What are the most frequent daily activities and the time spent in each activity?
   (i.e., daily schedule)
2. How does the individual plan daily activities?
3. Are there balanced activities including time for work, play, rest, and sleep?
   (i.e., time for shopping, time for social outings)
4. Does the individual meet his own goals? Does he meet family or societal expectations?

E. Feedback

1. Is the individual satisfied with his role performance? Can he identify strengths and weaknesses?
2. What changes would the individual like to make as a homemaker? Can he determine methods of implementing and evaluating the changes?

Other roles could also be examined using role theory as a model. In addition to assessing current role function, role performance during the occupational career yields past and present strengths and deficiencies. Moorhead has developed an assessment, the Occupational History, to assist in this process. By examining the decisions made in order to move from one role to another or in the acquisition of habits, weaknesses in the choice process are revealed (16). The role-occupant plans daily activities with a balance in time among work, play, rest, and sleep. Effective planning requires the decision-making skills of recognizing and evaluating alternatives. Westphal has developed the steps in basic decision-making into an assessment tool (17).

With information on past successes and failures, decision-making skills, and current expectations and functioning, an occupational therapy program can be specific enough to ensure that the individual acquires the relevant skills (that is, ability to prepare a meal), and general enough to allow the individual to build the skills of decision-making and response to feedback into flexible habits necessary for competent role performance.

Summary

The President of the American Occupational Therapy Association and the 1974 Task Force on Target Populations have recommended that occupational therapy broaden its focus to consider the occupational role as a determinant of health. Occupational behavior is a model based on role theory and may be used to assess role performance. Role performance generalizes and each individual performs in a career of roles throughout his life. Each career is unique and guided by the decision-making process of occupational choice, which directs movement between roles.

The concepts of occupational behavior and occupational career are designed to supplement the extensive body of knowledge guiding current occupational therapy practice. By viewing clients as role occupants and assessing and treating them as homemakers or workers, occupational therapy can respond to a broadened focus without sacrificing the legacy of the profession. ●

REFERENCES

1. Johnson JA: Occupational therapy: A model for the future. *Am J Occup Ther* 27: 1-7, 1973
2. Task force on target populations, I. *Am J Occup Ther* 28: 158-163, 1974
3. Reilly M: A psychiatric occupational therapy program as a teaching model. *Am J Occup Ther* 20: 61-67, 1966
4. Reilly M: The educational process. *Am J Occup Ther* 23: 299-307, 1969
5. Meyer A: The philosophy of occupational therapy. *Am J Occup Ther* 1: 1-5, 1922
6. White RW: Strategies of adaptation: An attempt at systematic description. In *Coping and Adaptation*. GV Coelho, Editor. New York, Basic Books, 1974
7. Churchman CW: *The Systems Approach*, New York, Dell Publishing Company, 1968
8. Sarbin TR: Role theory. In *Handbook of Social Psychology*, G. Lindzey, Editor. Menlo Park, CA, Addison-Wesley Publishing Company, 1968
9. Smith MB: Competence and socialization. In *Socialization and Society*, J Clausen, Editor. Boston, Little, Brown and Company, 1968
10. McCall CJ, Simmons JL: *Identities and Interaction*, New York, The Free Press, 1966
11. Matsutsuyu J: Occupational behavior—A perspective on work and play. *Am J Occup Ther* 25: 291-294, 1971
12. Linton R: *The Science of Man in the World Crisis*, New York, Columbia University Press, 1945
13. Ginzberg E, et al: *Occupational Choice*, New York, Columbia University Press, 1951
14. Maurer P: Antecedents of work behavior. *Am J Occup Ther* 25: 295-297, 1971
15. Ginzberg E: Toward a theory of occupational choice: A restatement. *Vocational Guidance Q* 20: 169-172, 1972
16. Moorhead L: The occupational history. *Am J Occup Ther* 23: 329-332, 1969
17. Westphal MO: A study of decision making. Unpublished master's thesis, Department of Occupational Therapy, University of Southern California, 1967

R30403

Comprehensive Occupational Therapy Evaluation Scale

Sara J. Brayman
Thomas F. Kirby
Aletha M. Misenheimer
M.J. Short

This paper presents the Comprehensive Occupational Therapy Evaluation Scale (COTE Scale) for use by occupational therapists in short-term, acute-care psychiatric facilities. The scale defines 25 behaviors that occur in and are particularly relevant to the practice of occupational therapy. The scale is used as an initial evaluation, as a record of patient progress, and as a means of communicating the evaluation, progress, and treatment to other hospital departments. Ratings of patients that indicate improvement and readiness for discharge are supported by the evaluations of other disciplines.

With the trend toward greater accountability in hospital care, professionals treating the mentally ill are being asked more frequently to define the behaviors they are treating. As members of this group of professionals, occupational therapists often have difficulty defining the patient behaviors involved in treatment programs in acute psychiatric settings. Lack of definition leads others to question what is occupational therapy and, more importantly, what is its value in the psychiatric therapeutic milieu.

Third-party payers often do not pay for services that are not defined, such as milieu therapy. As noted in *Psychiatric News* (1), Blue Cross has refused to pay some claims where milieu therapy was involved. In testimony before the House Subcommittee on Retirement, Insurance, and Health Benefits, Dr. Robert Laur, vice-president of the Blue Cross Association and the National Association of Blue Shield Plans, testified that one of the requirements mental health coverage should meet is that "the services to be covered must be capable of definition, so that subscribers, providers, and carriers will have a responsible understanding of what will be paid for." (2)

As an initial attempt to provide definition of its services, the occupational therapy staff at

The American Journal of Occupational Therapy
February 1976, Volume 30, No. 2

TABLE 1

COMPREHENSIVE OCCUPATIONAL THERAPY EVALUATION SCALE
(COTE SCALE)
FORM A

DATE	1	2	3	4	5	6	7	8	9	10	11	12	13	14	15
I. GENERAL BEHAVIOR															
A. APPEARANCE															
B. NON-PRODUCTIVE BEHAVIOR															
C. ACTIVITY LEVEL (a or b)															
D. EXPRESSION															
E. RESPONSIBILITY															
F. PUNCTUALITY															
G. REALITY ORIENTATION															
SUB-TOTAL															
II. INTERPERSONAL BEHAVIOR															
A. INDEPENDENCE															
B. COOPERATION															
C. SELF-ASSERTION (a or b)															
D. SOCIABILITY															
E. ATTENTION-GETTING BEHAVIOR															
F. NEGATIVE RESPONSE FROM OTHERS															
SUB-TOTAL															
III. TASK BEHAVIOR															
A. ENGAGEMENT															
B. CONCENTRATION															
C. COORDINATION															
D. FOLLOW DIRECTIONS															
E. ACTIVITY NEATNESS OR ATTENTION TO DETAIL															
F. PROBLEM SOLVING															
G. COMPLEXITY AND ORGANIZATION OF TASK															
H. INITIAL LEARNING															
I. INTEREST IN ACTIVITY															
J. INTEREST IN ACCOMPLISHMENT															
K. DECISION MAKING															
L. FRUSTRATION TOLERANCE															
SUB-TOTAL															
TOTAL															

SCALE 0 - NORMAL, 1 - MINIMAL, 2 - MILD, 3 - MODERATE, 4 - SEVERE

COMMENTS:

_____

_____

_____

_____

_____

_____

_____

_____

_____

_____

_____

_____

(THERAPIST'S SIGNATURE)

Marshall I. Pickens Hospital developed a behavioral rating scale that defines patient behaviors. The Comprehensive Occupational Therapy Evaluation Scale (COTE Scale) serves both as an initial evaluation and as a record of progress. It consists of 25 behaviors each of which are rated on a scale of from 0 to 4, representing degrees of departure from normalcy. The behaviors and their definitions are shown in Table 1.

In its function as a comprehensive community mental health center, Marshall I. Pickens Hospital provides a 50-bed inpatient program for acutely disturbed adolescents and adults. Each patient is under the care of a private psychiatrist and the average length of stay is 11 days. Patients routinely attend occupational therapy once a day for five days a week and attend occupational therapy an average of eight times. The occupational therapy department is staffed by two registered occupational therapists, one certified occupational therapy assistant, and one occupational therapy assistant.

Development of the Scale

Several objectives guided the development of the scale. The first was to identify behaviors that occurred in and were particularly relevant to the practice of occupational therapy, the basis of which were provided by Fidler and Fidler (3) and Mosey (4, 5). Most of the behaviors are those that are usually evaluated by occupational therapists and then reported in an evaluation or in progress notes.

The second objective was to define the identified behaviors in such a manner that they could be reliably observed and rated by two or more therapists. Again the works of Fidler and Fidler (3) and Mosey (4, 5) were used as a guide.

A third objective was to direct the information on the scale primarily to the referring, busy psychiatrist. A short, one-page form, without definitions, was selected (Table 2). In this way the psychiatrist could quickly see his patient's status on 25 different behaviors when the scale was used as an initial evaluation. Subsequently, the scale is used as a record of patient progress and provides the doctor with the affects of the total treatment process on each of the behaviors evaluated by occupational therapy.

Each of the 25 behaviors on the scale is rated from 0 to 4. A rating of zero indicates normal function or an absence of problem behavior, while a rating of 4 represents a severe problem. The totaled ratings could range from 0 to 100; higher ratings indicate more severe problems.

Reliability

To determine the reliability between therapists using the scale, percent agreement between the ratings of two therapists was computed in the following manner. After a one-hour session in occupational therapy, two therapists independently rated the same patient on the 25 behaviors of the scale. A criterion of ratings within one degree of each other (0 - 1, 1 - 2, 2 - 3, 3 - 4) for each behavior was considered acceptable. Percent agreement was calculated by dividing the number of agreements by the number of agreements plus disagreements. Percent agreements between therapists for 55 patients ranged from 76 percent to 100 percent and averaged 95 percent. Percent agreements were also calculated for exact agreement of ratings between therapists on the same patients. They ranged from 36 to 84 percent and averaged 63 percent. A total of five therapists, resulting in seven different pairings, were involved.

Validity

To determine the validity of the scale, the charts of 56 discharged patients who had attended occupational therapy on at least 4 days were randomly selected from a group of 400. Total scores on the COTE Scale for the first day and the last day of attendance were then compared. First-day scores averaged 31 and last-day scores averaged 17. This drop in total scores was interpreted as readiness for discharge. The drop in total scores also agreed with the improvement noted by staff in psychiatry, nursing, and other disciplines involved in treatment and discharge planning.

Discussion

Using the rating scale, occupational therapists can briefly and clearly relate or communicate a patient's progress to other team professionals. It can serve as an initial evaluation in occupational therapy and as a record of patient progress. Nursing, recreational therapy, social work, psychology, and occupational therapy departments contribute equally in the team meetings where each patient's treatment milieu is planned and assessed. Since numerical ratings only are required, the therapist needs little time to record behavior change and is free to write notes if he/she chooses, thus providing the patient's psychiatrist with a great deal of information that can be reviewed in a very short time.

Summary

With the current trend toward greater accountability and the need for clear definitions of milieu therapy, professionals treating the mentally ill must take steps to clarify the confusion that now exists in the field. The Comprehensive Occupational Therapy Evaluation Scale (COTE Scale) is a step toward clarifying this confusion for occupational therapists. The scale defines the behaviors that occupational therapy works with, provides a means for more objective evaluation of new patients on these behaviors, and then provides

TABLE 2

COMPREHENSIVE OCCUPATIONAL THERAPY
EVALUATION SCALE
DEFINITIONS

PART I. GENERAL BEHAVIOR

A. APPEARANCE
The following six factors are involved: (1) clean skin, (2) clean hair, (3) hair combed, (4) clean clothes, (5) clothes ironed, and (6) clothes suitable for the occasion.
0—No problems in any area.
1—Problems in 1 area.
2—Problems in 2 areas.
3—Problems in 3 or 4 areas.
4—Problems in 5 or 6 areas.

B. NONPRODUCTIVE BEHAVIOR
(Rocking, playing with hands, repetitive statements, appears to be talking to self, preoccupied with own thoughts, etc.)
0—No nonproductive behavior during session.
1—Nonproductive behavior occasionally during session.
2—Nonproductive behavior for half of session.
3—Nonproductive behavior for three-fourths of session.
4—Nonproductive behavior for the entire session.

C. ACTIVITY LEVEL (a or b)
(a) 0—No hypoactivity.
1—Occasional hypoactivity.
2—Hypoactivity attracts the attention of other patients and therapists but participates.
3—Hypoactivity level such that can participate but with great difficulty.
4—So hypoactive that patient cannot participate in activity.

(b) 0—No hyperactivity.
1—Occasional spurts of hyperactivity.
2—Hyperactivity attracts the attention of other patients and therapists but participates.
3—Hyperactivity level such that can participate but with great difficulty.
4—So hyperactive that patient cannot participate in activity.

TABLE 2

PART II. INTERPERSONAL

A. INDEPENDENCE
0—Independent functioning.
1—Only 1 or 2 dependent actions.
2—Half independent and half dependent actions.
3—Only 1 or 2 independent actions.
4—No independent actions.

B. COOPERATION
0—Cooperates with program.
1—Follows most directions, opposes less than one half.
2—Follows half, opposes half.
3—Opposes three-fourths of directions.
4—Opposes all directions and suggestions.

C. SELF-ASSERTION (a or b)
(a) 0—Assertive when necessary.
1—Compliant less than half of the session.
2—Compliant half of the session.
3—Compliant three-fourths of the session.
4—Totally passive and compliant.

(b) 0—Assertive when necessary.
1—Dominant less than half of the session.
2—Dominant half of the session.
3—Dominant three-fourths of the session.
4—Totally dominates the session.

D. SOCIABILITY
0—Socializes with staff and patients.
1—Socializes with staff and occasionally with other patients or vice-versa.
2—Socializes only with staff or with patients.
3—Socializes only if approached.
4—Does not join others in activities, unable to carry on casual conversation even if approached.

D. EXPRESSION

0—Expression consistent with situation and setting.
1—Communicates with expression, occasionally inappropriate.
2—Shows inappropriate expression several times during session.
3—Show of expression but inconsistent with situation.
4—Extremes of expression-bizarre, uncontrolled or no expression.

E. RESPONSIBILITY

0—Takes responsibility for own actions.
1—Denies responsibility for 1 or 2 actions.
2—Denies responsibility for several actions.
3—Denies responsibility for most actions.
4—Denial of all responsibility-messes up project and blames therapist or others.

F. PUNCTUALITY

0—On time.
1—5-10 minutes late.
2—10-20 minutes late.
3—20-30 minutes late.
4—30 minutes or more late.

G. REALITY ORIENTATION

0—Complete awareness of person, place, time, and situation.
1—General awareness but inconsistency in one area.
2—Awareness of 2 areas.
3—Awareness of 1 area.
4—Lack of awareness of person, place, time, and situation (who, where, what, and why).

E. ATTENTION-GETTING BEHAVIOR

0—No unreasonable attention-getting behavior.
1—Less than one-half time spent in attention-getting behavior.
2—Half-time spent in attention-getting behavior.
3—Three-fourths of time spent in attention-getting behavior.
4—Verbally or nonverbally demands constant attention.

F. NEGATIVE RESPONSE FROM OTHERS

0—Evokes no negative responses.
1—Evokes 1 negative response.
2—Evokes 2 negative responses.
3—Evokes 3 or more negative responses during session.
4—Evokes numerous negative responses from others and therapist must take some action.

for well-defined ratings that describe the patient's progress in the treatment program. By using the scale, the occupational therapist can develop a sharply focused treatment program and then clearly communicate what is taking place in treatment to other departments.

Table 2, Part III continues on page 142.

Acknowledgments
The authors wish to acknowledge the efforts of Carol Draeger, O.T.R., who developed the initial form, and Gerald Sharrott, O.T.R., Beth Robinson, O.T.A., Jill Richards, O.T.R., and Mike R. Buben, O.T.R., who assisted in developing the definitions and the final format.

REFERENCES
1. McDonald M: Blue Cross fights milieu therapy. *Psychiatric News* 10: 1-28, 1975
2. A Statement by the Blue Cross Association and National Association of Blue Shield Plans. Prepared for Subcommittee on Retirement, Insurance, and Health Benefits of the Post Office and Civil Service Committee United States House of Representatives, September 16, 1974, pp. 1-9
3. Fidler, G, Fidler J: *Occupational Therapy: A Communication Process in Psychiatry*, New York, The Macmillan Company, 1963
4. Mosey AC: *Three Frames of Reference for Mental Health*, Thorofare, NJ, Charles B. Slack, 1970
5. Mosey, AC: *Activity Therapy*, New York, Raven Press, 1973

TABLE 2

PART III. TASK BEHAVIOR

A. ENGAGEMENT
0—Needs no encouragement to begin task.
1—Encourage once to begin activity.
2—Encourage 2 or 3 times to engage in activity.
3—Engages in activity only after much encouragement.
4—Does not engage in activity.

B. CONCENTRATION
0—No difficulty concentrating during full session.
1—Off task less than one-fourth time.
2—Off task half the time.
3—Off task three-fourths time.
4—Loses concentration on task in less than 1 minute.

C. COORDINATION
0—No problems with coordination.
1—Occasionally has trouble with fine detail, manipulating tools or materials.
2—Occasional trouble manipulating tools and materials but has frequent trouble with fine detail.
3—Some difficulty in gross movement-unable to manipulate some tools and materials.
4—Great difficulty in movement (gross motor); virtually unable to manipulate tools and materials (fine motor).

D. FOLLOW DIRECTIONS
0—Carries out directions without problems.
1—Occasional trouble with more than 3 step directions.
2—Carries out simple directions-has trouble with 2.
3—Can carry out only very simple one step directions (demonstrated, written, or oral).
4—Unable to carry out any directions.

*E. ACTIVITY NEATNESS
0—Activity neatly done.
1—Occasionally ignores fine detail.
2—Often ignores fine detail and materials are scattered.
3—Ignores fine detail and work habits disturbing to those around.
4—Unaware of fine detail, so sloppy that therapist has to intervene.

*F. ATTENTION TO DETAIL
0—Pays attention to detail appropriately.
1—Occasionally too concise.
2—More attention to several details' than is required.
3—So concise that project will take twice as long as expected.
4—So concerned that project will never get finished.

G. PROBLEM SOLVING
0—Solves problems without assistance.
1—Solves problems after assistance given once.
2—Can solve only after repeated instructions.
3—Recognizes a problem but cannot solve it.
4—Unable to recognize or solve a problem.

H. COMPLEXITY AND ORGANIZATION OF TASK
0—Organizes and performs all tasks given.
1—Occasionally has trouble with organization of complex activities that should be able to do.
2—Can organize simple but not complex activities.
3—Can do only very simple activities with organization imposed by therapists.
4—Unable to organize or carry out an activity when all tools, materials, and directions are available.

I. INITIAL LEARNING
0—Learns a new activity quickly and without difficulty.
1—Occasionally has difficulty learning a complex activity.
2—Has frequent difficulty learning a complex activity, but can learn a simple activity.
3—Unable to learn complex activities; occasional difficulty learning simple activities.
4—Unable to learn a new activity.

J. INTEREST IN ACTIVITIES
0—Interested in a variety of activities.
1—Occasionally not interested in new activity.
2—Shows occasional interest in a part of an activity.
3—Engages in activities but shows no interest.
4—Does not participate.

K. INTEREST IN ACCOMPLISHMENT
0—Interested in finishing activities.
1—Occasional lack of interest or pleasure in finishing a long term activity.
2—Interest or pleasure in accomplishment of a short term activity—lack of interest in a long term activity.
3—Only occasional interest in finishing any activity.
4—No interest or pleasure in finishing an activity.

L. DECISION MAKING
0—Makes own decisions.
1—Makes decisions but occasionally seeks therapist approval.
2—Makes decisions but often seeks therapist approval.
3—Makes decision when given only 2 choices.
4—Cannot make any decisions or refuses to make a decision.

M. FRUSTRATION TOLERANCE
0—Handles all tasks without becoming overly frustrated.
1—Occasionally becomes frustrated with more complex tasks; can handle simple tasks.
2—Often becomes frustrated with more complex tasks but is able to handle simple tasks.
3—Often becomes frustrated with any tasks but attempts to continue.
4—Becomes so frustrated with simple tasks that he refuses or is unable to function.

---

* Rate either Activity Neatness or Attention to Detail, not both.

Comprehensive Evaluation of

Basic Living Skills

Jean Starr Casanova
Julie Ferber

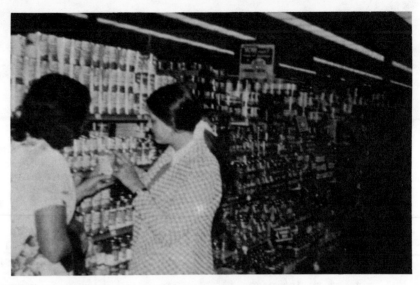

Figure 1 Observation of shopping skills for the *Practical Evaluation*

In this paper a rationale is established for an evaluation of basic living skills for chronic psychiatric patients living in mental institutions, and a comprehensive evaluation is presented. The advantages of this battery of tests over currently used activities of daily living scales are: it is specifically designed for psychiatric patients, it tests a wide range of skills, the items are graded in complexity, it can be administered in full or in part, and it has a scoring system and a summary that indicates the patient's functional status. The information gained from the evaluation improves staff communication about patient care and aids in the planning of the patient's future placement or treatment situation.

One of the primary functions of the occupational therapist is to minimize the disabling effects of a handicap. In the treatment of clients with physical disabilities concentration on basic living skills has long been recognized as an integral part of the rehabilitation process (1-7). Once a client has been evaluated in terms of these skills, the occupational therapist may, through activity or exercise, increase appropriate muscle strength and endurance; suggest, prescribe, and train the client in the use of adaptive equipment; and/or advise the client on the most simple or therapeutic procedure to follow in carrying out activities.

A review of current literature in psychiatry

reveals an increasing interest in the acquisition of basic living skills as an important part of the treatment of psychiatric clients. Many sources now contend that one of the primary reasons for the chronic psychiatric client's lack of adjustment to the community upon discharge is the inability to cope with the stresses of daily living (8-11). According to Broekema, Danz, and Schloemer:

> *"The chronic client is often unable to perform basic living skills appropriately . . . Basic living skill deficits are frequently seen in the areas of personal hygiene and appearance, money management, shopping skills, eating habits and cooking skills, use of public transportation, housekeeping skills, and the use of leisure time. For example, heavy application of makeup, torn hems, unshaven face, or inappropriate fashion makes the client appear out of place in the community and contributes to his isolation. Difficulty in performing these basic living skills adds further stress to the client's often tenuous adjustment and actively interferes with his integration into the community."* (11)

Thus, failure to acquire basic living skills can be considered a handicap in itself and must be dealt with as such. The importance of these skills is recognized and treatment in this area is offered in many psychiatric settings, but no detailed evaluation of basic living skills for psychiatric clinics has been published (2, 8-10, 12-16).

The Comprehensive Evaluation of Basic Living Skills (CEBLS) grew out of a practicum experience for a senior psychiatric occupa-

Jean Starr Casanova, O.T.R., is presently a staff therapist with Coordinated Health and Management Services, Milwaukee, Wisconsin.

Julie Ferber, O.T.R., is currently a staff therapist at Wassaic Developmental Center, Wassaic, New York.

TABLE 1

CHECK LIST FOR PERSONAL CARE AND HYGIENE

NAME _____

CLIENT NO. _____

SCORE _____

RATING

   Observe the client performing the following skills. Place the number corresponding to the client's correct level of function in the blank preceding each skill.

    4. Performs skill independently and correctly.
    3. Requires some assistance to perform skill correctly.
    2. Requires much assistance to perform skill correctly.
    1. Cannot perform skill independently or correctly.

Indicate N/A if the item is not applicable.

Toileting
____control of bowel and bladder needs
____get on toilet
____adjust clothing
____use of toilet paper
____get off toilet
____re-adjust clothing
____flush toilet

Brushing Teeth
____put toothpaste on brush
____proper brushing motions
____rinse mouth

Bathing
____operate faucets in sink
____operate faucets in tub or shower
____adequate use of soap
____adequate use of towel, wash cloth
____able to get in and out of bathtub
    or shower
____wash hands
____wash face

Hair Care
____shampoo hair
____dry hair
____set hair
____comb and brush hair in organized way

Dressing
____choose adequate clothing appropriate
    for physical/social situation
____put on undergarments
____put on shirts, blouses
____put on pants or dress
____operate fasteners
____put on loafer shoes
____put on and lace, tie shoes
____put on and buckle belt
____hang up clothing
____put on coat, hat, scarf, gloves
____glasses(clean, put back in case)

Make-Up
____apply base, powder, lipstick, eye make-up
____use proper amount when applying

Shaving
____adequate use of electric or safety razor
____use razor safely

Posture
____sit properly
____walk appropriately

Nail Care
____trim fingernails safely and neatly
____trim toenails safely and neatly

Housekeeping
____make a bed
____dust
____sweep/vacuum
____launder clothes
____iron clothes

SCORING

               sum of ratings_____
   number of N/A items X four_____
Personal Care and Hygiene Score_____

List any additional skills the client has difficulty performing.

administered by

_____
signature   title

_____
date

tional therapy course at the University of Wisconsin at Madison. The practicum took place at Mendota Mental Health Institute on a ward that operates a reality-oriented therapeutic milieu and in which the treatment emphasis is on dealing with the manifest problems of daily living. Before the development of the CEBLS, a battery used to evaluate chronic psychiatric clients, there was no established procedure for evaluating the broad spectrum of basic living skills, even though a client's deficits in these areas were the focus of treatment. At Mendota, the CEBLS improved occupational therapy treatment because it is based on specific areas of deficit exhibited by a client, thus eliminating trial and error or redundant treatment.

The occupational therapy program supports the treatment philosophy of reality orientation primarily by providing instructions in basic living skills, which include not only the traditionally perceived dressing, grooming, hygiene, and cooking activities, but also skills of intellectual and social functioning that are important in living a normal life. For example, intellectual skills include the ability to balance a checkbook, to budget money, to write a comprehensible sentence, to read, and to tell time. The social skills incorporate more subjective qualities such as the ability to relate to others in a group situation.

The occupational therapist uses discussion and role playing in simulated real-life situations to teach these basic living skills. The treatment approach is different for each client and depends upon his level of function and individual needs.

Description of the CEBLS

The content of the CEBLS resulted from a combination of many different evaluations of basic living skills from the treatment areas of physical disabilities (1, 2, 4-7, 17) and psychiatry (18, 19), as well as the common treatment concerns of psychiatric clinics. The skills are divided into three sections. The *Personal Care and Hygiene* section evaluates the client's ability to clothe, wash, and groom himself and to perform light housekeeping tasks. In the *Practical Evaluation* section, the client plans and prepares a meal and uses public transportation and the telephone. The *Written Evaluation* tests the client's ability to read, to write, to understand time, to solve math problems, and to manage money.

The skills in each section are scored on a rating scale from one to four, with four indicating the highest level of independence. The directions for scoring the *Personal Care and Hygiene* and the *Practical Evaluation* are shown on their respective checklists. Since the *Written Evaluation* is completed by the client, a separate *Written Evaluation Score Sheet* is used for scoring this section. If information is sought in only one area, then only that section of the battery need be given. For example, if

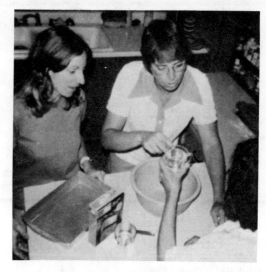

Figure 2 The ability to follow a recipe is evaluated during the *Practical Evaluation*

the client is a male and his wife will be cooking for him upon his return home, the *Practical Evaluation* may not reveal some of the deficits important to his successful re-entry into the home environment.

A client is encouraged to complete as many items as he can in each section, but if he is unable to complete the simple items, he need not answer the more complicated items. For example, if a client cannot solve any of the math problems, he will not be able to balance a checkbook, therefore, those problems need not be presented.

Administration of the CEBLS

Since the time involved in the administration of the CEBLS could take as long as eight hours, it is not intended for use with acute clients, in crisis intervention, or in short-term treatment facilities.

The nursing staff can complete *Personal Care and Hygiene Checklist* more efficiently since they generally have the most intimate contact with the client. They can fill out the checklist in a matter of minutes. Reliability of using ward staff to gather this type of data was obtained in a study of the retarded by Abelson and Payne (20), and by Dinnerstein, Lowenthal, and Dexter (2) in an evaluation of of daily living skills for the physically handicapped. Although a reliability study remains to be done for the entire CEBLS, it appears that reliability as shown in the above studies could be generalized to a psychiatric setting for the *Personal Care and Hygiene Checklist*.

The occupational therapy staff who administer the *Practical Evaluation* observes the client while he/she plans a menu, makes a shopping list, telephones a store, uses public transportation to get to the store, shops for groceries, prepares a meal, serves it to friends, and cleans up afterwards. The *Practical Evaluation Checklist* is completed as

The American Journal of Occupational Therapy

TABLE 2

CHECK LIST FOR PRACTICAL EVALUATION

NAME_____

CLIENT NO._____

SCORE_____

RATING

Observe the client performing the following skills. Place the number corresponding to the client's correct level of function in the blank preceding each skill.

    4. Performs skill independently and correctly
    3. Requires some assistance to perform skill correctly.
    2. Requires much assistance to perform skill correctly.
    1. Cannot perform skill independently.

Indicate N/A if the item is not applicable.

PART ONE: Meal Planning
_____knowledge of basic four
_____menu planning
_____formation of grocery list

PART TWO: Telephone
_____use of telephone book
_____depositing dime
_____dialing
_____asking information
_____use appropriate social behavior on phone ("hello," "thank you," etc.)
_____retaining information

PART THREE: Bus
_____what bus to take
_____location of bus stop
_____distance from bus stops to hospital and store
_____times bus arrives at bus stops
_____time it takes to walk to bus stop
_____how to board bus
_____how much money bus costs
_____where to stand at stop
_____how to tell which bus to get on
_____how long to stay on the bus
_____where to get off
_____how to inform bus driver to stop
_____how much time it takes to get to store, do shopping and get back
_____how much time at disposal
_____what bus to take back

PART FOUR: Shopping
_____comparative shopping
_____look for quality in fruits, vegetables, etc.
_____pay clerk
_____check change
_____put things away in proper place

PART FIVE: Meal Preparation
_____can follow recipe
_____get things from refrigerator
_____get utensils and pans from cupboard
_____handle milk carton
_____break eggs
_____operate small appliances (toaster, electric mixer, etc.)
_____adequate stirring techniques
_____peel, cut, fruits/vegetables
_____can prepare fried foods
_____can prepare baked foods
_____can prepare boiled foods

PART SIX: Serving and Eating
_____serve food appropriately
_____offer food to others
_____pass food at table
_____appropriate use of napkin
_____maintain suitable posture
_____appropriate use of utensils
_____drinking from cup or glass
_____pour from pitcher
_____adequate chewing motions

PART SEVEN: Meal Clean-Up
_____clear table
_____put away food
_____scrape and stack dishes
_____wash dishes
_____wash pots and pans
_____wipe off work areas, table
_____dry dishes
_____put dishes, pans, utensils, in proper storage areas
_____remove dishwater
_____clean dish cloth and sink
_____sweep floor

SCORING

           sum of ratings:_____
number of N/A items X four:_____
Practical Evaluation Score:_____

List any additional skills the client has difficulty performing.

administered by

_____
signature   title

_____
date

soon as possible after the observation period.

The *Written Evaluation* is also administered by a member of the occupational therapy staff and takes approximately one half to one hour. The presence of the therapist is necessary since some of the answers are given orally. This also allows the client to ask any questions he may have about the test. The problems on the *Written Evaluation* are graded from simple to complex. The ability to solve simple problems appear to be an incentive for trying other problems.

A *Summary Sheet* is included that provides space for the scores, for a concise summary of each of the three evaluation sections, and for comments on impressions made during the administration of the battery. The *Summary Sheet* can be inserted into the client's chart, and provides a gross picture of the client's current level of functioning, as well as the degree of independence, which can indicate the direction, and the amount and nature, of further care and treatment.

Conclusion

The primary advantage of the CEBLS are: a wide range of skills is tested; the items are graded in complexity; it is administered by the staff who work with the client in a given skill area, it is therefore efficient to administrate and relatively accurate in results; the evaluation may be administered in part or in whole; and the objective system makes scoring specific, accurate, and efficient. These advantages have implications for the effectiveness of the CEBLS as a tool for evaluation, treatment, and future research.

Given on admission and again before discharge, the CEBLS scores can be used to indicate a client's response to treatment and/or the effectiveness of treatment. It might also be used to correlate with the rate of success in independent living. Statistical data of this sort, that is, correlations between the acquisition of basic living skills and actual level of independence, are not only necessary to evaluate the effectiveness of treatment, but also to add validity to occupational therapy treatment already being carried out in many reality-oriented psychiatric clinics.

Acknowledgments

The CEBLS is an expansion of an evaluation developed by Kay Conzemius and Cheryl Thorsen while they were occupational therapy students at Mendota Mental Health Institute under the direction of Georgia Spielman, O.T.R.

NOTE: The complete CEBLS, including equipment list and specific procedures, can be obtained for $1 from Jean Casanova, 2185 North Hi Mount Boulevard, Milwaukee, Wisconsin 53208.

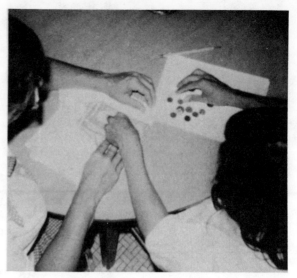

Figure 3 A client making money transactions during the *Written Evaluation*

REFERENCES

1. Sarno JE, et al: The Functional Life Scale. *Arch Phys Med* 54:214-220, 1973
2. Dinnerstein AJ, Lowenthal M, Dexter M: Evaluation of a rating scale of ability in activities of daily living. *Arch Phys Med* 46:579-584, 1965
3. Bruett TL, Overs RP: A critical review of 12 ADL scales. *Phys Ther* 49:857-861, 1969
4. Gauger AB, Brownell WM, Russell WW, Retter RW: Evaluation of levels of subsistence. *Arch Phys Med* 45:286-292, 1964
5. Schoening HA, Anderegg L, et al: Numerical scoring of self-care status of patients. *Arch Phys Med* 46:689-697, 1965
6. Schoening HA, Iversen IA: Numerical scoring of self-care status: A study of the Kenny self-care evaluation. *Arch Phys Med* 49:221-229, 1968
7. Stanfiel JD, Tompkins WG, Brown HL: A daily activities list and its relation to measures of adjustment and early environment. *Psychol Rep* 28:691-699, 1971
8. Marx AJ, Test MA, Stein LI: Extrahospital management of severe mental illness: Feasibility and effects of social functioning. *Arch Gen Psychiatr* 29:505-511, 1973
9. Hersen M: Independent living as a threat to the institutionalized mental patient. *J Clin Psychol* 25: 316-318 1969
10. Harrand G: Rehabilitation programs for chronic patients, I. Testing the potential for independence. *Hosp Community Psychiatry* 18:376-377, 1967.
11. Broekema MC, Danz KH, Schloemer CU: Occupational therapy in a community aftercare program. *Am J Occup Ther* 29: 22-27, 1975
12. Goering P: A bridge between: The transition from hospital to community. *Menninger Perspectives* 2:26-29, 1971
13. Bell G, et al: An ADL upgrading program for adolescent girls. *Can J Occup Ther* 39:137-141, 1972
14. Nussbaum K: Objective assessment of degree of psychiatric impairment: It is possible? *Johns Hopkins Med J* 133:30-37, 1973
15. Bolton BF, Butler AJ, Wright GN: Clinical versus statistical prediction of client feasibility. *Wisc Studies Voc Rehab Monogr*, No. 7: 68, 1968
16. Rosen M, Floor L, Baxter D: Prediction of community adjustment: A failure at cross-validation. *Am J Ment Defic* 77:111-112, 1972
17. Donaldson SW, et al: A unified ADL evaluation form. *Arch Phys Med* 54:175-179, 1973
18. Campbell AC: Aspects of personal independence of mentally subnormal and severely subnormal adults in hospital and in local authority hostels. *Int J Soc Psychiatry* 17: 305-310, 1971
19. Katz MM, Lyerly SB: Methods for measuring adjustment and social behavior in the community: Rationale, description, discriminative validity and scale development. *Psychol Rep* 13:503-535, 1963
20. Abelson RB, Payne D: Regional data collection in state institutions for the retarded; Reliability of attendant ratings. *Am J Ment Defic* 73:739-744, 1969

R30206

The Task-Oriented Group As A Context for Treatment*

GAIL S. FIDLER, O.T.R.†

ABSTRACT

Increasing recognition of the influence of man's social and cultural environment on behavior has extended the parameters of patient treatment. Such developments are manifested in the gradual melding of sociologic, psychoanalytic and learning theories and the emerging focus on ego functions and adaptive skills. This paper explores concepts of the task-oriented group within this context, offering a definition and delineation of purpose for its use in occupational therapy as a remedial-learning experience for the schizophrenic patient.

Returning the hospitalized psychiatric patient to an acceptable, productive role in the community and appreciably reducing the rate of recidivism is a complex problem. Such concern has led to intensive studies of both psychotherapeutic procedures and organizational structures of the mental hospital. The impact of sociologic inquiry into the mental hospital has been to add another dimension to our theoretical constructs regarding both individual feeling and behavior and conditions under which such behavior may be altered to the benefit of the patient.

Understanding the significance of the social matrix in which the patient functions has brought more sharply into focus factors influencing ego function in addition to the intrapsychic and interpersonal. As early as 1931 Harry Stack Sullivan[1] spoke of the importance of the social setting to the behavior of schizophrenic patients. Literature of the past fifteen years is replete with investigations and analyses of the import of environment on patient functioning.[2-4] This focus has inevitably led to theoretical and practical attempts to relate concepts of ego psychology to social theories of the environment.[5,6] Such linkage as well as the social scientists's interest in group phenomena has given impetus to increased exploration of the many facets of group process and group therapy

Group Process and Group Psychotherapy

Group psycotherapy is firmly established as a method of treatment of mental illness. It has its

and their applicability to patient care and treatment.

foundation in psychodynamic personality theories and emerged in America essentially from a psychoanalytic frame of reference stressing personality change through exploration of intrapsychic and interpersonal pathology believed to be at the root of conflicts and problems.[7-10] The group has been seen as a setting in which the individual with the help of the therapist and through sharing with other members could explore and work through those unconscious conflicts and problems which inhibited personality change and growth. Such a frame of reference places primary importance on unconscious phenomena and explores here-and-now feelings and behavior as a means to arriving at an awareness and understanding of intrapsychic conflict. The role of the therapist is to facilitate such awareness and elicit the involvement and help of members in exposing and working through personal conflicts and problems.

The social scientist's interest in groups emanated from a sociologic orientation rather than from personality theories. This frame of reference stresses the impact of society and the group on individual behavior and seeks to explain behavior on the basis of the nature of the society in which man lives. This ideology is exemplified by Lewin[11] who theorized that behavior was determined by the situation in which it occurred as well as by personality factors. The sociologist's beginning involvement with groups was via his interest in organizational structure and this was reflected in an early focus on the use of the group to accomplish a task or to effect a change in management.[12] Such experimentation inevitably led to the development of theories regarding the use of such groups in teaching and learning.[13]

*The work described here was carried out at New York State Psychiatric Institute from 1963-1966.

†Director, Activities Therapy, Hillside Hospital, Glen Oaks, N.Y. Associate in Rehabilitation Medicine, College of Physicians and Surgeons, Columbia University. Formerly, Director of Professional Education, Dept. of Occupational Therapy, New York State Psychiatric Institute.

Theories and practice in the field of group dynamics have focused on the group as a dynamic force in facilitating learning and behavioral change. Emphasis on "the group" as the primary change-producing agent thus accentuates the importance of exploring the dynamic forces within the here-and-now group to both understand and facilitate such change. Group structure and membership roles become significant and individual feeling and behavior is viewed only as it contributes to or deters from cohesive structure and contributory roles.

ayuh"

As the group therapist, the psychiatrist and social scientist work collaboratively in an attempt to resolve some of the complex problems of the mentally ill, these two seemingly disparate theories have moved closer together. There are increasing efforts to integrate not only practice of group psychotherapy and group dynamics but also the more apparently divergent concepts of each. One has but to survey current literature to be impressed with the ubiquity of these efforts.

Experimental Studies

In "Social Psychology In Treating Mental Illness,"[14] Fairweather describes an experimental approach combining the psychodynamic doctrine of patient treatment with theories of social psychiatry, sociology and the small group. This program focused around patient-led, small task-oriented groups for the chronic regressed schizophrenic. Such an approach, Dr. Fairweather points out, "called for an altered perception of the patient's role from that of a subordinate to that of a peer group member with responsibilities to himself and his group members, and away from that of a passive recipient of treatment to that of an active participant within the limits of his abilities, despite existing psychopathology."[15] Tasks around which these autonomous patient-led groups were organized concerned the current and future living of each member. Thus task levels ranged according to the capacity of the patient from personal care and ward responsibility to responsibility for vocational planning and placement. These groups provided opportunity for patients to explore and develop their capacities for independent function, creating patient roles within the hospital which were more consistent with those of the outside community.

This study makes an important contribution to patient programming and treatment. Although it concerned itself entirely with problems of the chronic regressed schizophrenic, there is much that would seem to be directly applicable to other patient categories and most certainly to patient groups in rehabilitation settings.

Marshall Edelson's experimental study[6] at the University of Oklahoma was concerned with "making possible the meaningful integration of both group experience and individual psychotherapy in an intensive treatment program designed to accomplish fundamental alteration in characterological disorder rather than solely rapid relief of acute secondary symptomatology and restoration of an ability to function marginally in the community." This work combines ego psychology and group dynamics in a therapeutic community as the basis for intensive psychotherapy. The focus of this study is aptly stated by Dr. Edelson in these words, "The therapeutic community (and small group) is organized to provide opportunities for the appearance of the patient's characterological difficulties or way of life as these are expressed in activities and other aspects of group living and for the confrontation of the patient and the group with these difficulties and their consequences to the life of the (hospital) community."

A third innovative experiment is Robert Morton's use of the laboratory method with psychiatric patients.[17] This study describes the design and use of a group process laboratory training program for hospitalized mental patients. The laboratory is a structured, small group experience designed to bring about change by establishing conditions whereby participants are forced to test their assumptions regarding interpersonal and group relations. Not only is the application of the laboratory experience to hospitalized psychiatric patients a creative innovation, but it is even more provocative to learn that these were autonomous, staff-leaderless, patient groups. Morton agrees with Fairweather that cohesive, decision-making groups with psychotics cannot be explored if a professional leader is present. It is their contention that even the most permissive therapist-leader reenforces dependency for the psychotic to a detrimental extent. This experiment provides some useful and creative postulates regarding small group experiences for psychiatric patients and should stimulate further research and study in the adaptation of this technique in treatment and rehabilitation programs.

It is interesting to note that in follow-up studies on the Morton experiment only two findings seemed to be suggestive.[18] Training laboratory patients were employed a mean of 5.92 months during the nine months' follow-up period whereas the group therapy patients were employed 4.70 months ($p > .10$). In the Fairweather study, patients participating in the small-group program were significantly better than the control group in community adjustment with regard to areas of employment, verbal communication with others and friendships.

These three experimental studies are examples of the way in which the small group is being used and adapted to meet treatment needs and essentially bridge the apparent gap between theories of individual psychodynamics and sociology.

The Task Group in Occupational Therapy

Development of task-oriented treatment groups approximately four years ago within the occupational therapy program at New York State Psychiatric Institute emanated from several not unrelated observations. First, the increasing conviction that as patients engaged in activities or created objects they expressed characterological difficulties and that attention to these problems as they emerged and were operant in the here and now seemed to be of benefit to the patient. Second, a seemingly evident relationship between problems evidenced by the patient in his activity experiences and difficulties he encountered in the work-a-day world. Third, the nature of the occupational therapy setting which expects active involvement in doing, provides a microcosm of life-work situations which can be seen and explored as they occur rather than in retrospect. Fourth, recognition of the relationships between verbal skills and learning and our experience which indicated that learning and concomitant growth were enhanced when problems in doing were identified and explored. Finally, our belief that the shared, small group experience is conducive to the exploration and amelioration of some problems in ego function.

Groups were organized with approximately eight members selected on the basis of their particular difficulties in doing and being productive as well as their readiness and need for a small group experience. All patients admitted to these early groups were male schizophrenics and placement in a given group was determined by the level of ego function. Meetings were held three to four times a week for periods of one and one-half hours. Each group was responsible for choosing its own common task and arriving at a consensus regarding procedures for accomplishing that task.

Definition and Purpose

Task as it relates to such groups is defined as any activity or process directed toward creating or producing an end product or demonstrable service for the group as a whole and/or for persons outside of the group. Some examples of

tasks chosen by these groups were: publishing a newspaper, cooking, building a playhouse for the childrens' service, gardening, organizing a patient council, play reading and ward decoration and improvement.

The intent of the task-oriented group is to provide a shared working experience wherein the relationship between feeling, thinking and behavior, their impact on others and on task accomplishment and productivity can be viewed and explored. Alternate patterns of functioning can be considered and tested within the context of the here and now, to the end that such learning may induce ego growth and improve function. Task accomplishment is not the purpose of the group but hopefully the means by which purpose is realized. It is seen as the catalytic agent which elicits behavior and interaction, brings into focus both functional capacities and limitations, facilitates collaboration in working through problems and provides a concrete reality factor against which to measure learning and achievement. Furthermore, the task provides a frame of reference which helps to keep in focus what is relevant to explore and work through and what conflicts and issues belong more appropriately in other treatment settings. In such a group, issues and problems which directly effect the cohesiveness and/or task accomplishment are the appropriate agenda items.

Such groups are not unique in eliciting or diagnosing conflicts of the schizophrenic but it would seem that use of a common task within a small group setting does facilitate delineation of certain problems and their amelioration. Responsibility for selecting and accomplishing a task provides opportunity for the group to explore problem-solving and decision-making skills, to have concrete evidence of their ability to function as well as to identify those expectations which give rise to conflict. The expectation that an activity needs to be chosen and implemented makes it necessary for the group to look at concepts regarding self and others that have impaired problem-solving skills and gives impetus to working toward their resolution.

The ability to perceive cause and effect relationships is a well-recognized problem of the schizophrenic and learning in this area requires consistent, repeated opportunities to see and have evidence of cause and effect. The task-oriented group with its focus on the relationship between feelings, thinking, behavior and task achievement thus creates excellent learning opportunities. Following through on a task procedure, the nature of doing or not doing, gives ample confirmation of cause and effect regarding behavior and function. When task responsibility must be shared and when the nature of one's doing is viewed in terms of its contribution to the group, such learning is further amplified.

Reality testing through consensual validation is an essential process in every group and is of particular value to the schizophrenic. In addition to the shared reality indigenous to group structure and interaction, a clearly delineated task with standard procedures and techniques provides a shared reality from which perceptions can be tested and shared. Shared participation in an activity, the necessary interdependence makes possible an objective, demonstrable assessment of one's capacities and limitations. One of the values of the task-oriented group is the consensual validation of the patients' capacity to grow and change as evidenced in the accomplishment of a task.

The need to work together as well as talk together about one's doing contributes to learning to conceptualize and verbalize more accurately and directly. Identification of problems in functioning, discussion of these as well as exploration of alternatives, combines feeling, behavior and cognition and provides the necessary components of learning and change. The shared decision-making, working experiences available in these groups and the opportunity to explore and work through problems that interfere with satisfactory function make integrated learning possible. If we are to teach new and better ways of functioning then we need to combine the patient's doing with his thinking and bring such relationships into awareness in order that he may integrate such learning.

Collaboration on a concrete, clearly defined task encourages more direct and clear communication and coupled with group support provides a safe area in which to practice such skills. In addition, experiences in working and sharing help the schizophrenic to begin to perceive and conceptualize his needs within the context of gratification potential with increasing awareness of his own potential for obtaining gratification rather than the expectation of rejection or frustration outside himself.

The task-oriented group with its focus on function related to here-and-now tasks and doing their corresponding responsibilities bears a closer resemblance to living in the outside community and provides learning which correlates more directly with those skills and expectations required in community adjustment.

It would seem useful at this time to make some distinction between these groups and verbal psychotherapy and delineate some values to the patient when both experiences are cor-

related. Within the task-oriented group setting, issues concerning feelings, perceptions and behavior are discussed and explored only insofar as they are shared by others and impede or contribute to the problem-solving and/or activity accomplishment of the group. Personal, intra-psychic and historical determinants are not emphasized but are reserved for investigation in psychotherapy. Many personal and interpersonal perceptions and responses are elicited but not dealt with in the group. Psychotherapy provides an opportunity to explore these in depth, interrelating the unconscious, the historical, the personal and interpersonal to the here and now. Likewise, the task-oriented group provides a life-like action and doing setting in which insights gained in psychotherapy can be tested and consolidated through performance. The extent to which the task-oriented group and psychotherapy is correlated, the degree to which the purpose of each and their relationship is understood by both staff and patients, may well determine the extent to which treatment potential will be realized.

Leadership

The role of staff leader or therapist is an important determinant in the group. The function of the leader is to facilitate a process and milieu which will be conducive to the kind of learning and growth to which these groups are directed. The role of the leader is to make learning possible and not to assume responsibility for the group. Fulfillment of objectives will depend in good measure upon the leader's concepts of the mental patient and himself, as well as his skill in group and interpersonal processes.

Confidence in the inherent capacity of the group to be constructively self-determining, in its ability to ultimately recognize problems and reach realistic solutions to these, is a basic requirement. The foundation for such an attitude is belief in the right of the patient to be self-determining and a trust sufficient to allow exercise of freedom in exploring and testing his capacities. The group needs to be perceived as a therapeutic agent in its own right and leadership not as giving treatment but rather as the agent which helps to maximize the therapeutic and learning potential of the group.

It would seem that we tend to see patients as more fragile and thus needing more guidance and direction than seems warranted, at least on the basis of our experience. Perhaps this view of the patient is sustained by our need to be needed and important to the patient and to be recognized as having expertise. Autocratic leadership confirms for the patient his dependent position and tends to reaffirm his concept of self as inept and inadequate, while hesitant, aloof, permissiveness increases his sense of vagueness, unpredictability and limitlessness. Jay W. Fidler[19] defines the nature and extent of leader activity as it pertains to working with groups of psychotics, emphasizing the importance of active interventions based on sensitivity and understanding of the schizophrenic's particular problems with reality testing and other ego functions.

Such understanding and attitude sets however, are not the only basis of leadership skills for these groups. An intimate knowledge of and skill in problem-solving procedures is essential if the group is to be helped toward learning and developing such capacities. The extent to which problem-solving skills are an inherent part of the leader's way of thinking and functioning, his ability to make these appropriately apparent in identifying and dealing with issues will, by and large, determine the extent to which the group will be able to learn these processes and incorporate them into their functioning.

The extent and quality of the leader's receptivity to looking at himself and his relations to others, his freedom to participate in the learning and growth process, his ability to share perceptions and his openness to exploring all aspects of his functioning in the group, will either make learning and growth possible and a less threatening expectation for members, or confirm the many doubts and distortions they bring to the experience. The leader cannot expect from his group what he is not willing or able to do himself.

Problems of the Schizophrenic

Several aspects of the task-oriented group seem to bring into focus particular problems of the schizophrenic patient. *First*, decision-making is particularly difficult, especially the decision regarding task choice. There seems to be little question that groups expect the staff leader to make the choice for them. Some groups have insisted that this be done while others have behaved as though this was what they both wanted and expected. Groups have discussed their anxieties and conflicts about decision-making and these discussions suggest that problems in this area are related to dependency needs, fear of responsibility and the ultimate unacceptability of any decision they might make. It would seem that since they conceptualize themselves as worthless and "bad," any decision they make as well as its implementation will be worthless and "bad" and reflect basic ineptness and inadequacy. It would also seem they expect authority (the parental figure) to find any decision they make

unacceptable and inadequate. However, groups resent and many forcefully reject any task choice suggestion made by the leader. Ambivalence with regard to dependency, coupled with problems related to self concept compose one of the major conflictual areas which need to be worked through before meaningful growth can occur. Some of these findings would seem to support Fairweather's hypothesis that the dependency needs of the psychotic contraindicate staff leadership in task-oriented groups.

More recently we have been experimenting with a standard task for each beginning group in an effort to assess the extent to which decision-making problems may be altered or reduced when task choice is not an initial requirement. It is further hoped that such a procedure may lead to the development of a group diagnostic implement. However, the issue is not so much whether we deny or gratify the patient's dependency needs but rather how we can teach decision-making. It seems reasonable to conjecture that teaching such skills is a problem because of our limited understanding of the full nature of blocks to learning and thus our inability to identify and utilize techniques and procedures which facilitate learning.

Second, expectations of a shared group are frightening. It is as though fluid ego boundaries and difficulties in perceiving self as separate from others makes the closeness inherent in the small group an additional threat to identity. For some patients there is also the expectation that narcissistic needs will be frustrated and that sharing in a group will deny dependency needs. In addition, anticipation of shared doing seems to represent a threat to the schizophrenic's defenses and orientation. However, the structured, predictable aspects of the task and engagement with non-human objects increase opportunities for supportive consensual validation of observable abilities and facilitates identification of those perceptions which they share in common.

Third, great difficulty is experienced in problem-solving. Although some of the dilemmas operant in problem-solving are obviously related to dependency needs and authority relationships, difficulties which emerge in these groups suggest also that many patients have never learned even the basic procedures for identifying problems and exploring possible solutions, or have lost the ability to appropriately perceive and organize perceptions into logical concepts.

The combined thinking and doing, the cognitive perceptual skills at both the motor and verbal level inherent in the product of these groups, seem to bring clearly into focus disturbances and abilities in thinking and learning.

Fears associated with learning and related conflicts, disturbances in cognition and resultant dysfunction become readily evident. By the same token, the structure and focus of these groups make possible a sense of competence and learning less conflictual, the task providing evidence of movement toward achievement. Task activity furthermore creates opportunities to engage and relate in a more concrete way making it possible to be involved at a conceptual level commensurate with current capacities rather than consistently requiring a higher symbolic thinking order. The task also facilitates gradation of learning. As we become more knowledgeable about blocks to learning and their impact on function we should be able to articulate more meaningfully related learning experiences and use more fully the potential of the task-oriented group.

Finally, two generalized responses have been evident in these groups. There are those who find expectations of doing, the intrinsic action, learning and responsibilities, very threatening. These patients place a high premium on talking about their problems and intellectualization is used as a way of avoiding the more hazardous and fearful doing of a task. These groups have great difficulty arriving at a choice of task and such a decision may be prolonged for an inordinate period of time. Other patients seem driven to an excessive emphasis on the task, to a flight into activity as a means for avoiding bringing problems into awareness and working them through. Furthermore there would seem to be a correlation between the leader's characteristic way of functioning, what he perceives as the more important "therapeutic set" and a group's sustained focus or movement toward a more equitable balance between these two responses.

One further observation would seem to be useful and this relates to the kind of task choices made by groups. There seems to be an identifiable relationship between the task selected by a group, the level and nature of their primary emotional needs and the conflicts surrounding these needs. Furthermore, task choice seems to reflect the group's progress or regression. Further study of this phenomenon should increase our understanding of need-gratifying processes and enhance our ability to make growth potential opportunities available to patients.

Returning the schizophrenic patient to the community as a potentially productive, contributing member with an increased capacity to sustain such a role, is a many faceted, complex problem. The task-oriented group represents one of many attempts to reduce the problem. It seems that at least it provides a structure wherein

dysfunction can be observed and explored. Hopefully these and other explorations will make it possible to ultimately articulate more clearly the essential factors of remedial processes. As we become increasingly able to inter-relate psychodynamic and sociologic concepts, as we enhance our knowledge of the cognitive process and its relationships to intrapsychic phenomena and overt behavior, our efforts may come closer to realizing the ultimate goal of satisfactory community living for our patients.

ACKNOWLEDGMENT

The author is indebted to Dr. Lothar Gidro-Frank and Dr. Eugene Friedberg for their interested support and to Miss Patricia Mayer, O.T.R., whose creative thinking and skillful leadership contributed so much to our learning.

REFERENCES

1. Sullivan, Harry Stack, "Socio-psychiatric Research: It's implications for The Schizophrenic Problem and mental Hygiene," *Amer J Psychiat* Vol. 10 (1931).
2. Stanton, A. H. and Schwartz, M. S., *The Mental Hospital*, Basic Books (1954).
3. Caudill, William, *The Psychiatric Hospital As a Small Society*, Harvard Univ. Press (1958).
4. Jones, Maxwell, *The Therapeutic Community: A New Treatment Method in Psychiatry*, Basic Books (1953).
5. Cummings, John and Cummings, Elaine, *Ego and Milieu*, Atherton Press, N.Y. (1963).
6. Edelson, Marshall, *Ego Psychology, Group Dynamics and The Therapeutic Community*, Grune & Stratton, N.Y. (1964).
7. Slavison, S., *Group Psychoanalytic Psychotherapy*, International Univ. Press, New York (1964).
8. Wolf, A., "The Psychoanalysis of Groups," *Amer J Psychother* Vol. 3 (1949).
9. Bach, George, *Intensive Group Psychotherapy*, The Ronald Press, N.Y. (1954).
10. Mullan, Hugh and Rosenbaum, Max, *Group Psychotherapy, Theory and Practice*, Glencoe Free Press (1962).
11. Lewin, Kurt, *Dynamic Theory of Personality*, McGraw Hill (1945).
12. Schien, Edger H. and Bennis, Warren, G., *Personal and Organizational Change Through Group Methods*, John Wiley & Sons, N.Y. (1965), 357-368.
13. Bradford, L., Gibb, Jack and Benne, K., *T-Group Theory & Laboratory Method*, John Wiley & Sons, N.Y. (1964).
14. Fairweather, George W., *Social Psychology In Treating Mental Illness*, John Wiley & Sons (1964).
15. *Ibid.* 14
16. *Ibid.* 6
17. Morton, Robert B., "The Uses of the Laboratory Mehtod in a Psychiatric Hospital," in *Personal and Organizational Change Through Group Methods*.
18. Johnson, D. L., Hanson, P. G., Rothaus, R., Morton R. B., Lyle, E. and Moyer, R., "Follow Up Evaluation of Human Relation Training for Psychiatric Patients," in *Personal and Organizational Change Through Group Methods*.
19. Fidler, Jay W., "Group Psychotherapy of Psychotics," *Amer J Orthopsychiat* Vol. XXXV, No. 4 (1965).

Structured Learning Therapy:

Development and Evaluation

Arnold P. Goldstein **N. Jane Gershaw** **Robert P. Sprafkin**

This paper describes the procedures, materials, and evaluation of Structured Learning Therapy, one of several skill training therapies to emerge in recent years. A number of issues are considered in regard to enhanced outcomes for such therapies, particularly means for more successful transfer of newly learned skills from therapy to real-life settings, and prescriptive use of such psycho-educational treatments.

Arnold P. Goldstein, Ph.D., is Professor of Psychology, Syracuse University, Syracuse, New York.

N. Jane Gershaw, Ph.D., is Psychologist, Veterans Administration Mental Hygiene Clinic, Veterans Administration Hospital, Syracuse, New York.

Robert P. Sprafkin, Ph.D., is Director of Veterans Administration Day Treatment Center, Veterans Administration Hospital, Syracuse, New York.

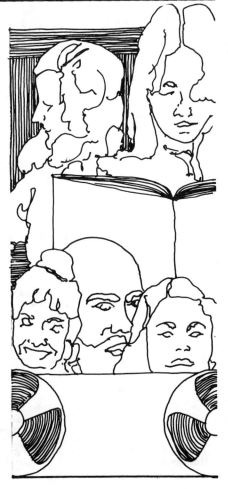

Occupational therapy has long been concerned with the training of diverse types of individuals in the skills and activities necessary for effective and satisfying daily living. This concern has variously focused upon teaching adaptive prevocational skills (1); enhanced problem-solving skills (2); new behavioral repertoires (3); organizational skills (4); social skills (5); adaptive skill training (6); and similar skill-enhancement targets. This emphasis upon building strengths to directly enhance real-life functioning, contrasted with the focus on undoing the psychopathology inherent in most dynamic psychotherapies, has become a recognized psychotherapeutic movement. Stimulated in large part by the behavior modification therapies in which treatment is viewed as a teaching-learning process, several *psycho-educational* approaches to altering behavioral deficiencies have emerged. These typically are sets of behavioral learning techniques that possess a clearly didactic emphasis designed to teach an array of social, coping, intrapersonal, and related skills. Psychotherapists implementing these approaches are often called "trainers," where patients are treated as "trainees" who meet in "classes" or "instructional groups," rather than "psychotherapy groups." Skill enhancement goals tend to focus on skills necessary for effective daily living. Although they have all appeared since 1970, these psycho-educational psychotherapies have firm roots in earlier works in which psychotherapy is more implicitly viewed as an educational process (7). These therapies or training programs, which are literal attempts at adult education, include the Adult Development Program (8), Conjugal Relationship Enhancement Program (9), Life Coping Skills Project

(10), Media Therapy (11), Personal Effectiveness Training (12), the Step Group Program (13), Structured Learning Therapy (SLT) (14, 15), and more focalized attempts to alter dating behavior (16), marital conflict (17), and the social skills of depressed individuals (18). These skill enhancement programs constitute a significant new direction within the broader behavior modification movement.

Yet these programs are far from equivalent. They differ in the specific techniques they use, the trainees they assist, the skills they enhance, and the quality and depth of their empirical support. This paper describes the nature, development, and research base for SLT—both as an illustration of the psycho-educational movement described above, and as an aid to the potential user in determining whether SLT is or is not prescriptively appropriate for a given patient population.

Development of Structured Learning Therapy

Unlike several of the other skill training programs, our interest in skill enhancement as treatment did not grow primarily from an involvement in social learning or behavior modification. Most notable was the consistent failure of almost all psychotherapeutic approaches when offered to lower social class clients. The failure was a result of an erroneous treatment strategy. Therapeutic efforts with such patients typically reflected a "conformity prescription." That is, the treatment offered remained unaltered from that typically offered most psychotherapy patients—traditional, insight-oriented, and verbal psychotherapy. The patient was expected to conform to the role demands of this prescription, either "naturally," or via efforts at conformity

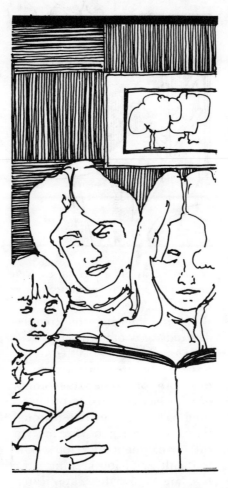

enhancement made by expectancy-altering (19), or relationship-improving interventions (20). The general failure of these attempts to make the patient fit the therapy led to a contrasting strategy, a "reformity prescription" in which efforts were to develop therapies to fit the (lower social class) patient. In implementing this latter strategy, the authors sought information about social class-linked preferred learning styles, and found it in literature dealing with comparative child-rearing practices. Middle-class child rearing, with its emphases upon feelings, intentions, self-regulation, motivation, and inner dynamics appeared to be excellent basic training for participation in insight-oriented therapies. In marked contrast, a

focus upon compliance with external authority instead of self-regulation, concern with consequences and not intentions, emphasis upon action and not introspection, all seemed to characterize child rearing in the lower social class home. Such a learning style, it was reasoned, would better prepare the lower-class person for a therapy that was concrete and behavioral; that relied heavily upon the use of external, authoritative example; that encouraged "learning by doing"; and that provided immediate feedback. With these considerations in mind, SLT was initiated.

Procedures and Materials

SLT consists of modeling, role playing, social reinforcement, and transfer training. Small groups of patient-trainees listen to audiotapes of a person (the model) performing the skill behaviors the patient is to learn (i.e., *modeling*); they are given considerable opportunity and encouragement to rehearse or practice the behaviors that have been modelled, in a manner relevant to dealing with the patient's own real-life problems (i.e., *role playing*); provided with positive feedback, approval, or reward as their role playing behavior becomes more like the behavior of the model (i.e., *social reinforcement*); and exposed to these three processes so that what the patient learns in the training setting will in fact be applied in a reliable manner on the job, on the ward, at home, or elsewhere in his real-life environment (i.e., *transfer training*).

Before developing specific training materials, such as modeling audiotapes, certain trainees had to be chosen for the initial focus. Adult, chronic psychiatric inpatients and outpatients were chosen for two reasons. First, the vast majority of hospitalized psychotic patients in the United States are of the lower social class. Second, to increase the likelihood of both their being discharged from the hospital and functioning successfully in the community, a training program emphasizing the development of effective daily living skills seemed most appropriate. In response to these considerations, the audio modeling tapes developed were of two types: basic skills and application.

Each basic skill tape is a vignette portraying the concrete behavioral steps that constitute a given skill. The 37 vignettes or tapes cover a broad spectrum of content areas relevant to the interpersonal, situational, social, and vocational demands faced by both psychiatric inpatients and those living in the community. They are organized into five groups: Conversations—beginning skills; conversations—expressing oneself; conversations—responding to others; planning skills; and alternatives to aggression.

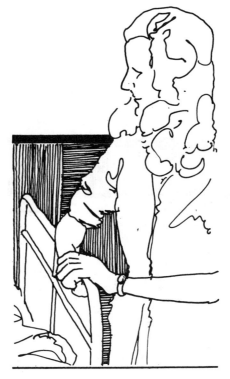

The 22 application tapes were developed to help patients bridge the gap between mastering basic skills and meeting the complex demands of community living. In these, combinations of three to eight Basic Skills are portrayed in sequences appropriate to the solution of a variety of real-life problems. Finding a place to live (through formal channels); moving in (typical); managing money; job seeking (difficult); and job keeping (strict boss) are just 5 of the 22 application tapes available.

In the SLT approach, a modeling tape is played, usually one per session, to a group of eight patients selected for their common skill deficits. The patients are aided by two trainers to enact the behavioral steps of the modeled skill as it applies to their real-life environment with significant others. Feedback procedures follow, emphasizing the effectiveness with which the patient employed the skill being taught. Such feedback is largely a function of how well the enactment portrayed or departed from the behavioral steps that constitute the skill. Finally, homework assignments are made in which patients are asked to practice their newly learned skills outside the training setting, in their real-

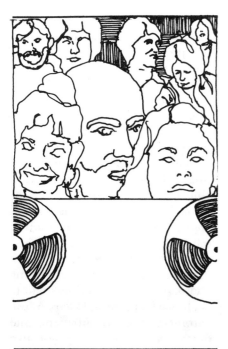

life environment. These assignments are systematically reported upon in the subsequent session.

In addition to the primary goal of teaching a variety of community living skills to clinical populations, another concern has been the selection and training of SLT trainers. Since its inception, many persons from a variety of disciplines were trained in a format that incorporates the four major components of SLT. Trainers are shown examples of SLT groups being led by experienced trainers (i.e., modeling); given an opportunity to practice leading SLT training groups (i.e., role playing); given feedback and corrective criticism regarding their performance as trainers (i.e., social reinforcement); and instructed on applications to actual trainee groups (i.e., transfer of training). Many of the trainers have been occupational therapists.

Evaluation

Several studies were conducted to evaluate the effectiveness of SLT for skill enhancement purposes. In many of these studies, changes in both the immediate post-therapy and later real-life (transfer) skill levels were examined. In two such investigations, Gutride, Goldstein, and Hunter (21, 22) found significant immediate post-therapy and later transfer changes in an array of social interaction skill behaviors in samples of withdrawn, asocial, psychiatric inpatients. Similarly significant findings were obtained in another series of studies that sought to increase patient assertiveness (23). Only immediate post-therapy (not transfer) changes were found in an investigation of the effects of SLT on patient level of role-taking skills (14). The immediate and transfer effects of SLT with adult psychiatric patients, for a number of the other expressive, responsive, planning and application skills are under study.

A second evaluation effort involved adolescent trainees, with special attention to teaching prosocial alternatives to aggression. Specifically, youngsters were taught self-control (24), negotiation (25, 26), empathy (27), perspective-taking (28), instruction-following (29), assertiveness (30), and cooperation (31). On-going studies with children and adolescents focus on such "alternative-to-aggression" skills with juvenile delinquent, emotionally disturbed, and mentally retarded youngsters. Others are studying the effectiveness of SLT with geriatric patients.

In addition to this research, a parallel concern has been the training of *helpers*. If many working class and middle class individuals develop daily living skills in their natural environment via procedures akin to modeling, role playing, and social reinforcement, perhaps an effective and efficient means of teaching helper skills to such persons might be SLT. Working primarily with working class persons employed in helper or potential helper capacities, SLT was used successfully to teach a wide array of relevant skills. These include teaching affective sensitivity to nurses (32-34); empathy to parents (35), home aides (36), and nurses (37); crisis intervention skills to police (38); confrontation skills to counselors (39); contingency management skills to hospital aides (40) and to teachers (41); and certain human relations-oriented managerial skills in an industrial context (42, 43).

These adult psychiatric, child, and adolescent, and helper skill development studies using SLT yield a number of conclusions that in general may be relevant for the

psycho-educational psychotherapy movement.

Conclusions

Skill Acquisition. SLT is a rapid and effective means of developing immediate skill acquisition. On post-tests *immediately* following training sessions, skill enhancement is evident across almost all types of trainees and types of skills.

Transfer of Training. It is only partially effective in developing enduring skill performance. The durability of skill enhancement is a function of skill complexity, adequacy of trainer attention to the transfer training procedures, and most importantly, the trainee's real-life reinforcement contingencies, i.e., the level of reward or payoff received by the trainee when be uses a given skill.

It is common for a therapy to succeed in the training setting, yet fail to succeed in transferring positive outcomes to the patient's real-life environment. The means of correcting this failure of transfer can be studied in several ways: greater use of in vivo training in which the training and application settings are identical or highly similar, greater use of real-life significant others as co-actors with the participants: for example, one's friends, employer, spouse; heavier reliance upon self-instructional and self-reinforcement procedures; and more concern with "rewarding the rewarder," that is, with discovering means for sustaining the continued interest and involvement of whoever in the patient's world—spouse, parent, friend, nurse—is serving as reinforcement dispenser.

Prescriptive Utilization. In order to enhance the effectiveness of this approach to either acquisition or transfer criteria, its procedures must be implemented in a manner pre-

scriptively tailored for *that* population. For example, with chronic schizophrenic trainees—whose attention span is short and whose motivation for skill enhancement is low—it is important to adapt the procedures to have 1. more active trainers 2. more social reinforcement and for lesser skill increments, 3. thinning reinforcers later, 4. shorter and more repetitive sessions, 5. fewer patients per group, 6. more relative attention to simpler levels of a given skill, 7. more total time per skill, and 8. less demanding homework assignments. Analogously prescriptive use of SLT with other trainee samples is recommended.

Prescriptive Outcome Research. The several psycho-educational therapies consist of a few dozen distinguishable didactic, social learning, and audiovisual procedures. The separate and combined contribution of these procedures to patient skill acquisition is a continuing research question. Not only must "instant traditionalism" and premature hardening of therapeutic packages be avoided, but new and varying procedural combinations must also be examined for their effectiveness with diverse groups of trainees and with diverse types of trainers.

Acknowledgment
The program reported in this paper was supported in part by PHS Grants No. MH 16426 and MH 13669 from the National Institute of Mental Health. Basic skills tapes, application tapes, the new trainer preparation tapes, and written materials may be obtained from Pergamon Press, Inc., Fairview Park, Elmsford, NY 10523.

Theses listed in references 24-41 are available through Syracuse University Interlibrary Loan, and the dissertations from Dissertation Abstracts, University of Michigan.

REFERENCES

1. Stein F: Ego-functioning in schizophrenia. Paper presented at the Fourth International Congress, World Federation of Occupational Therapists, London, 1966
2. Reilly M: Occupational therapy can be one of the great ideas of 20th century medicine. *Am J Occup Ther* 16:1-9, 1962
3. Diasio K, Jones M: The role of prevocational services in the rehabilitation of the young adult psychiatric patient. Paper presented at the Fourth International Congress, World Federation of Occupational Therapists, London, 1966
4. Smith AR, Tempone VJ: Psychiatric occupational therapy within a learning theory context. *Am J Occup Ther* 22:415-420, 1968
5. Fidler GS, Fidler Jay W: *Occupational Therapy*, New York: Macmillan, 1963
6. Mosey A: *The Three Frames of Reference in Mental Health*, Thorofare, NJ: Charles B. Slack, 1970
7. Authier J, Gustafson K, Guerney B, Kasdorf JA: The psychological practitioner as teacher: A theoretical-historical and practical review. *J Couns Psychol* 5:31-49, 1975
8. Armstrong H, Bakker C: Day hospitals or night school? Unpublished manuscript, University of Washington, 1971 (available from author)
9. Guerney B, Stollak G, Guerney L: The practicing psychologist as educator—an alternative to the medical practitioner model. *Prof Psychol* 2:271-282, 1971
10. Adkins W: Life skills. Structured counseling for the disadvantaged. *Pers Guid J* 49:108-116, 1970
11. Ivey A: Media therapy: educational change planning for psychiatric patients. *J Couns Psychol* 20:338-343, 1973
12. Liberman RP, King LW, DeRisi WJ, McCann M: *Personal Effectiveness*, Champaign, IL: Research Press, 1975
13. Authier J: A step group therapy program based on levels of interpersonal communication. Unpublished manuscript, University of Nebraska College of Medicine, 1973 (available from author)
14. Goldstein AP: *Structured Learning Therapy: Toward a Psychotherapy for the Poor*, New York: Academic Press, 1973
15. Goldstein AP, Sprafkin RP, Gershaw NJ: *Skill Training for Community Living: Applying Structured Learning Therapy*, New York: Pergamon Press, 1976
16. Christensen A, Arkowitz H: Preliminary report on practice dating and feedback as treatment for college dating problems. *J Couns Psychol* 21:92-95, 1974

17. Weiss R, Hops H, Patterson G: A framework for conceptualizing marital conflict: A technology for altering it, some data for evaluating it. In *Behavior Change: Methodology, Concepts and Practice*, L Hamerlynck, L Handy, E Mash, Editors. Champaign, IL: Research Press, 1973
18. Lewinsohn P, Weinstein M, Alper T: A behavioral approach to the group treatment of depressed persons: A methodological contribution. *J Clin Psychol* 26:525-532, 1970
19. Hoehn-Saric R, Frank JD, Imber SD, et al: Systematic preparation of patients for psychotherapy. I. Effects on therapy behavior and outcome. *J Psychiatr Res* 2:267-281, 1964
20. Goldstein AP: *Psychotherapeutic Attraction*, New York: Pergamon Press, 1970
21. Gutride M, Goldstein AP, Hunter G: The use of modeling and role playing to increase social interaction among asocial psychiatric patients. *J Cons Clin Psychol* 40:408-415, 1973
22. Gutride M, Goldstein AP, Hunter G, et al: Structured learning therapy with transfer training for chronic inpatients. *J Clin Psychol* 30:277-279, 1974
23. Goldstein AP, Martens J, Hubben J, et al: The use of modeling to increase independent behavior. *Behav Res Ther* 11:31-42, 1973
24. Swanstrom C: Training self-control in behavior problem children. Unpublished doctoral dissertation, Syracuse University, in progress.
25. Fleming D: Teaching negotiation skills to pre-adolescents. Unpublished doctoral dissertation, Syracuse University, 1976
26. Golden R: Teaching resistance-reducing behavior to high school students. Unpublished doctoral dissertation, Syracuse University, 1975
27. Berlin RJ: Teaching acting-out adolescents prosocial conflict resolution through structured learning training of empathy. Unpublished doctoral dissertation, Syracuse University, 1976
28. Trief P: The reduction of egocentrism in acting-out adolescents by structured learning therapy. Unpublished doctoral dissertation, Syracuse University, 1976
29. Fleming L: Training passive and aggressive educable mentally retarded children for assertive behaviors using three types of structured learning training. Unpublished doctoral dissertation, Syracuse University, 1976
30. Raleigh R: Individual versus group structured learning therapy for assertiveness training with senior and junior high school students. Unpublished doctoral dissertation, Syracuse University, 1976
31. Cobb FM: Acquisition and retention of cooperative behavior in young boys

through instructions, modeling, and structured learning. Unpublished doctoral dissertation, Syracuse University, 1973
32. Berlin RJ: Training of hospital staff in accurate affective perception of fear-anxiety from vocal cues in the context of varying facial cues. Unpublished master's thesis, Syracuse University, 1974
33. Healy JA: Training of hospital staff in accurate affective perception of anger from vocal cues in the context of varying facial cues. Unpublished master's thesis, Syracuse University, 1975
34. Lopez MA: The influence of vocal and facial cue training on the identification of affect communicated via paralinguistic cues. Unpublished master's thesis, Syracuse University, 1974
35. Guzzetta RA: Acquisition and transfer of empathy by the parents of early adolescents through structured learning training. Unpublished doctoral dissertation, Syracuse University, 1974
36. Robinson R: Evaluation of a structured learning empathy training program for lower socioeconomic status home aid trainees. Unpublished master's thesis, Syracuse University, 1973
37. Goldstein AP, Goedhart AW: The use of structured learning for empathy enhancement in paraprofessional psychotherapist training. *J Commun Psychol* 1:168-173, 1973
38. Davis C: Training police in crisis intervention skills. Unpublished manuscript, Syracuse University, 1974
39. Rosenthal N: Matching counselor trainees' conceptual level and training approaches: A study in the acquisition and enhancement of confrontation skills. Unpublished doctoral dissertation, Syracuse University, 1975
40. Lack DZ: Problem solving training, structured learning training and didactic instruction in the preparation of paraprofessional mental health personnel for the utilization of contingency management techniques. Unpublished doctoral dissertation, Syracuse University, 1975
41. Schneiman R: An evaluation of structured learning and didactic learning as methods of training behavior modification skills to lower and middle socioeconomic level teacher-aides. Unpublished doctoral dissertation, Syracuse University, 1972
42. Goldstein AP, Sorcher M: *Changing Supervisor Behavior*, New York: Pergamon Press, 1974
43. Moses J: *Supervisory Relationships Training: A New Approach to Supervisory Training. Results of Evaluation Research*, New York: Human Resources Development Department, AT&T, 1974

Occupational Role Acquisition:

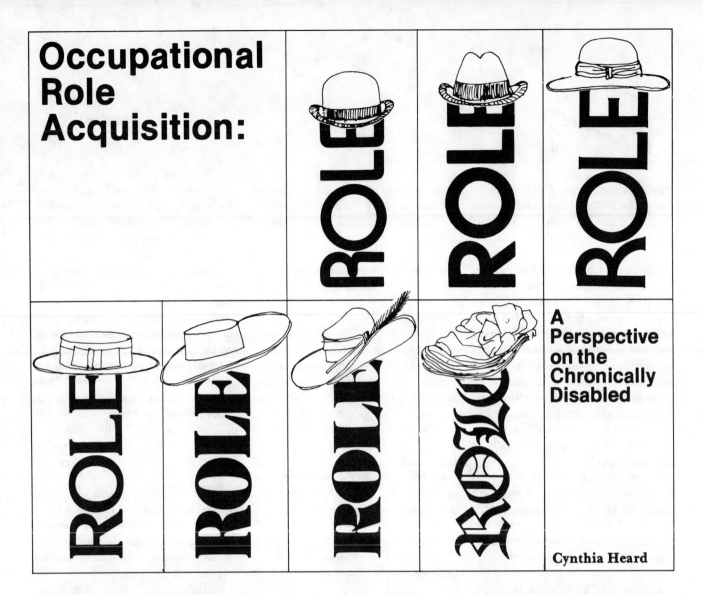

A Perspective on the Chronically Disabled

Cynthia Heard

Occupational therapists are aware that chronic disability restricts not only physical and mental skills, but also social skills and the resulting ability of the patient to function in society. The issue of quality of life for the chronically disabled requires assisting them in the acquisition of new, although not always remunerative, occupational roles. The occupational role defines daily activity and appropriation of time, as well as the contribution to society and societal worth. This article presents the sociological concepts of role, three critical points in conceptualization of the occupational role acquisition process, a model for evaluating and monitoring a patient's progress, and a case study.

Cynthia Heard, M.A., OTR, is director of special services for groups on-site occupational therapy program at California Youth Homes, Inglewood, California.

In the last decade, nearly half of all Americans have been been burdened with at least one chronic disease or impairment. Eighty-three percent of American deaths are the result of chronic disease (1,2). In Dubos' words:

The very process of living is a continual interplay between the individual and his environment, often taking the form of a struggle resulting in injury or disease . . . complete and lasting freedom from disease is but a dream. (3, p 18)

Throughout this paper, *chronic disease* refers to the presence of any physical, mental, or social handicap that disrupts or lessens man's capacities for participation in and adaptation to his environment.

With the steady increase in the chronically disabled population, the health system should have produced highly visible models of care to respond to the consumer's changing needs. However, the current medical system continues to invest the major part of its time, fiscal resources, and intervention strategies in the treatment of the acute phases of the disease process. Physical discomfort is reduced, pathological affects are lessened, and life is rescued and prolonged. There is a narrow focus on the latest life-saving devices or techniques without interest or foresight given to the *end of the hospital ramp* for the patient. Such a focus ignores the overwhelmingly traumatic and devastating changes in the lifestyle of the chronically disabled (4-6).

Occupational therapists have traditionally assisted chronically dis-

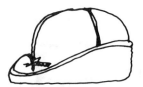

abled patients in their adaptation to daily life. They are aware that chronic disability restricts not only physical and mental skills, but also social skills and the resultant ability of the patient to function in society. Physical capacities are reduced, and the past lifestyle becomes fragmented. Many are permanently removed from the marketplace, a low value assigned them as a societal member not remuneratively employed, and marginal existence is begun. The skills and capacities of the chronically disabled as nonentities become lost in society and further reduce the opportunities for meaningful societal participation (5).

In response to the total health needs, occupational therapists are obligated to assist in adaptation to daily living in three areas—the physical function, the pscyhological image, and the social worth (7). Physical function is improved by the reactivation of daily living strategies with limited skills, and the psychological image is rebuilt and supported to form a new self-concept. Most overlooked is the societal worth, the contributory activities contained within the occupational role (8-10). The occupational behavior framework provides a perspective of chronic disability to include the occupational role, in addition to physical dysfunction and psychological processes.

Purpose

The purpose of this article is to identify knowledge in the area of occupational role acquisition. When the issue of quality, rather than quantity, of life for the chronically disabled arises, the disabled will require assistance in the acquisition of new, although not always remunerative, occupational roles. The following sections present a global description of role, and three points

necessary for placing the process of occupational role acquisition within the context of clinical application. A conceptual framework allows the ordering of occupational role acquisition into a model. Clinical applications of the material are also presented through a case study (*below*).

Role

The term *role* originated in the theatre and denoted conduct that adhered to certain "parts." The performer was expected to animate a certain ascribed social position (i.e., doctor, mother), with its unique characteristics, to make the character believable to the audience. The concept of role, most recently developed by social psychologists, is defined as the expected pattern of behavior associated with occupancy of a distinctive position in society (11). As Ralph Linton describes further:

A role represents the dynamic aspect of a status. The individual is socially assigned to a status and occupies it with relation to other statuses. When he puts the rights and duties which constitute the status into effect, he is performing a role . . . . Every individual has a series of roles deriving from the various patterns in which he participates and, at the same time, a role, general, which represents the sum total of these roles and determines what he does for his society and what he can expect from it. (12,p114)

Just as roles define one's societal status (worth) and expected behavior, our activity and time usage are equally defined and relegated according to the role demands. Kielhofner further defines the correlation between these areas. Roles are classified into three major categories—sexual, familial, and

occupational. Occupational roles include preschooler, student, worker, volunteer, homemaker, and retiree and serve as the boundary for this paper. Roles are not static, but dynamic, and change within both the context of a day and of the life cycle. Within a given 24-hour period, the roles may change frequently and include parent, spouse, worker, volunteer, and sibling. By contrast, the major lifetime roles are associated with developmental tasks and age-appropriate function. The occupational role becomes the activity in an individual's life that contributes to society and, thereby, defines the person's societal worth (8-10).

Three critical points for the clinical application of role were identified through a literature review. These points provide the background information for viewing occupational role acquisition as a process.

1. Habits and skills are components of role. The fulfillment of roles requires the presence of skills and habits. Skills are conscious manipulations of the environment and become action sequences for role. Habits are mastered skills that, with repetition, become automatic routines. Generalized habits serve to routinize behavior so that attention is directed only toward novel demands for skills. As new roles are acquired, skills are integrated into the habit structure. For example, a student hopefully learns promptness during classroom training. In this role, time management is a skill. In remunerative employment, the employer expects promptness as a habitualized routine. The employee's attention may be directed to the skills specialized for the job (13,14).

2. Role is the organizing component for competence in daily life. The performance of certain service tasks is unique to an occupational

Figure 1 The model of occupational role acquisition

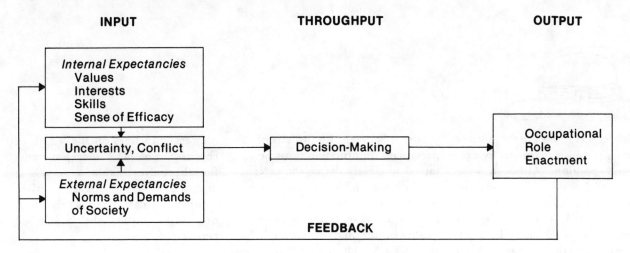

role. The ability to perform those tasks adequately comprises competent role performance. There is an orderly progression of occupational roles in the lifespan from player to student to worker, volunteer, or homemaker, and then retiree. The lifetime sequencing of occupational roles is similar to the process of metamorphosis. Life begins in the caterpillar stage, retreats into the cocoon, and emerges a butterfly. At each stage, the basic materials present are rearranged and transformed to adapt to the new functions of the next stage. Occupational role acquisition, then, is an ongoing process that transforms and builds on previously acquired skills to enable the individual to assume the demands of a new occupational role.

The transition between roles, particularly from the student to the worker, represents crisis points for the individual. The presence of a chronic disability hinders the ease of role acquisition and often provides an additional burden, particularly if former roles were not successfully mastered. The knowledge of occupational role acquisition will enable a therapist to develop strategies for assisting patients toward satisfactory role enactment.

3. The ease of occupational role acquisition is dependent upon the adaptive nature of the individual. Adaptation requires individuals to amend or elaborate on their skill pool and habit structure to meet the demands of the new role with the best advantage to themselves. In occupational role acquisition, adapta-

tion means the organization of behavior for role performance. With the increase in the number of role-taking and role-filling experiences, and individual acquires more ease and flexibility in entering into roles. The skilled role player is more flexible than the less skilled in adjusting to sudden, unforeseen changes in external role demands. The chronically disabled, with their impaired capacities, are restricted in exposures, and are also less flexible in their behavior strategies.

The Model
The process of occupational role acquisition and its components will be identified and ordered into a model to allow the clinician to evaluate and monitor a patient's ability to assume the proposed role. *General Systems Theory* provides conceptual models with which to organize relevant information (7). According to systems theory, a process consists of information inputs, a transforming throughput, an output, and feedback. In assuming a job, employees are provided with instructions (inputs) for filing records. They decide (throughput) the extent to which they can and will follow these instructions, and do so (output). They receive messages (feedback) from their supervisor, peer, or themselves regarding their progress. In this fashion, the necessary ingredients for occupational role acquisition, the throughput transformation, the output of actual role behavior, and the feedback for acceptability of the behavior, are identified (Figure

1).

Inputs. In the acquisition of an occupational role, the inputs include internal and external expectations of the role.

Internal Expectancies. Individuals bring their skills and habits to the role acquisition process. Internal expectations of the role are based on values, interest, skills, and a sense of efficacy (15,16). Values represent the goals and commitments for acquiring a particular role and are responsible for differences in interpretation of role demands (17,18). The individuals' interests determine the commitment to internalization of external role demands and indicate choice states for a course of action (19).

Individuals acquiring a new role are faced with the task of fulfilling, optimally, the role expectations. How well the task is performed is dependent on the available relevant skill pools and habit structure, and the ability to generalize the skills into a new role. Skills, then, determine the role that may be fulfilled. Individuals who believe in and use their skills to effect a change feel a sense of power in the control of their destiny (20). This sense of efficacy determines the amount of role making or change in external demands the individual attempts. The person who feels incompetent is less likely to assume new roles, as elaborated by Burke.

External Expectancies. External expectations of a role are both implicitly and explicitly stated and serve to prescribe the role behavior.

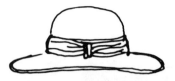

Implicit expectations are the rules or norms culturally determined by age, sex, and position. Although wide latitude of behavior is allowed by norms, a certain degree of conformity is expected (16,21). Explicit demands may be detailed in a job description or verbal exchange. They represent the necessary skills and tasks that must be performed to fulfill minimal role requirements (19).

Transactions. Because a role represents only one segment of the total man, the interrelationship between the role and the man affects and transforms them both. When the norms and demands of the role differ from the expectancies of the individual, a bargaining series begins to lessen the differences. Conflict and uncertainty in meeting given role demands is the usual state in the acquisition of a role. Conflict, and its alter state, curiosity, are further defined in Robinson's paper.

Each individual manages many roles that demand different obligations, activities, and responses. These roles may be familial and sexual, as well as occupational. Because of the other role demands, the individual, before acquisition of the role, arbitrates and prioritizes the internal and external demands of the role. The differences in the internal and external expectations may be due to value systems or fluctuations in commitment to norms. The lessening of conflict between internal and external expectations is attempted so that behavior becomes more consistent. The input, then, represents one of conflict in role expectations and behavior (15,19).

Throughput. Decision-making behavior serves as the transforming process in role acquisition. Decision-making organizes behaviors as it sorts and selects the eventual role behavior. For a decision that com-

promises between the two sets of expectancies, information must be obtained to clearly define the external expectations and the internal goals. Alternative courses of action are identified and are limited only by the quality of information-seeking behavior. Each alternative is then weighted by the values and arranged in order of priority. The optimal alternative behavior is an attempt to meet the role demands with the best advantage to the individual (22,23).

Output. The output is the actual role behavior implemented or enacted from the selected alternatives. The enactment represents a trial period subject to feedback and revision. This trial period allows individuals to *try on* the role and determine the degree to which its obligations enhance or conflict with their other roles. During this *trying on* or enactment period, the role expectancies are made explicit so that they create, modify, and bring the role to life (19). This is a critical period for the disabled, whose needs for support are high because conflicts frequently occur. The arthritic homemaker who trys on the role of volunteer must be able to respond both to the volunteer demands as well as to her own for joint protection.

Feedback. Feedback from internal and external sources may validate the selected role enactment behavior. The obligations and norms within the role serve as the standards for feedback (22). If the behavior is unacceptable, further transactions may occur for a more suitable enactment behavior or the individual may decide not to assume the role (15). External messages may include more explicit information on the boundaries of the expected behavior or tasks. Individuals may decide that their selected enactment creates excess conflict or difficulties in meeting their other role demands. Supervisors

may set guidelines on the length of charting time and therapists may find themselves unable to meet those demands. They would initiate another alternative to meet the charting tasks within the prescribed period.

Empirical Evidence

An assessment battery and strategy for monitoring the readiness for occupational role acquisition was devised and implemented in a study conducted by the author (24). A case study is presented here to illustrate the data obtained and the usefulness in clinical practice.

C.J. is a 17-year-old female with a diagnosis of cerebral palsy and adolescent adjustment reaction. She ambulates with a slight limp and has poor control of the right hand. She is verbal, independent in self-care, and failing her high school classes. At the time of assessment, C.J. was beginning the occupational role acquisition of worker.

C.J.'s strongest interests are selected discriminately and supported by skills. The prioritizing of values is within normal limits, although conflicting areas were present. Test scores indicate an internally controlled individual who does believe in using feedback to modify behavior. She does not request feedback but responds when it is given. In decision-making behavior, C.J. lacks the ability to seek information about external expectations and to assess her own skill level to meet role demands. Consequently, C.J. has not mastered most adolescent tasks.

Historically, C.J. has difficulty enacting occupational roles where expectations are not concretely stated. This was clearly delineated in the student role where C.J. felt she had no advance notice of failing, was unaware of any difference in study habits between herself and her peers, and was unable to state classroom expectations and assignments. Her optimal functioning has been in a structured environment (MacDonald's Hamburgers) where her tasks were listed, assigned, and scheduled for her. Consistent feedback is necessary for maximal task performance. C.J. was currently attempting the role acquisition of a sales clerk. She listed her tasks as standing at the cash register and speaking to customers as they enter the store.

C.J.'s strengths in the occupational role acquisition process were identified as sense of efficacy and control over the environment, interests based on skills, and the ability to monitor behavior when given feedback. Her deficits were identified as information-seeking behavior for clarification of external expectations and demands, self-evaluation and monitoring, and internalization of norms. C.J. was given consistent feedback to increase her awareness of meeting external demands, which required the matching of external requirements with personal skills, and was presented tasks in segments to encourage information-seeking behavior as well as explicit presentation of role demands. Following these treatment sessions, C.J. was able to acquire the role of worker, a salesperson, after repeated attempts to clarify expectations.

Conclusion

Occupational role acquisition has been identified as an aspect of daily living that has been overlooked in occupational therapist's treatment of the chronically disabled. Critical to the middle-aged man who must adjust his work role after a stroke, or the depressed housewife whose chidren are grown and is trying to acquire the worker role, the information on occupational role acquisition also identifies normal transition points from student to worker to retiree as stressful periods possibly requiring occupational therapy intervention. Although the acquisition process is more difficult for the disabled, use of this model in clinical application with marginal groups such as the unemployed, juvenile delinquents, and low-normal adults will make opportunities for productive participation possible.

Acknowledgment

This article is based in part upon material submitted in partial fulfillment of the requirements for the Master of Arts Degree, University of Southern California, Los Angeles. Partial financial support for this study was provided by the Division of Maternal and Child Health, Department of Health, Education and Welfare.

REFERENCES

1. Metropolitan Life Insurance Company Statistical Bulletin. Anne R. Somers, quoted in *Health Care In Transition: Directions for the Future,* Chicago: Hospital Research and Educational Trust, 1971
2. *National Center for Health Statistics: Current Estimates from the Health Interview Survey.* Anne R. Somers, quoted in *Health Care in Transition: Directions for the Future,* Chicago: Hospital Research and Educational Trust, 1971, p 20
3. Dubos RJ: *Mirage of Health,* New York: Harper Publishing Company, 1959, p 18
4. *Life, Death and Medicine,* Edited by Time-Life. San Francisco: W.H. Freeman and Company, 1973
5. Sussman MB: *Sociology and Rehabilitation,* Washington, DC: Department of Health, Education and Welfare, 1965
6. Glazier W: Task of medicine: The problem of chronic illness. *Sci Am* 228:13-17,1973
7. von Bertalanffy L: *General Systems Theory,* New York: George Braziller, 1969
8. Chapple D: *Rehabilitation: Dynamics of Change,* Ithaca, New York: Cornell University Publications, 1970
9. Meyer A: The philosophy of occupational therapy. *Arch Occup Ther* 1:1-10, 1922
10. Reilly M: Occupational therapy can be one of the great ideas of 20th century medicine. *Am J Occup Ther* 16:1-9, 1962
11. Sarbin TR: Role theory. In *Handbook of Social Psychology,* Gardner Lindzey, Editor. Menlo Park, California: Addison-Wesley Publishing Company, 1968, pp 491-530
12. Linton R: *The Study of Man,* New York: Appleton-Century, 1936, p 114
13. Bruner JS: The skill of relevance or the relevance of skills. *Saturday Rev* April 18, 1970, pp 66-74
14. Koestler A: Beyond atomism and holism—The concept of the holon. In *Beyond Reductionism,* Arthur Koestler, Editor. Boston: Beacon Press, 1969
15. Turner RH: Role-taking: Process versus conformity. In *Human Behavior and Social Processes,* Arnold M. Rose, Editor. Boston: Houghton Mifflin Company, 1962
16. Schein MB: On the meaning of alienation. *Am Soc Rev* 24: 782-791, 1959
17. *Metropolitan Life Insurance Company Statistical Bulletin.* Anne R. Somers, quoted in *Health Care in Transition: Directions for the Future,* Chicago: Hospital Research and Educational Trust, 1971, p 20
18. Buhler C, Brind A, Horner A: Old age as a phase of life. *Human Dev* 11: 53-63, 1968
19. Goode WJ: A theory of role strain. *Am Soc Rev* 25: 483-491, 1960
20. Rotter JB: Generalized expectancies for internal versus external control of reinforcement. *Psychol Monogr* 80: 609-636, 1966
21. Williams RM: The concept of norms. In *International Encyclopaedia of the Social Sciences,* New York: Crowell Collier and Macmillan, Inc., 1968
22. White RW: Strategies of adaptation: An attempt at systematic description. In *Coping and Adaptation,* George V. Coelho, David A. Hamburg, and John E. Adams, Editors, New York: Basic Books, Inc., 1974, pp 47-68
23. Simon HA: *Administrative Behavior: A Study of Decision Making Processes in Administrative Organization,* New York: Macmillan Company, 1961
24. Heard CL: *Adaptation in the Chronically Disabled: A Model of Occupational Role Acquisition,* unpublished master's thesis, Department of Occupational Therapy, University of Southern California, Los Angeles, California, 1975

Temporal Adaptation:

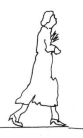
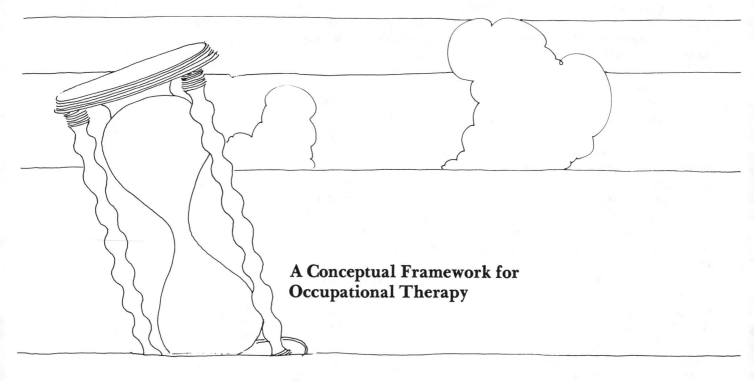

A Conceptual Framework for Occupational Therapy

Gary Kielhofner

Gary Kielhofner, M.A., OTR, is Coordinator of Training in Occupational Therapy, University of California at Los Angeles Neuropsychiatric Institute, in the University Affiliated Facility.

The concept of temporal adaptation was introduced into the field of occupational therapy early in its development; however, it has not been developed as part of the theoretical backing of the field. This paper re-introduces the theme and provides both a general perspective for the clinician in thinking about patients' temporal behavior and a preliminary framework for application. Temporal adaptation when applied in clinical practice should add a wider perspective to existing clinical interventions. It is proposed as a generically applicable theoretical perspective appropriate across all dysfunctional categories of patients. Two case histories are presented to demonstrate the application of the theoretical framework to intervention.

In 1922, Adolf Meyer proposed a philosophy of practice for the newly formed profession of occupational therapy. He maintained that the key to successful application of occupational therapy would lie in an awakening to:

...a full meaning of time as the biggest wonder and asset of our lives and the valuation of opportunity and performance as the greatest measure of time . . . . (1)

Eleanor Clarke Slagle pioneered the application of Meyer's proposal that occupational therapy should view patients within the context of time through the unfolding of their daily lives. She implemented a program of "habit training" based on the principle that the normal use of time in a purposeful daily routine would exert

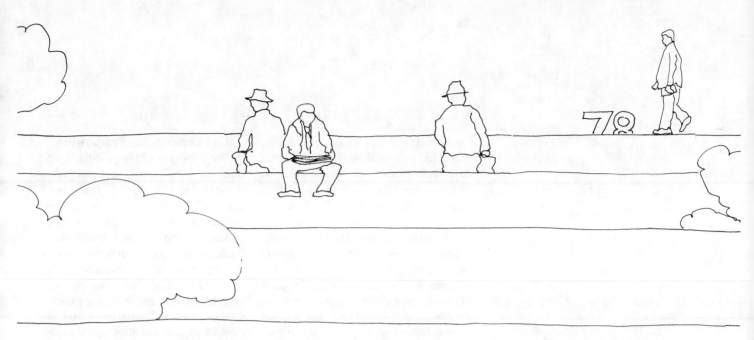

an organizing force on even the most regressed, unmedicated mentally ill patients (2). Slagle intuitively recognized habit as a critical regulator of man's use of time and consequently as a significant component of his adaptation.

From Meyer and Slagle the profession received the proposition that in the richness of man's daily routines and his purposeful use of time, there was both health-maintaining and health-regenerating potential. Further, the way in which disabled individuals used and organized their time in daily life was revealed as a measure of their adaptiveness. Health was revealed in how patients functioned on a day-by-day, hour-by-hour basis. The temporal dimension in human adaptation was installed as a legitimate concern for occupational therapists. This temporal perspective gave to occupational therapy a special caretaker position for patients' activities of daily living.

However, occupational therapy practice has subsequently evolved away from a concern for patients' temporal functioning (3). The full appreciation of the meaning of time, which Meyer so strongly advocated, never came to pass in occupational therapy. Consequently, the broad humanistic theme of activities of daily living suffered a substantial loss of content. Presently, the concept of activities of daily living conveys little more than a checklist for self-care (4).

At a time when occupational therapy must face the reality of its "derailment," as Shannon suggests in his paper, it is imperative that the profession scrutinize its underpinnings and carefully examine its philosophy and practice for critical concepts that have been lost. The task that lies before the profession is to reclaim and revitalize those elements which made occupational therapy such a viable and energizing idea for the founders and early leaders of the profession.

The theme of temporal adaptation is a valuable scheme for practice and should be reintroduced to occupational therapy. Therefore, this paper first provides support for temporal functioning as a useful conceptual base from which human adaptation and dysfunction of the disabled can be better understood. Second, it proposes a temporal conceptual frame-

work that serves as a background from which to generate evaluations and interventions.

The Temporal Dimension in Adaptation

The elderly person whose abundant leisure has become painful monotony, the physically disabled person whose self-care has been expanded into a long and tedious procedure, the psychiatric patient whose personal helplessness makes the future an unwelcome burden, and the mentally subnormal person for whom the string of events in time seems a jumble . . . each represent a special difficulty in temporal adaptation. Although occupational therapists are thoroughly acquainted with such temporal problems, the systematic application of clinical intervention aimed at temporal dysfunction is not formally or consistently part of the clinician's treatment. In order to reintroduce temporal adaptation to clinical practice, this section provides a general theoretical overview. *Temporal adaptation* serves in this paper as a descriptive term for integration of an entire spectrum of activities, the organization of which supports health on an ongoing daily life basis. *Temporal dysfunction* will refer to problems that arise in this daily life organization. Temporal adaptation and dysfunction represent descriptive

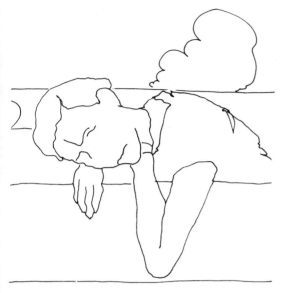

terms for talking about complex daily activity from the specific but universal dimension of time.

Time. Time is the inescapable boundary for human existence and activity. Hall describes it as the "unconscious determinant or frame upon which everything else is built," (5) and Henry states that for man time is a universal dimension, guiding and structuring his experience and his activity (6). Human adaptation is inextricably bound up in the conscious experience of time. Man's conscious placement in time is a function of the capacity to symbolize internally that which is perceived externally (7). Each man bears a complex symbolic model or image of himself located in time (8). His initial awareness of time results from the experience of change in the self and the environment (9). The model or image of external temporal reality is generated and continuously reorganized through the accumulated experience of changing events.

Armed with temporal consciousness, man is a supreme actor in time. Not only is he aware of changing events, but he is likewise conscious of the fact that he can have some effect on that course of events. The perception of the self as a cause comes from experiencing the results of one's own actions in time (10). Man's awareness of time, the awareness of his causative ability, and its potential for consequences are interrelated phenomena. The human condition is transformed by the awareness of the individual that he or she has acted, is acting, and will continue to act. Man's awareness of time makes possible this continuity of experience that transforms the nature of his adaptation. In John Dewey's words:

Man differs from the lower animals because he preserves his past experiences . . . . With the animals, an experience perishes as it happens and each new doing or suffering stands alone. But man lives in a world where each occurrence is charged with echoes and reminiscences of what has gone before, where each event is a reminder of other things. Hence he lives not, like the beasts of the field, in a world of merely physical things, but in a world of signs and symbols. (11)

Although overt experiences occur as disconnected and episodic events, the inner symbolic experience is an uninterrupted flow in which past and future are orienting reference points for human adaptation. Man draws upon his past experiences as an information source for future action. He projects himself into the future, planning events, and setting goals that may not be realized for days, months, or even years. Through imagination, he can test alternative courses of action and contemplate their consequences (7). Once placed consciously in time, the human organism adapts through purposeful action. Man adapts through awareness of his own agenthood and placement in time that makes possible the conscious planning of action. Action and time are concomitant components of the human experience linked to purpose through hindsight and foresight.

The Conceptual Framework

The concepts of temporal adaptation can be put into operation through a conceptual framework designed to generate strategies of evaluation and treatment in occupational therapy. A preliminary framework was constructed as a series of propositions about temporal adaptation. The first four concern external factors and learning that influence temporal experience and activity. Propositions five and six concern the internal organization of temporal behavior. The seventh proposition concerns pathologies or dysfunctions of time.

Proposition 1: Each person bears a temporal frame of reference that is culturally constituted. Individuals carry an image of their placement in time that is a unique product of their culture (12). Their temporal frame of reference is maintained and transmitted within the culture in the form of norms and values and contains the basic notion and valuation of time (13).

In American society the notion of time is that of a straight line or path extending into the future. Time is experienced as a "supersensible medium or container, as a stream of infinitely extended warp upon which the woof of human happenings is woven . . . . " (14) It is sectioned off and takes on the nature of enclosed or finite space, the segments of which are to be filled with activity (12, 13). This notion of time is exhibited in the American habit of scheduling events. Random behavior that lacks a pattern of organization is not functional in the mainstream of American society (6). The American culture values time as a commodity; it can be bought, sold, saved, or wasted (13). This sense of time is captured in the phrase *time is money* and, understandably, wasting time has a strong negative connotation in

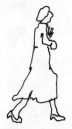

the culture.

Although the orderly, punctual life of Americans is not an innate feature of human existence, it is largely considered a fact of nature. This notion and valuation of time is the framework of the culture that sets boundaries for competent action in daily life. In order to adapt to the society the individual must to some degree internalize and order behavior according to the culture's temporal frame of reference.

Proposition 2: A unique temporal frame of reference is accumulated through learning and socializing experiences that begin in childhood. Although the basic ability to perceive time is a cognitive developmental phenomenon, the particular culture frame of reference is a product of socialization (6). The transmission of the temporal frame of reference has been classified by Hall into three levels of socialization or learning: technical, informal, and formal (13).

The technical learning of time occurs in a didactic framework, as when a child is taught to tell time and to comprehend the division of seconds, minutes, and hours. Informal time is learned through imitation of role models and the learning comprises activities and mannerisms that are so much a part of daily life that they are performed almost unconsciously. An example of informal time is knowing that being 5 minutes late for an appointment is acceptable, whereas 20 minutes is not. Formal learning is taught by precept and admonition, and concerns traditions and values transmitted through the expectations and prohibitions of each culture. As an example, the prohibition of wasting time is passed on in American culture as an important value.

From this teaching, modeling, precept, and admonition, children's socialization is accomplished through the internalization of a complex temporal frame of reference. It is within the family that children first learn to organize time under this framework toward fulfillment of a social role. The role of children or siblings within the family bears with it a whole set of activities ordered in time. Learning to be on time for meals, to do chores when assigned, to habitually care for themselves, and to periodically clean their rooms are all part of the complex schema children must incorporate. Learning temporal organization, which occurs within the family, generalizes to other roles children must take on later. Children not only know a particular set of behaviors ordered in time, but more importantly, also learn to organize activity in time.

In addition to learning how and when to behave, children learn a complex set of temporal expectations; Toffler gives the following poignant description.

From infancy on the child learns, for example, that when Daddy

. . . leaves for work in the morning, it means that he will not return for many hours . . . . The child soon learns that "mealtime" is neither a one-minute nor a five-hour affair, but that it ordinarily lasts from fifteen minutes to an hour. He learns that going to a movie lasts two to four hours, but that a visit with the pediatrician seldom lasts more than one. He learns that the school day ordinarily lasts six hours. He learns that a relationship with a teacher ordinarily extends over a school year, but that his relationship with his grandparents is supposed to be of much longer duration. Indeed some relationships are supposed to last a lifetime. (15)

Where the household temporal patterns are chaotic, children's learning of the temporal frame of reference may be maladaptive (6). Consequently, competent participation in the culture may be hindered as they falter in organizing time to respond to other successive social institutions, such as school and the job setting.

Proposition 3: There is a natural temporal order to daily living organized around the life-space activities of self-maintenance, work, and play. Adolph Meyer pointed out that there is a natural rhythm in the organization of daily life around life spaces (1). These life spaces are assigned to activities that represent a social order, determining appropriate times for role behavior. Reilly conceptualized daily living as divided into life spaces of existence, subsistence, and discretionary tim (16). Existence is that time spent for eating, sleeping, personal hygiene, and other aspects of self-maintenance; subsistence is the life space devoted to working for an income; and discretionary time is that life space reserved for recreation and leisure. Recreation and leisure comprise dual aspects of play in adult life. Recreation is the period of time when man is made ready for the next cycle of work through relaxation. Leisure is earned time made possible by the satisfying performance of work.

Health consists of the proper balance of the life spaces that is both satisfying to individuals and appropriate for their roles within society. Balance refers to more than just so much work, play, and rest. Rather, balance recognizes an interdependence of these life spaces and their relationship to both internal values, interests, and goals, and external demands of the environment. It is the interrelated balance of self-maintenance, work, and play that comprises health.

While homeostasis is used to describe the biological health of the organism, a broader concept of

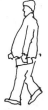

balance in daily life describes the conditions for psychosocial health of the human organism. Occupational therapists are in a position to make critical statements about the health of their patients from **both** interrelated dimensions of homeostasis and balance. Far from being limited to the idea of self-care, activities of daily living refer to man's total state of health, which depends on both biological and psychosocial factors.

Proposition 4: Society requires its members to organize their use of time according to ascribed social roles. While cultural norms and values provide a contextual framework for man's use of time, his individual daily pattern must be organized around his occupational roles (17). Heard expands on this theme of role behavior in her paper. The sum total of man's activity within his life spaces has been referred to as occupational behavior (18). Life spaces are filled according to the occupational roles to which they are assigned. Within the daily routine, an individual's life spaces may be divided between several occupational roles such as the father, worker, and community volunteer. Adaptation requires individuals to use their time in a manner that supports their roles. The student must organize time for attendance at classes and homework, the worker for the job schedule, and the retiree for effective and satisfying use of leisure time.

The organization of time around one's roles is not a static skill. Occupational roles change and overlap; each individual passes through a succession of roles in a lifetime (19). Taking on a new role requires a new strategy for organizing one's time. When role change is abruptly forced upon an individual through an incurred disability, developing new temporal skills is a critical factor in adapting to the disability.

Proposition 5: An individual's use of time is a function of internalized values, interests, and goals. Values are commitments to action that organize an individual's use of time by establishing an internal order of what comes first and how much time will be allotted to various activities (20). An individual's values set priorities of actions, and their consequences create a personal valence that is ultimately translated into a life style. Values serve an important function in the choice an individual makes to take on various roles. Although values reflect more serious commitments, interests also guide the commitment process. They are states of readiness for choices and action (21). Interests sustain action and serve thereby to maintain commitments over time. Like values, interests prioritize activities and lend organization to temporal behavior.

Goals represent strategies toward the fulfillment of values and interests. Values and interests yield automatic goal-setting and consequent adjustment and organization of daily patterns of time use. This process occurs at various levels of awareness and is necessary for ordering daily life. The individual who has no goals or has difficulty setting goals cannot organize daily life to use existing skills effectively and will, consequently, feel frustrated or helpless (22, 23). Further, an individual must be able to identify and execute appropriate actions for goal-attainment. Problems arise when an individual cannot identify and carry out in proper sequence those activities that lead to successful goal achievement (23, 24). Robinson expands this notion, sequencing action in time, in her paper on rules.

Proposition 6: Habits are the basic structures by which daily behavior is ordered in time and psychosocial health is maintained. While habits are traditionally thought of in terms of vices and virtues, they extend a more subtle and profound influence on daily temporal functioning. All that is familiar, routine, and predictable in daily life bears a relationship to habit. Without habit structure, an individual's daily life would be a chaotic series of disjointed events.

Habits are instantaneous, automatic choices of action made throughout the day (3). Although organized into unconscious routines, they are the products of once conscious choices made until they become automatic (3). Habits reflect actions related to values and interests cemented over time in daily patterns. Further, habits provide a crucial service to adaptation by organizing temporal behavior to meet societal requirements for competence. Consequently, habits perform an important role in assuring that skills are used in an adaptive manner. Skills must not only be present, but also organized into a daily routine.

Proposition 7: Temporal dysfunction may exist in relationship to categories of pathology. Temporal dysfunction may occur as an integral part of some mental illness or as a consequence of imposed physical disability.

When viewing individuals from the perspective of temporal adaptation, it becomes obvious that strategies for intervention cannot begin and end with the physical, mental, or emotional pathology. Each may be integrally related to a broader and often more difficult set of problems in the person's temporal adaptation.

Persons who are so disoriented in time that they cannot give the day, month, or year are readily suspected of being afflicted with amentia, senility, or some psychotic disorder (12). Actual distortions of the perception of time have been shown to occur in some cases of mental ill-

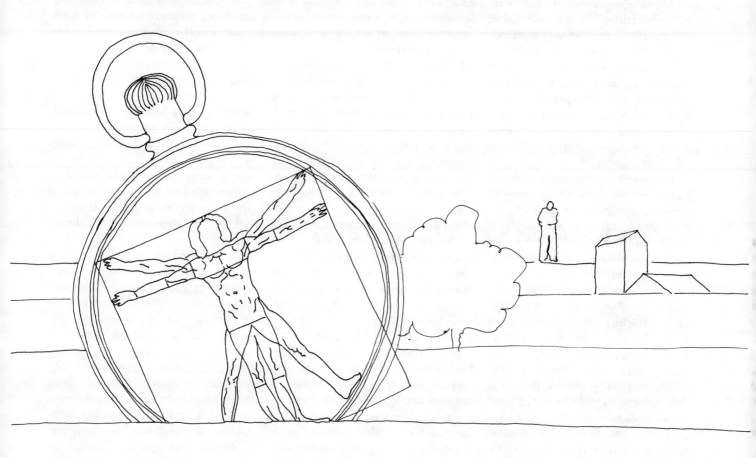

ness (9). Further, when individuals cannot organize their time toward fulfillment of their social roles, they may become candidates for psychiatric care (24). Disorganization of time is associated with the subjective sense of helplessness and incompetence seen in mental illness.

Disorganization of temporal adaptation may also be identified in the reaction of an individual to residual physical disabilities. Maintaining a pace of life comparable to individuals without disability may be impossible for some persons whose motor performance is dysfunctional. The impact of sudden disability often imposes tremendous distortions of daily life spaces by increasing the amount of time required for routine activities. Further, where one or more roles change or end as a result of acquired physical disability, the individual may be unable to find new meaningful activities and roles to fill the life-spaces formerly occupied by old ones.

Implementation

Propositions were formulated as a guiding framework for incorporating temporal adaptation into clinical evaluation and treatment. The clinician may use the framework for integrating clinical data with points raised in the propositions. The framework gives the clinician another dimension for viewing patient problems and for generating and interpreting data. It thereby serves as a basis for developing new treatment strategies. Three principles should be adhered to in applying the conceptual framework to evaluation. First, data should be collected on several variables contained in the propositions. Relevant data include the patient's values, interests, goals, balance of play and work, habit structure, and temporal frame of reference. Second, the evaluation should take into consideration internal constraints on time as revealed in the nature of the patient's physical, mental, or emotional disability. Third, the evaluation should also consider the external factors influencing time use: the patient's roles, family expectations, cultural background, and the demands of time and physical space that affect the patient's daily living.

Treatment intervention will be based on the particular pattern of temporal dysfunction revealed by the evaluation. As data is interrelated and considered in light of the conceptual framework, dysfunctional patterns should become evident. For example, one patient's chaotic day may be a reflection of a lack of ability to prioritize interests and to set goals. Without the ability to set priorities and goals, the patient cannot generate habits for a normal, satisfactory daily routine. By using the conceptual framework of temporal adaptation, the clinician should be able to formulate a more comprehensive treatment plan.

Case Examples

Two case histories, together with examples of clinical interventions that follow the principles above, are presented to serve as examples of how the temporal adaptation framework can be applied. Treatments described speak only to the temporal framework and assume the inclusion of other traditional occupational therapy interventions.

Case H.B. H.B. is a 24-year-old, single male psychiatric patient. When admitted to the hospital, his presenting problems included depression and chronic repeated failures in work settings. H.B. graduated from college with a degree in music with plans to re-enter college for graduate study in musicology. He not only has definite

skills as a musician but has also demonstrated a strong commitment by voluntarily organizing a teenage choir in a local church.

However, H.B. has not managed during the last three years to hold down a steady job and save enough money to re-enter college. His recent occupational history includes such jobs as working in an electrical shop repairing fans, driving a school bus, and doing maintenance work in apartment complexes. H.B. was fired from each of these jobs because of his inability to concentrate on the work. He found the jobs uninteresting and had difficulty applying himself. He attempted to save money toward college, but used up his savings during periods of unemployment between jobs.

H.B. describes his daily life as highly variable and without routine. He has been unable to maintain any schedule and often finds himself late for work and appointments. Further, social activities have taken up a large part of his schedule so that he is negligent in doing many basic self-maintenance tasks. His housekeeping recently became so disorganized that he was evicted from his apartment. H.B. perceives his daily life as chaotic and complains that "there is so little time with so much to do, that I often get stuck on things and never get around to what I set out to do." He feels helpless and depressed since he is not close to his goal of re-entering college and does not feel he is progressing toward it. At this point his response to this subjective state is to become inactive. He is without a job and recently does not even pursue his interests in music on a leisure basis.

When considered in light of the conceptual framework, H.B.'s temporal dysfunction can be outlined as follows. H.B. has internalized values and goals. He considers further

education important and realistically has chosen an area of study within his capacities. His temporal dysfunction lies in the areas of: (a) identifying and pursuing reasonable short-term objectives that will bring him closer to his overall goal; (b) maintaining a satisfying daily schedule that would balance activities of work, play, and self-maintenance; and (c) organizing his time around present necessary role of being a worker. The temporal dysfunction that has eroded his competence in several areas augments his feelings of depression and helplessness.

Recommendations for treatment should include: 1. assisting H.B. in identifying how his present worker role will lead to the eventual goal of re-entering college and developing a strategy that balances his interest in music with the necessity of working on a daily basis; 2. practice in formulating a basic, balanced daily routine and adhering to it consistently; and 3. making beginning steps toward his overall goal, by gathering information on graduate programs in music, their requirements, and possible scholarships. By subdividing each of these goals into subroutines such as finding a new job or ways of pursuing his interest in music on a leisure basis, he may be able to overcome the vicious cycle of daily life incompetence, helplessness, and depression. Treatment would occur in graded steps toward the eventual reconstruction of daily living skills.

Case T.J. T.J. is a 17-year-old male who sustained a spinal cord injury in an automobile accident. Five months after the injury, T.J., a paraplegic, remains depressed and withdrawn. When approached about his depressed state, T.J. responds that his life-plans have been destroyed. Prior to his injury he was an excellent athlete with a promise of an athletic scholarship to a university.

Beyond his college training, T.J. had hoped to become a high school coach. Further, T.J. points out that he is now forced to spend days in bed or a wheelchair, whereas formerly he was active in a variety of intramural and varsity sports. He describes the present as boring and sees little prospect for change in the future. Also, data from his family points out that T.J.'s former positive self-image revolved around his physical appearance and athletic prowess; he now views himself as an invalid.

In T.J.'s case it should be noted that: (a) his former values and interests focused on activities he can no longer engage in or he must learn to participate in with some modifications; (b) his self-image and prospects for the future revolved around skills and capacities no longer intact; (c) his former daily routine revolved around his athletic role. In summary, those values and habits that formerly maintained a satisfying daily routine and those skills and goals which made the future desirable are no longer intact.

T.J.'s treatment under the framework of temporal adaptation would focus on the following sequence of treatment strategies: 1. reconstruction of the self-image through successful experiences in areas related to his past interests; 2. exploration of new activities to develop interests (in the clinic and his own community); 3. reconstruction of his daily routine, which will have to accommodate different life spaces—such as the expanded space necessary for self-care and personal hygiene; and 4. refocusing on his career goals so that a viable and acceptable objective could at least be tentatively pursued.

Conclusion

Temporal adaptation was iden-tified as an early theme in occupational therapy that has been dropped out of clinical practice. The concept of temporal adaptation was reintroduced and formulated in a preliminary framework for clinical intervention. Temporal adaptation serves as a conceptual schema to broaden the clinician's current perspective and repertoire of skills and, as such, does not replace traditional therapeutic efforts but expands them into a more comprehensive framework. Temporal adaptation is a rich conceptual schema for occupational therapy because it speaks to a class of dysfunction found in the entire range of patients seen by occupational therapists.

Acknowledgment

This article is based in part upon material submitted in partial fulfillment of the requirements for the Master of Arts Degree, University of Southern California, Los Angeles. Partial financial support for this study was provided by the Division of Allied Health Manpower, Department · of Health, Education and Welfare.

REFERENCES

1. Meyer A: The philosophy of occupational therapy. *Arch Occup Ther* 1:1-10, 1922, p 9
2. Slagle EC: Training aides for mental patients. *Arch Occup Ther* 1:11-16, 1922
3. Kielhofner GW: The evolution of knowledge in occupational therapy-understanding adaptation of the chronically disabled. Master's Thesis. Department of Occupational Therapy, University of Southern California, Los Angeles, 1973
4. Reilly M: The modernization of occupational therapy. *Am J Occup Ther* 25:243-247, 1971
5. Hall ET: The paradox of culture. In *In the Name of Life*, Bernard Landis and Edward S. Tauber, Editors. New York: Holt, Rinehart, and Winston, 1971, p 226
6. Henry J: *Pathways to Madness*, New York: Vintage Books, Random House, 1971
7. White R: Strategies of adaptation: an attempt at systematic description. In *Coping and Adaptation*, George Coelho, David Hamburg, and John E. Adams, Editors. New York: Basic Books, 1974
8. Boulding K: *The Image*, Ann Arbor: University of Michigan Press, 1961
9. Larrington G: An exploratory study of the temporal aspects of adaptive functioning. Master's Thesis. Department of Occupational Therapy, University of Southern California, Los Angeles, California, 1970
10. DeCharms R.: *Personal Causation*, New York: Academic Press, 1968
11. Dewey J: *Reconstruction in Philosophy*, New York: H. Holt and Company, 1920, p 36
12. Hallowell I: *Culture and Experience*, New York: Schocken Books, 1955, p 217
13. Hall ET: *The Silent Language*, Greenwich: Fawcett Publications, Inc., 1959
14. Parkhurst HH: The cult of chronology. In *Essays in Honor of John Dewey*, New York: H. Holt and Company, 1929, p 23
15. Toffler A: *Future Shock*, New York: Random House, 1970, p 360
16. Reilly M: A psychiatric occupational therapy program as a teaching model. *Am J Occup Ther*, 20:2-10, 1966
17. Newcomb T: *Social Psychology*, New York: Henry Holt and Company, 1959
18. Matsutsuyu J: Occupational behavior: a perspective on work and play. *Am J Occup Ther* 25:291-293, 1971
19. Arensenian J: Life cycle factors in mental illness. *Ment Hyg* 52:19-30, 1968
20. Kluckhohn C: Values and value orientations in the theory of action: an exploration in definition and classification. In *Toward a General Theory of Action*, T. Parsons and E. Shils, Editors. Cambridge: Harvard University Press, 1951
21. Matsutsuyu J: The interest checklist. *Am J Occup Ther* 23:323-326, 1969
22. Lakein A: *How to Get Control of Your Time and Your Life*, New York: The Signet, The New American Library, Inc., 1974
23. Kiev A: *A Strategy of Daily Living*, New York: The Free Press, 1973
24. Black MM: The evolution of social roles—a perspective on fantasy. Master's Thesis. Department of Occupational Therapy, University of Southern California, Los Angeles, California, 1973

Neighborhood Extension of Activity Therapy (NEAT) is a structured transitional-discharge activity program for psychiatric patients which uses existing community resources. A series of collaborative interviews between client and therapist are used to ascertain the client's activity preferences, abilities, and the amount of structure and support he needs to attend activity sessions. The program includes an extensive search of specific activities available in the client's immediate community, recommendations of appropriate activity choices, and a graduated supportive follow-up procedure. In the past two years the NEAT program has reinforced and broadened clients' spheres of competence by providing them with successful activity experiences in their communities.

NEIGHBORHOOD EXTENSION OF ACTIVITY THERAPY

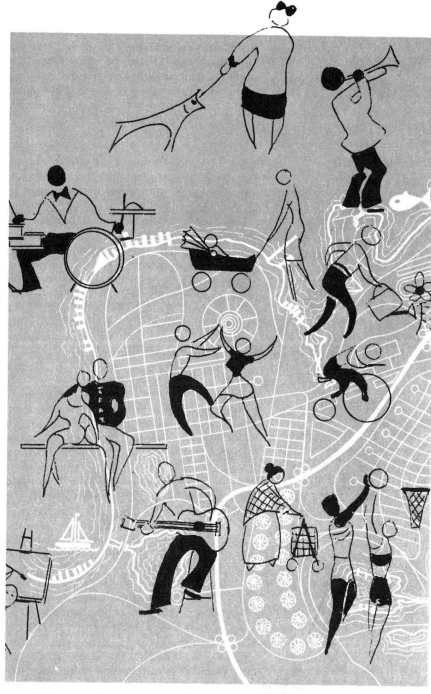

Ellen L. Kolodner, O.T.R.

Competence, the ability to interact effectively with one's environment, requires "substantial contributions from activities which, though playful and exploratory in character, show direction, sensitivity, and persistence in interacting with the environment." The experience that is produced from successful interactions with both the human and nonhuman environments has been termed a "feeling of efficacy."[1]

Occupational therapists have long recognized that each man's perceptions of his own ability to cope with his environment are constantly altered as a result of his daily successes and failures. If the skills of an individual are consistently insufficient for the situations encountered, the individual begins to doubt his competence. Occupational therapy often aims to "improve self-concepts" through the use of success or efficacious experiences. Therapists choose and structure activities which use skills already mastered by the patient. These, then, produce a feeling of efficacy and help the individual to identify and develop his sphere of competent functioning. The Neighborhood Extension of Activity Therapy (NEAT) program extends this competence by structuring patient participation in appropriate community activities.

The Problem

Avocational activities which individuals use as release mechanisms for anger or tension, as well as those which provide input to support a positive self-image, are often neglected during times of illness. Such mechanisms must be practiced in order to become assimilated.[2] During inpatient treatment pa-

Ellen Kolodner, formerly staff therapist in the activities department at Eastern Pennsylvania Psychiatric Institute, is now director of education and training, Occupational Therapy Department, Norristown State Hospital, Norristown, Pennsylvania.

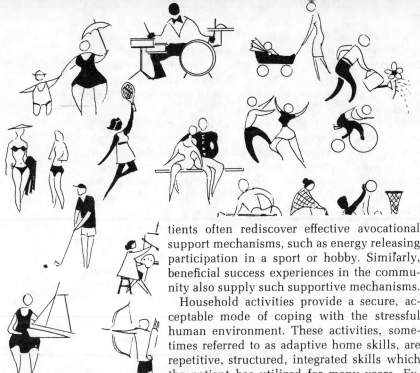

tients often rediscover effective avocational support mechanisms, such as energy releasing participation in a sport or hobby. Similarly, beneficial success experiences in the community also supply such supportive mechanisms.

Household activities provide a secure, acceptable mode of coping with the stressful human environment. These activities, sometimes referred to as adaptive home skills, are repetitive, structured, integrated skills which the patient has utilized for many years. Examples of such activities are ironing, washing floors and cars, or cleaning closets. The patient is not taught these activities; he is merely encouraged to utilize them more frequently, especially during times of stress.

It is the goal of the NEAT program to sustain and reinforce avocational support mechanisms and adaptive skills until these become genuine interests which are utilized by the patient to his best advantage.

During hospitalization, rehabilitation staff make a concerted effort to provide daily constructive, therapeutic programming. As discharge approaches and the individual begins to spend less time in the hospital, an emphasis is placed upon returning to work. Avocational or recreational planning is usually left to the patient's discretion. The NEAT program uses a combination of activity structure and support to meet this specific need.

The NEAT Program

A patient is referred to the NEAT program by the occupational therapist, recreation therapist, social worker, or psychiatrist on the ward. Referrals include information about the client's activity skills, differential learning abilities, motivation, group functioning, and discharge plans which include his probable place of residence. Clients are selected for participation in the program on a basis of interest and motivation for activity. It is assumed that when the patient becomes involved and attends activities, the positive input becomes a motivating force.[3]

The Initial Interview

The intake therapist in an informal interview outlines the purpose of the program to the patient. The program is presented with an emphasis on involvement in the home and community. The feeling-tone of the interview is one of impending independence and a complete "breaking of ties" with the hospital. Activities are presented as being separate from the hospital; reassurance is given that the patient will utilize known or mastered skills. It is emphasized that expectations of competence will not be above those of his present level.

During this interview, the therapist ascertains the client's interests and skills. The patient and therapist jointly complete an interest inventory based upon "The Interest Checklist" (Table 1).[4] Possibilities for pursuing adult

TABLE 1

Interest Checklist

The interest checklist is an extensive list of specific activities, grouped under the following general categories: music-related; games; sports; home-related; crafts; educational; and social. The following is a *partial* example:

Interest Checklist

Name and Ward_____ Date_____

Please check each item below according to your interest:

Activity	Interest			Previous Participation
	Strong	Casual	None	
Music-Related: Dancing				
Guitar				
Popular Music				
Classical Music				
etc.				

forms of the activity are explored and recorded. The therapist attempts to identify the repetitive, structured activity the patient could develop for use as an adaptive home skill. The client is urged to continue to utilize the skills within his repertoire. Many patients need validation for their action; they may recognize that activities such as cleaning or sewing are "therapeutic" but may not have accepted the emotional importance of the frequent use of these skills.

Resources and Activity Choice

The activity identification is limited to those agencies which are geographically accessible to the client. Activities are chosen to meet individual patient's needs for structure, support, competition, group interaction and work tolerance including attention span and concentration span. A minimum of two activities are investigated to afford flexibility of choice and to facilitate involvement in more than one activity group.

Local Y's, evening schools, art centers, and

other neighborhood agencies are approached by a volunteer, aide or the therapist. Contacts are located through the telephone book, department of recreation listings, or the *Directory of Community Resources—Health and Welfare Council* publication. Inquiry is made concerning the activities offered, the type of instruction, expected participation, fees, and the size of the group. Whenever possible the name and status of the client are kept confidential. Contacts are recorded in the patient's file and a card is prepared for the neighborhood file. Brochures are requested and a file of agencies is compiled according to neighborhoods.

Information concerning the programs offered by agencies is evaluated and the client and therapist select an appropriate activity. Choices are usually listed in order of preference in the patient's file.

Preparatory Interviews

In the second interview the patient is urged to begin routinely utilizing the adaptive home skills in the hospital and while he is at home.

In the third interview the client is shown the results of the survey which consists of agencies, programs, dates, and fees. Together, the patient and therapist select the activity group and plan the starting date. Patients are urged to visit the facility prior to the start of the activity group. The client is given written instructions concerning the time and address of the activity, travel route, the phone number of the therapist and the date of the next interview. If the client is hesitant to attend the first session, the therapist may ask another client who has previously attended community activities to accompany him. If this option is not available, the therapist may accompany the client. During this interview, his successes are discussed and the patient is urged to continue utilizing his adaptive home skills. Further preparatory interviews may be indicated if the patient appears reluctant to attend the first activity.

In preparation for attendance at the activity, the fourth interview should take place immediately before the activity. This interview may be conducted in person or over the telephone. It provides crucial additional support at a stressful time.

Follow-Up

The follow-up interview takes place the day after the client's first attendance at the activity. The client and therapist discuss the experience. Support is offered concerning the difficulty of meeting a new group of people. If the experience was successful, the client is encouraged to continue attending the activity. An appointment is arranged immediately following the next activity session. If the session was unsatisfactory, the therapist explores which aspects were unpleasant and evaluates whether the patient should be urged to return

to that group. The best course is discussed with the patient and appropriate action is taken. If a new activity is needed, the therapist will turn to the second activity choice. The patient is encouraged to continue practicing his adaptive home skills.

It is important that additional follow-up be provided to encourage continued activity participation. Either the client or the therapist contacts the other each week, by telephone or in person. During these brief interviews, the therapist explores how frequently the client is attending the activity and his success and failure experiences. She also investigates his life-style adjustment and use of adaptive home skills since leaving the hospital. It is during this stage that the therapist may recommend new activities or do an activities configuration to determine how the client is utilizing his leisure hours.[5]

As the patients become more skillful in their use of activities, their feelings of competence increase and their desire for independence deepens. Less support is needed. Contacts are made through the use of the telephone and interviews are brief. Clients may now become increasingly independent and search out their own activities. Phone contacts become limited to support of the clients' interest and activity.

Summary

This paper outlines a program that extends occupational therapy to patients in their community and home environment. Its basic assumptions are that patients have difficulty utilizing their leisure time constructively, and that these periods of unstructured time lead to the extinction of essential adaptive skills. As these skills diminish, the patient's ability to interact effectively with his environment also diminishes.

Feelings of efficacy and competence are crucial to the emotional well-being of a person. During the time that the Neighborhood Extension of Activity Therapy Program has been in effect, more than 75 clients have participated. The program has reinforced and broadened their activity skills by providing them with successful experiences in their own communities. A follow-up study of this program will assess continued activity on the part of clients and the value of their extended use of this program towards achieving a sense of competence. ■

REFERENCES

1. White RW: Early Childhood Play: Selected Readings to Cognition and Motivation, New York, Simon and Schuster, 125, 1968
2. Ginsburg H, Opper S: Piaget's Theory of Intellectual Development, Englewood Cliffs, New Jersey, Prentice-Hall Inc, 31, 1969
3. Ayllon T, Azrin N: The Token Economy—A Motivational System for Therapy and Rehabilitation, New York, Appleton-Century Crofts, 60, 1968
4. Matsutsuyu JS: The interest checklist, Am J Occup Ther 23: 327, 1969
5. Willard H, Spackman C: Occupational Therapy (fourth edition), Philadelphia, J B Lippincott Co, 88–89, 1971

A Planning Group for Psychiatric Outpatients

Gail Kuenstler

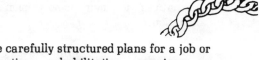

Planning leisure time successfully can contribute to a patient's ability to function in the spheres of work and family as well. A leisure-time planning group for psychiatric out-patients is described in this article and includes the treatment principles upon which the group is based, the format of the sessions, and the goal-setting techniques employed. A concrete, highly structured, and self-actualizing approach was used to help patients discover and develop their interests. Members often encountered similar problems in their attempts to plan leisure time despite their varied backgrounds and skills in planning, which led to the use of specific approaches in dealing with these common problems, and also suggested a wider application for the Planning Group.

Despite carefully structured plans for a job or for daytime rehabilitation, evenings or weekends can still present a problem for the newly discharged psychiatric patient. Since difficulty in planning for leisure time can be a stumbling block in the patient's successful return to society, a planning group was developed to deal with this problem. The Planning Group helps patients to focus on their interests and to integrate them into their leisure hours. The approach to the problem of what to do with free time is concrete, highly structured, and self-actualizing. This paper discusses the criteria for group membership; the treatment principles upon which the group is based; the method and format of the group sessions; the importance of setting goals; the approaches to dealing with the shared problems routinely experienced by those in the Group; the value of the Group; and the possibility of wider application.

Group Membership

The Planning Group is held once a week for one and a half hours. All participants in the group are psychiatric outpatients who had been hospitalized on a short-term unit (average stay is five weeks). The patients are introduced to the Group during their last week of hospitalization and remain members of the Group as long as they perceive some difficulty in structuring their leisure time and as long as they are willing to set goals. The ability to function in a group setting without being too disruptive and the motivation to return week after week are the criteria for group membership. Patients are referred to the Group by their activities therapist or by their doctor. These patients lacked friends, had difficulty leaving the house, lived in an isolated fashion, or expressed a particular interest in the Group.

The Group chosen to illustrate the concepts of the program has six members; four have been in the Group for nearly one year. Their difficulties in living with or relating to others are quite varied and representative of the inpatient population as a whole. Their lives contain few focal points—a therapist, one family member, a TV, and perhaps a job. The task of this Group is to explore interests however tentative that might provide alternatives to their impoverishment and alienation.

Treatment Principles

The Group is based upon the central premise that people must take the responsibility for what goes on in their lives. DeCharms supports this premise in a discussion of the importance of internal motivation. The fact that "a person perceives his behavior as determined by his own choosing . . . is more important motivationally than objective facts." (1, p. 273) In terms of the Group, this means that even very "sick" people are expected to take responsibility for what they do in their leisure time. Taking responsibility means that everyone has choices: they can choose in an active way to make plans, or they can choose to drift passively through an evening or a day. Planning decisions are made more difficult by feelings of inadequacy and fear, but the Group assumes that its members will nevertheless make a serious attempt to plan.

Another treatment principle is that everyone needs a variety of things to do in their leisure time. The human need for variety is fully described by Pearce and Newton (2). Active manipulations of the physical world — gardening or straightening the living room — may be combined with swimming or intellectual activities. Although watching TV and going to the movies are often an exclusive leisure-time diet, they are generally not felt to be satisying because both activities are quite passive and isolating, with little sense of mastery and no possibility of offering something of one's self. Members of the Group admit that all isolation, all childrearing, or all work makes them unhappy, even though they are not able to act on this knowledge because they do not know where to begin. Therefore, members figure out what might be realistic in terms of each member's tolerance. For example, a mother finds that Saturday mornings are peaceful enough, but if plans are not made for the afternoon, she and her children begin to fight.

Because balance and variety are considered crucial in the activities of the patient's life, it is helpful for the group leader to have a command of the nature and usefulness of different categories of activity. For example, arranging and playing a game of tennis requires a quite different set of social skills than those required when attending a sewing class. A ceramics class or a massage may be ideal for one patient, but very frightening for another. A knowledge of the stages or steps involved in an activity and the developmental skills essential for taking each step enables the therapist to offer a realistic short-term goal for a particular need. Llorens established a helpful table of developmental levels of activities drawn from several theoreticians (3).

Members are often lonely, and they confuse this feeling with many other feelings, particularly depression. In the Group, they are encouraged to distinguish betweeen wanting to be alone and when they are lonely and wanting to be with people. People may or may not need time to be alone, but they should not be alone by default. They need to choose to make time for taking a long bath or for resting. They also need to recognize loneliness (a more accurate word might be "deprivation"), the need for movement, contact, an exchange of feelings, or for stimulation in the environment. For example, if members can make it to the street from their apartments, they may find their spirits lifting. A shift is made from the "refuge-prison" of the house to the possibilities of the street. The transition from being "stuck in one's feelings" at home to beginning an activity is one that members are often unable to make. One way of getting "unstuck" is to call someone and talk about the feelings that are getting in the way of moving.

A third treatment principle of the Group is that, despite the enormous fear of intimacy experienced, members need human contact. H.S. Sullivan's discussion of the disorganizing aspects of the need for intimacy was helpful in understanding this contradiction (4). A member's search for a boyfriend or a friend is rarely approached directly. Instead, an interest in tennis or photography involving new people is discussed. The need for—and the terror of—people can be modulated through the structure of the interest because both the class in photography and the game of tennis include others with similar inclinations. The activity protects the member from an unstructured encounter, but also supports the need to make contact. Members of the Group seem to understand this. No one ever sets the specific goal of getting together with another person; but they often talk about how helpful it is to make plans with someone else — it is easier to leave the house if they are meeting someone. Pearce and Newton explore aspects of this need for support in their discussion of the juvenile era (2). It is emphasized in the Group that some task or activity, with or without concrete material or a product, is **always** a part of the meeting of two human beings.

Method

The method used in the Group combines elements of behavioral and intrapsychic approaches. Behavior is the focus, and the social, active behaviors are emphasized. Sitting alone in front of the TV a great deal is replaced by going to a pottery class or getting together with a friend for dinner. It is assumed that members want to change, to be happier, and that they have within them both the motivation for this task and an interest or the memory of an interest that can be nurtured. Smith, a psychologist now working on this hypothesis, sees the therapist's faith in the client's human potential as an important strategy (5). In a strictly behavioral approach, on the other hand, nothing is assumed about the internal motivation of the subject.

A desire to fulfill a need for gratifying activity with other people, at whatever developmental level, is assumed. Intrapsychic conflicts of feelings are not dealt with except when they interfere with the accomplishment of the member's goal. Often the members argue for an intrapsychic approach: "If my

head was in the right place, I would know how to organize my life and have friends." However, the premise used in the group is that people change their ideas about themselves by learning how to plan to be in a new situation and then getting support to manage, and later enjoy, the new experience. By planning step-by-step goals whereby new behavior is substituted for old, members get a taste for a new way to being in the world that may later be repudiated if it becomes too threatening, but it can never be erased (2).

This experimenting or trying out new behaviors is an important aspect of the Group. Patients are encouraged to suspend judgment and to try out things. The Group is designed to offer the possibility of experiencing control, and finally mastery, by emphasizing the demystification of the process of making friends, by learning realistic expectations for one's performance, and by common sense rules of social planning.

The Format

Members in the Group begin by writing a report of their schedules for an average week, hour-by-hour. Participants are instructed to choose an average week in terms of their functioning — not, for instance, the week before they were hospitalized. The schedule includes such details as: who was present for dinner on a particular night, when the laundry was done, and what happened on a typical Thursday evening. The participant then presents the schedule verbally to the group and includes an impression of how the whole week felt and a brief inventory of the "good" parts, including pleasures (making lasagna noodles).

Using the weekly schedule as a method of approaching leisure time allows the members to organize an idea of the past. The weeks or months before hospitalization may appear to members as a painful, vastly confusing time. Making the schedule is reassuring because they see that the behaviors of which their lives consist are describable. The schedule also suggests that planning is best done in time segments: Saturday is composed, for planning purposes, of a Saturday morning, a Saturday afternoon, a Saturday around dinner time, and a Saturday evening.

Because the therapist insists on details, members see that activities like going to the dry cleaners are part of a larger category of "self-maintenance," and that these activities are an important part of coping normally. Also, the detailed presentation helps members become aware of the smallest pleasures, the recognition of which might be lost with a vague, "I never do anything." Members begin to recognize and take seriously preferences or likings that constitute the beginnings of stronger interests or enthusiasms.

After the schedule is presented, the members have a chance to respond. Often they mention the most obvious and important aspects: "Well, you spend too much time with your kids. . . ." "I wish I had a roommate to talk to. . . ." "You told us you weren't functioning, but you cooked the meals, cleaned, and got the laundry done." Describing behavior can simplify psychologically complicated situations in a way that is helpful. For example, one member was literally spending every waking hour with her two-year-old twin boys. The Group pointed out that she could not be happy without some pleasures of her own. Her exclusive focus on the children is not dealt with as a manifestation of anything. Instead, the mother is encouraged to think of an interest of her own, something she likes to do, and to arrange to do it by setting small realistic goals. When she found she had the group's permission and support, she looked relieved and went on to make plans to join a cooperative play group and to ask a cousin to babysit in order to learn to knit. Feelings are discussed only as far as they actively interfere with the task. Often discouragement or frustration must be dealt with before members can focus on continuing and expanding the "good" parts of their lives.

Between the first and second meetings, participants try to define their interests and the areas they want to explore. One member's interests may help another to clarify his direction, or they may suggest new possibilities to him. Often it is possible for members to do all the necessary ground work in planning a strategy, like finding out where one can learn to crochet, or which agency needs volunteers, or where one can swim in the evenings.

Goal Setting

After a discussion with the other Group members, whose roles are to share experiences, test reality, and encourage, each participant sets a goal for the week. Failure to reach the goal is treated as an interesting problem to be explored. Perhaps the person did not really want to do the task or there were factors, which no one appreciated, that made it too difficult. The member is reminded that he is in charge and can set another goal. With the therapist's knowledge of task components, the task can be broken into more manageable short-term goals that are developmentally appropriate for the goal setter. Houts and Scott explain specific techniques of goal setting in their book, *Goal Planning in Mental Health Rehabilitation* (6). For example, if a member equates all socialization with a demand for sexual performance, goals should be set that take this into consideration. In this case, where his fearful yet eager attempts to meet people are focused on a mixed discussion group at a local church, the goal is to go, look around, participate in the discussion, and skip the coffee hour afterwards. Permission and support is thus given by the group to do nothing outside the "contract"—getting there is the first step.

Problem-Solving Approaches

As the group progressed, it became apparent that, despite varying backgrounds, the members had many problems in common in planning leisure time. The most recurrent problems were tackling difficult tasks, meeting people, planning for the time spent with new people, and changing one's own unfriendly behavior. A set of techniques was therefore developed to deal with these particular areas of behavior.

Arranging for Support. Members are taught that some tasks are too hard to do alone, and that they are hard for everyone. Consciously reaching out and arranging for support is presented as a desirable — not a weak — thing to do. Members learn to anticipate that they might not be able to get themselves to look for a job in the paper on a particular day or may not be able to visit a new "Y" program alone. Thus they can plan to avoid failure by arranging the support they need. One person may need to go to the library with a friend in order to get anything done. Someone else may be able to study if they know that they will have a good time after finishing the task. This knowledge helps them tolerate the isolation of their own feelings of inadequacy.

Meeting People. Patients usually cite the

time spent with husbands, wives, or friends as the most enjoyable. Often members ask, "Where did you meet that person?" A discussion follows about where the people in one's life come from: work, school, interest groups. Various ways of meeting people are discussed. Singles bars, dances, excursions to the "Village" to pick up someone are talked about in terms of their high-risk, high-anxiety potential. Over and over again, group members report having a better time when they plan activities: study dates during which one can learn to know the person and do some work, too; poker games that are not a disaster, even if one does not like the other players well enough to want to see them again.

What happens in the group can be used as an example of how people get together around a project. After two or three meetings, the members begin to relax with one another, share their fears and feelings of inadequacy, pressure each other to get to work, share their interests, and even express warmth and liking for each other. The therapist can say, "Look, it's not so impossible, it's happening here. Let's see how we can make sure it happens on the outside."

Learning to be with People. Terrors of getting to know people are explored, not on an intrapsychic level but with a view to learning social skills. Group members often share their obsessions about having nothing to say or feeling judged by others. Curiosity is encouraged as an alternative to private thoughts about personal inadequacy, and members practice "being curious" about others through role playing and in the group discussions. The Group discusses how people get to know each other: Members learn that it is easier to spend time successfully with another person who shares a common interest or activity. The leader or a group member can offer an example from his or her life of the historical development of a friendship. White discusses identification or "modeling behaviors" in the context of ego psychology in *Ego and Reality in Psychoanalytic Theory* (7).

The idea that friendships start with a simple conversation, that the first overtures can be learned and rehearsed, is a revelation. After role-playing situations — the meeting of two strangers on a train or two people in class — members get the idea that it is not the correct question that is essential to successfully begin and maintain a conversation, but rather, conversation consists of a flow of ideas, associations, and questions.

Substituting One Behavior for Another. Obviously, distorted perceptions of themselves and others often created problematic interpersonal behavior for the Group members. These problems, in turn, made change difficult. The same patterns of behavior that made group discussion and sharing difficult are the patterns that keep people lonely.

For example, for a member going through a

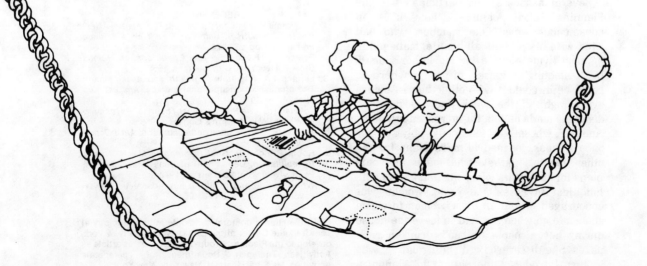

period of sharing endless obsessions with the Group, the therapist suggests setting a goal that would involve replacing the isolating, delusional behavior with another, more appropriate one. In this case, the member might talk about a current project of an exhibit of some photographs and needlepoint. No attempt is made to point out why she might need to share her delusions — to ask what is happening to make her upset — or to shut her up. Instead, the group helps her "catch" herself when she begins to use her "crazy" obsessions as a conversational gambit. When the group speaks to her about her behavior in a workmanly, "professional" way, they contribute to the mitigation of the fear and discrete condescension with which, because of her inappropirate behavior, she is met in her contact with others.

Each member discovers that he or she has subvocal obsessions: "My slip is showing, I'm sure it is." ". . . I have nothing to say. What am I going to say?" They begin to see that these subvocalizations interfere with responding in social situations, and learn that if they are busy in their heads with thoughts like "What am I going to say?" they are not listening and are therefore quite alone. If the function of this "crazy talk" is made clear, the members take hope, in spite of their impressive diagnoses and myriads of messages from others about their "chronicity."

The Value of the Group for Its Members

Several members who participated in the Planning Group changed their lives in conspicuous ways. One member, who had lived with his parents all his life, managed to support living alone after his father's death by "collecting" a variety of groups where he could be in contact with other human beings every night of the week and yet have no demands made on him for increased intimacy. Another, whose boyfriend could only see her once a week, learned to make plans for the other nights, and even to make alternate plans for the nights when she had a date with him, just in case. One young woman was encouraged to find an older woman to whom she could go when she had to leave the house during her alcoholic father's drunken rampages. She discovered a distant relative, who in turn introduced the patient to Alanon, a program for the families of alcoholics. Another

member began to write magazine articles about activities she had discovered in the process of doing research for the Group and experimented with getting together with the Group members outside the Group meetings.

Possible Applications

A planning group seems useful particularly for elderly people who need help in restructuring meaningful lives after retirement. Men and women who have participated in few activities that were purely for their personal pleasure in the years before retirement need support in finding interests that are in keeping with their sense of themselves as serious, worthwhile, and mature people. Women who have devoted themselves for a number of years to their children and homes may also benefit from a planning group, since they have particularly poignant problems in developing interests that allow for self-determination. However, the broad nature of the common problems encountered by the members of the planning groups suggest that the principles behind such a group have wide applicability. In fact, the constructive and satisfying use of leisure time is a generally neglected area and deserves more research into its dynamics.   •

Acknowledgments

The author thanks Ann G. Keill, M.D., George Hogben, M.D., Tony Hollander, O.T.R., and Ann Snitow for their support and helpful suggestions.

REFERENCES

1. DeCharms R: *Personal Causation: The Internal Affective Determinants of Behavior*, New York: Academic Press, 1968, pp. 273-274
2. Pearce J, Newton S: *The Conditions of Human Growth*, New York: Citadel Press, 1969
3. Llorens LA: Facilitating growth and development: The promise of occupational therapy. *Am J Occup Ther* 24: 1-9, 1970
4. Sullivan HS: *The Interpersonal Theory of Psychiatry*, New York: W.W. Norton & Co., Inc., 1953
5. Smith MB: Competence and adaptation. *Am J Occup Ther* 28: 11-15, 1974
6. Houts P, Scott R: *Goal Planning in Mental Health Rehabilitation*, Department of Behavioral Sciences, Pennsylvania State University, 1972
7. White R: Ego and reality in psychoanalytic theory. *Psychol Issues* 3: 190-192, 1963

•

Gail Kuenstler, a doctoral candidate in anthropology at The Graduate Center of the City University of New York, developed the Planning Group described in this article as Activities Therapist, Department of Therapeutic Activities, Mt. Sinai Hospital, New York, New York.

R30104

The Interest Check List

Janice S. Matsutsuyu, M.A., O.T.R.

The selection of patient activities in occupational therapy should be supported by a studied knowledge about the nature of interests as a differentiating human characteristic. Six propositional inferences are drawn from the literature to found a theoretical framework for an Interest Check List. This clinical datagathering instrument is described and its relation to other instruments is discussed. Its usefulness is implied as being explanatory of the commitment process underlying a patient's reconstitution of his daily living pattern.

Introduction

"To interest is to attract and hold the attention, to occupy and engage a patient's concern to the extent of employing his time, . . . This is one of the basic principles upon which occupational therapy is applied."[1]

From casual social encounters to erudite research endeavors statements can be found which reflect interest. "My interest is . . .," "I prefer . . ." or "I dislike . . ." are common expressions of interest that can be as precise as the one expressed by George Bernard Shaw who is purported to have said that he could never engage in any activity or thought that did not interest him. Whether deliberately or unwittingly, man, by his nature, commits himself to the world around him through his interests.

The Problem

Although the principle of holding and attracting a patient through his interest is commonplace in occupational therapy practice, the literature does not yield any studied approach to a systematic application of interest concepts to patient treatment. In this sense, the earliest question asked of a patient, namely "what are you interested in," is more of a social gambit than a technical inquiry. It has often been left to the intuitive powers of the occupational therapist, or to a blatant imposition of activities either to evoke or to force interest. An activity so selected may meet the treatment objectives but often leaves questionable the investment and commitment to the task at hand on the part of the patient.

The Purpose of the Study

The intent of this presentation is to identify the nature of interest as a differentiating human characteristic, propose criteria for an interest assessment instrument, and to describe an instrument for use in the assessment of interest by the occupational therapist.

Review of the Literature

There is much to support the view that whenever man concerned himself with the affective nature of activity, a productive approach has been made through interest. William James identified the main criteria of interest as attention, and Dewey wrote of the process of the identification of self with some object or idea for the maintenance of self-initiated activity.[2]

The description of interest seems to depend on whether the investigators approached the study of this phenomenon through methods of measurement or as a variable in personality development. When approached through measurement, interest is described as a task, an activity or description of an event.[3] Others support the view of interest within the dynamic forces of personality development. Interests are described as feelings, drives or reactions which are interest states and related to attitudes, values and other motivational indices such as attention, direction and sentiments.[3,4,5,6,7,8]

The more familiar use of interest terminologies appears in the literature around interest inventories as used in vocational testing, such as the Strong Vocational Interest Blank and the Kuder Preference Record. The development of interest measurement was an outgrowth of the difficulties encountered in making vocational predictions merely from general intelligence and

The American Journal of Occupational Therapy
July-August, 1969, Vol. XXIII, No. 4

aptitude tests.[3,9] That other factors contributed toward predicting vocational success led investigators into this area. Typically the interest inventory items are both vocational and avocational in nature and for the purpose of the inventory are grouped and considered as patterns of interest for evidence in supporting vocational choice. The client responds to the items as likes, dislikes, indifferences, or as preferences. The underlying factors are generally identified as mechanical, science, business system, persuasive, literary, musical, social service, and clerical.[10] Other factors include adventure vs. security, cultural conformity, need for diversion, for attention and such characteristics as nurturance and abstract thinking.[11,12]

The greater yield for occupational therapy practice seems to this writer to be the study of interest as an affective phenomena within personality constructs. Freyer early described the criterion of interest as that of a feeling. Feeling of pleasantness is interest and feeling of unpleasantness, aversion.[9] From this rather simplistic point of view subsequent investigators began to build a case for interest as by-products of personality and a special case in general motivational theory.[3,8,13,14]

Allport points to the mature personality as possessing "sophisticated and stable interest" and a "characteristic and predictable style of conduct." "Convictions and habits of expression are definitely centered, evaluations are sure, actions are precise, and the goals of the individual's life are well-defined." (p. 190)[5] For him, interest embodies two components: (1) a cognitive relationship of the person to the environment, and (2) a subjective relationship to his ego values. In addition, he views interest as more central to the person and therefore leading to his active participation in pertinent activities and contents. Interest satisfaction is not predominately "emotional" in the sense of tension reduction. "Learning proceeds because it is relevant to an interest system: (1) it adds to knowledge, (2) differentiates items within the system, and (3) broadens the range of equivalent stimuli" (p. 120).[15]

Roe and Seligman's study of the origin of interest was based on the premise that interest, as an aspect of personality should be subject to the same developmental principles as any other aspect of personality. They spoke of interest as meaning "any activity (action, thought, observation) to which one gives effortless and automatic attention." (p. 3)[4]

A further description of interest is offered by Gardner Murphy who defines interest as "the attitude with which one attends to anything; the feeling accompanying attention; . . . interests are dispositions defined in terms of objects which one easily and freely attends to or which one regards as making a difference to oneself" (p. 197).[16]

A most cogent conceptualization within motivational schemes can be found in Robert White's concept of competence which refers to an organism's capacity to interact effectively with his environment. This need for the organism to deal effectively with his environment is characterized by behavior that is directed, selective and persistent, and satisfies an intrinsic need to deal with the environment even after basic needs are in abeyance. White proposed the term effectance to the motivational aspect of competence.[7]

The term "feeling of efficacy" is ascribed to the subjective and affective aspects of effectance. It implies satisfaction where organisms have had behavioral transaction with the environment that produced changes in the stimulus field and led to competent interaction through exploration or mastery. Effectance transaction with the environment means directing attention to part of it, and interest is aroused when the stimulus can provide variability and novelty.

The Frame of Reference

Propositions of Interest

After a fairly exhaustive review of the interest literature, the author drew a series of inferences about this phenomenon. These were formulated as six propositions. A proposition in this sense means the relationship of variables which can be indirectly tested by means of its implications.[17]

Proposition 1. Interests Are Family Influenced.

Interests are determined by early developmental contingencies that are primarily localized in the family unit where early intra-familial experience influences direction.

The family, as the primary social agent, has considerable influence on the enculturation of the child in learning about himself and others. It is in the family that the child first receives the foundation for group living, for understanding social roles, and for learning about other social institutions. It is also in the family organization that the child's ego is directed into certain patterns, where other potentials are redirected, drives and interests are channeled, certain dependencies are permitted and other independent capacities according to age, sex and position in the family, are required.[18] The Roe and Seligman study of the origin of interest was based on the premise that "one of the earliest and greatest differentiation of interests develops from the degree to which attention is focused on persons and primarily as a result of early experience. Further differentiation follows throughout life" (p. 44).[4]

Proposition 2. Interests Evoke Affective Response.

Interest can evoke affective response with persons, things, and ideas and can be expressed as likes, dislikes, indifferences or as preferences.

The affective nature of interest can serve either to attract attention or to repel. Both the negative and positive poles of interests are critical factors in determining the capacity of the individual to state preferences for either the presence or absence of interest. This state may be related to age, sex, opportunities and experiences.

Proposition 3. Interests Are Choice States.

The capacity to make interest choices serves the process of commitment to life roles for work, through occupational choice, and for play, through recreation and leisure.

Adolescence as a critical period in preparing for the tasks of adulthood is well confirmed. Ginzburg and his associates identified interest, capacity, value and reality as major factors during this period for making occupational choice.[19] The integration of adolescent attitudes, interest and abilities with opportunities for trial and error, mastery and competition in relevant social settings of home, school and community with peers and meaningful adults are crucial events that guide the level and course of commitment.[20]

Proposition 4. Interests Can Be Manifest in Effective Action.

Interest as a subjective experience can lead the individual to engage in pertinent activities that can be satisfying and have adaptive value.

Effectance motivation embodies the characteristics of direction, selection and persistence. This occurs when an individual interacts with his environment and learns that he has had some effect on the environment as well as experienced the environment's effect on him. The association of interest with learning tasks related to work and play contributes to effective and rewarding ways of transacting with one's environment.[5,7]

Proposition 5. Interest Can Sustain Action.

Degree or strength of interests varies according to the level and type of interaction with the event and can serve to sustain action during the learning stages or to maintain functional achievement.

Beyond the point that interest attracts and directs attention is the issue of sustained or persistent transaction. White contends that once an effective action occurs, i.e. tasks are learned, ritualization or habituation incorporates certain of our daily activities without the intensity of the original interest that initiated the activity, or sustained it during the learning phase. Persistency is present when an activity can be maintained through novelty or when other levels of skill remain to be learned in a given transaction with person, things or ideas.[4,7]

Proposition 6. Interests Reflect Self-Perception.

Expressed interests are subjective statements which reflect self-perception.

In expressing an interest an individual is calling attention to the fact that he has a certain awareness about himself and about his environment.[3,8,13] Super postulates that interests reflect self-concept and that answers given to interest questionnaires are "I am" statements. Roe contends that this awareness of oneself and the surrounding world permits man to make reasonable rational choices either to realize or not to realize one's potentials.[21]

Operational Policy

A basic assumption of this investigator's interest study was that clinical validity and reliability is directly related to the frame of reference of the users. The above six propositions therefore, establish the theoretical basis upon which the Neuropsychiatric Institute Interest Check List was constructed. In addition, it is recommended that the operational policy be defined in order to make the use of such an instrument operative.

The operational policy is based on the conceptualization of occupational behavior as the balance between work, rest and play with the concomitant interpersonal and task skills that integrate and support the life roles of any socialized individual.[22,23,24,25,26] Interest is but one of the components to be assessed within this total concept.

Reilly has identified six specifications for an occupational therapy program that directs itself towards the assessment of occupational behavior and allows for reconstitution of the old behavior and for practice of newly acquired skills. The sixth of these specifications is accepted as the operational policy for this study. Specification No. 6 identifies a program structure for a rehabilitation milieu which presses for the exercise of life skills in a balanced pattern of daily living, takes into account individual interests and abilities, tailors daily events to age, sex and occupational role, and is guided by the knowledge of the proper objectives of each subdivision of daily life space.[22]

The Instrument

The Proposed NPI Interest Check List

The Neuropsychiatric Institute (NPI) Interest Check List (Fig. 1) is based on the impressionistic philosophy of assessment for providing a description of typical behavior and for differentiating individuals according to a set of variables. Its limitation is that it is not a test meeting the rigid requirements of psychometric testing. It is a data-gathering instrument within the range of the questionnaire class called "check lists."[27]

This NPI Interest Check List is an empirically derived instrument first introduced in 1961 for use with the adult psychiatric inpatients by the occupational therapy department at the Neuropsychiatric Institute, University of California at Los Angeles. Revisions for the instrument were based on the finding of this author and were guided by the interest assessment tools as devised and used by Roe and Seligman and by Tyler. [4,14]

The use of this instrument is dependent on its integration with other data-gathering tools being used or currently being designed by graduate occupational therapy students for assessing occupational behavior.[26,28] It is imperative that the users of this instrument understand the body of knowledge that supports the six propositions advanced as the underlying premise of the instrument. The NPI Interest Check List by itself merely provides gross findings of the subjective expressions of interests.

Purpose

The purpose of the NPI Interest Check List is to classify and describe the interest state of psychiatric patients by: (1) classifying the intensity of interest according to item responses, (2) classifying types of interest according to the category system, (3) describing the individual's ability to express personal preference, and (4) describing the individual's capacity to discriminate type and intensity.

NPI INTEREST CHECK LIST

Name: .... Unit: .... Date:........

Please check each item below according to your interest.

ACTIVITY	CASUAL	STRONG	NO
1. Gardening		✓	
2. Sewing	✓		
3. Poker	✓		
4. Languages		✓	
5. Social Clubs	✓		
6. Radio	✓		
7. Bridge			✓
8. Car Repair	✓		
9. Writing		✓	
10. Dancing		✓	
11. Needlework	✓		
12. Golf	✓		
13. Football	✓		
14. Popular Music	✓		
15. Puzzles		✓	
16. Holidays		✓	
17. Solitaire	✓		
18. Movies		✓	
19. Lectures		✓	
20. Swimming		✓	
21. Bowling	✓		
22. Visiting		✓	
23. Mending	✓		
24. Chess			✓
25. Barbeques	✓		
26. Reading		✓	
27. Traveling		✓	
28. Manual Arts		✓	
29. Parties	✓		
30. Dramatics	✓		
31. Shuffleboard			✓
32. Ironing	✓		
33. Social Studies	✓		
34. Classical Music	✓		
35. Floor Mopping	✓		
36. Model Building		✓	
37. Baseball	✓		
38. Checkers			✓
39. Singing	✓		
40. Home Repairs	✓		
41. Exercise	✓		
42. Volleyball	✓		
43. Woodworking	✓		
44. Billiards	✓		
45. Driving	✓		
46. Dusting	✓		
47. Jewelry Making	✓		
48. Tennis	✓		
49. Cooking	✓		
50. Basketball	✓		
51. History	✓		
52. Guitar			✓
53. Science	✓		
54. Collecting			✓
55. Ping Pong	✓		
56. Leatherwork	✓		
57. Shopping	✓		
58. Photography	✓		
59. Painting	✓		
60. Television	✓		
61. Concerts	✓		
62. Ceramics	✓		
63. Camping		✓	
64. Laundry			✓
65. Dating		✓	
66. Mosaics	✓		
67. Politics			✓
68. Scrabble			✓
69. Decorating	✓		
70. Math			✓
71. Service Groups			✓
72. Piano			✓
73. Scouting	✓		
74. Plays		✓	
75. Clothes		✓	
76. Knitting	✓		
77. Hairstyling			✓
78. Religion			✓
79. Drums	✓		
80. Conversation	✓		

Please list other special interests:

Rehabilitation
NPI/UCLA

FIGURE I

Description of the Instrument

The NPI Interest Check List is in three parts. Part 1 includes eighty (80) items to which affective responses could be made. These items were selected on an a priori and empirical basis by a cumulative panel of occupational therapists and graduate registered occupational therapy students. The final selection was based on the following criteria: (1) that the items be commonly understood items within the range of general knowledge; (2) that the items be categorically appropriate; the categories are Manual Skills, Physical Sports, Social Recreation; Activities of Daily Living and Cultural/Educational; (3) that there be some feasibility of translating the expressed interest activity into manifest action within the existing program.

The items are numbered 1 to 80 with columns to be checked under the headings of Casual Interest, Strong Interest, and No Interest.

Part II is the section at the end of the check list to add any special interests not listed.

Part III is on the reverse side where the respondent is asked for a written narrative report to the question, "Could you describe your interests, hobbies, pastimes, giving a historical summary of how you spent your leisure time from grammar school days to the present. Indicate what kind of thing you like to do best and least."

Classification and Description

The NPI Interest Check List primarily gives information about the expressed interests of the patient. The raw data can be systematized into a pattern of interests according to the five categories of Manual Skills, Physical Sports, Social Recreation, ADL and Cultural/Educational, and the three expressions of strength of interest.

The numerical scores provide the data for classification purposes.

The intensity of interests are classified according to item responses of Casual, Strong, and No.

All three responses are considered significant in reflecting the choice state of the individual.

The expressed responses will indicate the affective quality of attraction or aversion to an activity item. (Proposition 3). The number of items checked will indicate casual, strong or no focus of attention and gives a reading as to the type or direction the individual's interests take. (Proposition 2). The findings can provide the basis for a descriptive analysis of the interest state of the individual (Proposition 1).

The occupational therapist can derive a summary note from the findings of the classification system and the written historical narrative by the patient. This note will necessarily be descriptive since the data to this point has been taken directly from the self-reports of the expressed interests of the patient.

Interview

Further clarification and more definitive information about the interests of the patient can be gained through a follow-up interview. The systematized data and interest state description can lead to formulations of questions that can be directed to the patient for elaboration or clarification. It would be pertinent to ask questions regarding the recency of the individual's participation in any of the special interest activities in which he hopes to participate in the future or about which he would like to gain more information. Activities with negative responses can be questioned concerning the issues of low satisfaction, ineffective performance or lack of opportunity, with implications of non-supportive environment or deficits in capacity. (Proposition 1, 4, 5, 6).

Summary

Limitations imposed on a patient by injury or disease process may alter the course of his life-role function and cause the patient to reconsider his usual modes of behavior and performance. A critical issue to be considered in such cases is whether the motivational process of directed attention, selectivity and persistence are present, absent or in abeyance in the individual. Evoking interest on a day to day basis through treatment activities for limited and/or long term goals is a responsibility the occupational therapist assumes. Understanding the antecedent factors which evoke or sustain interest enhances the commitment process of the patient in reconstituting functional behavior through adaptation of old patterns or learning new or different modes of performance. It is hoped that a systematic collection of data will provide the occupational therapist with valid information from which to build an environment that sets standards for skilled instruction and protects a patient's right to hope and to learn.

BIBLIOGRAPHY

1. Hinsie, L. E. and Campbell, R. J. *Psychiatric Dictionary.* 3rd ed., p. 400. New York: Oxford University Press, 1960.
2. Berdie, R. F. "Factors Related to Vocational Interests," *Psychol Bull* 41 (1944): 137-157.
3. Super, D. E., Stariskevsky, R., Matlin, N., Jordaan, J.P. *Career Development: Self Concept Theory.*

New York: College Entrance Examination Board, 1963.

4. Roe, A. and Seligman, M. *The Origin of Interests.* Washington, D.C.: American Personnel and Guidance Association, 1964.

5. Allport, G.W. *Personality and Social Encounter.* Boston: Beacon Press, 1960.

6. Cattell, R.B. "Personality and Motivation Based on Structural Measurement". In *Psychology of Personality,* edited by J.L. McCary pp. 109-120. New York: Logos Press, 1956.

7. White, R.W. "Motivation Reconsidered: The Concept of Competence". In *Sourcebook in Abnormal Psychology,* edited by L.Y. Rabkin and J.E. Carr, pp. 77-101. Boston: Houghton Mifflin Co., 1967.

8. Carter, H.D. "The Development of Vocational Attitudes," *J Consult Psychol* 4, (1940) :185-191.

9. Freyer, D. *The Measurement of Interests.* New York: Henry Holt and Company, 1931.

10. Buros, O.K., ed. *The Sixth Mental Measurements Yearbook.* Highland Park: The Gryphon Press, 1965.

11. Guilford, J.P., Christensen, P.R., Bond, Jr., N.A., Sutton, M.A. "A Factor Analysis Study of Human Interests," *Psychological Monograph* 68, 1954.

12. Ronning, R.R., Stellwagen, W.R., Stewart, L.H. *Application of Multidimensional and Scale Analysis to Interest Measurement.* Berkeley: University of California, 1963. United States Office of Education.

13. Bordin, E.S. "A Theory of Interest as a Dynamic Phenomena," *Educ Psychol Measmt* 3, (1943) :46-66.

14. Tyler, L.E. and Sundberg, N.D. *Factors Affecting Career Choices of Adolescents.* Eugene: University of Oregon, 1964. Cooperative Research Project #2455.

15. Sheerer, M. "Cognitive Theory". In *Handbook of Social Psychology,* edited by G. Lindzey. Cambridge: Addison-Wesley Publishing Co., Inc., 1954.

16. Hahn, M.E. and MacLean, M.S. *Counselling Psychology.* New York: McGraw-Hill Book Company, Inc., 1955.

17. Marx, M.H., ed. *Phychological Theory: Contemporary Readings.* New York: The Macmillan Co. 1959.

18. Lidz, T. *The Family and Human Adaptation.* New York: International Universities Press, 1963.

19. Ginzberg, E., Ginsburg, S.W., Axelrad, S., and Herman, J.L. *Occupational Choice.* New York: Columbia University Press, 1951.

20. Erikson, E.H. "The Problem of Ego Identity." In *Psychological Issues* 1, (1959):101-164, Monograph.

21. Roe, A. "Man's Forgotten Weapon". In *Human Values and Abnormal Behavior,* edited by W. D. Nunokawa, pp. 140-147. Chicago: Scott Foresman and Co., 1965.

22. Reilly, M.A. "A Psychiatric Occupational Therapy Program as a Teaching Model." *Amer J Occup Ther* 20 (1966):61-67.

23. Silberzahn, M. A. "A Study of Human Adaptation as Skill Competency Process". Unpublished master's thesis, Occupational Therapy Department, University of Southern California, 1967.

24. Takata, N. N. "Development of a Conceptual Scheme for Analysis of Play Milieu". Unpublished master's thesis, Occupational Therapy Department, University of Southern California, 1967.

25. Shannon, P. D. "Work Adjustment and the Adolescent Soldier". Unpublished master's thesis, Occupational Therapy Department, University of Southern California, 1966.

26. Moorhead, L. "The Occupational History in Occupational Therapy." Unpublished monograph, Occupational Therapy Department, University of Southern California, 1967.

27. Sellitz, C., M. Jahoda, M. Deutsch, and S. W. Cook. *Research Methods in Social Relations.* New York: Holt, Rinehart and Winston, 1965.

28. Westphal, M.O. "A Study of Decision Making". Unpublished master's thesis, Occupational Therapy Department, University of Southern Calif., 1967.

The Occupational History

Linda Moorhead, O.T.R.

The phenomenon of occupational behavior is defined as a long process of developmental experiences. The inclusion of this theoretical framework requires the occupational therapist to assume responsibility for history-taking. Role experiences accumulated in the occupational developmental process are seen as important definitions of a patient's strengths and deficits as well as a major explanation of current functioning. The critical variables of occupational role performances are described and the difficulties of the history-taking method are discussed. The history-taking instrument is applied to a case and the usefulness of the method in drawing inferences for treatment planning is illustrated.

Introduction

The occupational therapist is reaching the stage in professional growth where he must assume the role of historian in his efforts to trace, analyze and explain the functional deficits and strengths of the patients.

Before examining clinical history-taking as a scientific method and demonstrating its application to case material, a brief explanation of occupational function is presented.

Occupational Behavior

The phenomenon of occupational behavior is so basic to human life and so broad in constituant components, that it defies simple analysis. It is most appropriately conceptualized as social behavior, that is, behavior molded and defined by the social institutions in the service of group needs.[1,2] It is active productive behavior that earns for man his membership in society and satisfies his needs for involvement.

It has been observed that handicapped people and discharged patients often have a particularly difficult time assuming useful roles in the community, roles in which their skills are needed and they can feel a part of productive society.[3] This fact is made all the more significant in view

Linda Moorhead is Staff Occupational Therapist at the Neuropsychiatric Institute of the University of California, Los Angeles.

July-August, 1969, Vol. XXIII, No. 4

of the general belief that involvement in occupational functions is a major contributor to mental health and provides structure and meaning for what would otherwise be, at best, marginal lives. It appears that patients returning to the community are probably more in need of structure and meaning than most, and that those in the helping professions have an obligation to assume larger responsibility in the matter.

This difficulty, so frequently blamed on residual pathology, or on a resistant and prejudiced public, seems to have more to do with the fact that many patients are ill-prepared for the occupations they seek. They are, in fact, ill-prepared for community membership in several spheres and it is the nature of that preparation this study seeks to uncover.

Occupational Role

One of the most helpful techniques for investigation of occupational function and the preparation behind it has been to view it in terms of social role theory. Role concept has been constructed as a frame of reference for conceptualizing man's interaction with his human and task-oriented environment. Social roles are viewed as institutionally prescribed and proper ways for an individual to participate in society and thus satisfy his needs and wants.[4]

This study has accepted the sociological generalization that human adult roles can be divided into three major role groups; (1) family roles, i.e. parental or sibling, (2) personal sexual roles, and (3) occupational roles.[5] The third group has been accepted as the most pressing and appropriate concern of occupational therapy.

Occupational roles are identified as much by the positions they afford people in their social context as by the actual tasks connected with them. It is possible to broaden the term occupation from its usual limited definition regarding paid employment, to include a number of major social roles such as homemaker, volunteer, and student. The overriding commonality between these roles is their meaning and importance to individuals as vehicles for social involvement. People identify each other by the occupational roles they perform and these roles become incorporated into personal self-identification systems.

Occupational Development

Occupational behavior can be viewed as a manifestation of an individual's response to the demands of his environment and the assumption can be made that his participation in earlier social roles supplied crucial experience for adult role performance. Developmental literature in the psycho-social fields supports this assumption and indicates that the child's experience in the roles of family member, student, peer group member, and beginning worker influences, almost totally, his ability to function occupationally as an adult. Researchers in the field of vocational development emphasize the necessity for children to explore and experience many task-related positions in order that they learn to appreciate their own assets and particular characteristics.[6,7,8] As they mature, they translate this self-knowledge into occupational choice. These authors indicate that the process of socialization can result in either a positive or negative assessment of one's capacities and potential. Developmental experiences dominated by success lend themselves to expectation of success and self-confidence, whereas repetition of failure after failure leads to negative expectations and severe limitations upon the individual's ability to make the translation into a satisfactory adult occupational role. In addition to the actual experiences the growing child encounters, he absorbs many cultural values and attitudes from the role models in his environment and incorporates these into his perceptions as well.

The developmental process is complex and not yet fully understood. Enough is known, however, to make occupational history-taking possible and provide reasonable clues to the conditions underlying functional deficits.

The following outline is a breakdown of skills and qualities seen as emerging through social learning and considered essential to occupational role performance. They are offered as variables helping to identify the behavior sought to describe.

Critical Variables to Occupational Function

A. Autonomy and Independence
   a. Realistic perception of one's own assets and liabilities
   b. Ability to make stable decisions and implement them effectively
   c. Competence in management of time, space, and personal needs

B. Implementation
   a. Motivation
   b. Orientation to:
      1. own interests, choices and preferences
      2. own requirements for rewards and satisfactions
      3. range of possibilities for implementation, some appreciation for alternatives
   c. Job or position seeking ability, possession of training, education, etc.

C. Maintenance
   a. Adequate task/work behavior
      1. continuity
      2. stability
      3. quality of performance
   b. Capacity to accept failure, perform under stress and maintain flexibility
   c. Adequate interpersonal competence
   d. Balancing skills in work-play, activity-rest, etc.
   e. The capacity to handle conflicting role expectations

History

The gathering of history is the essence of scientific method. Research itself is basically the art of recording, as nearly as possible, exactly what has occured in a certain situation. Whether the researcher sets up an experiment or examines naturally occuring phenomena he arrives at his findings through his record of historic events. Therefore, as historians, occupational therapists must assume responsibility for adherence to the rules of research protocol. These rules dictate what conditions must be met for findings to be reliable and valid and therefore useful as contributions to known fact.

In gathering occupational history the investigator is concerned with discovering how and under what conditions the individual patient has learned to perform occupationally as he does; how the patient has learned to approach tasks and role expectations as he does; and whether, he was ever more competent than he now appears? Can the therapist expect that the patient will be able to improve his role skills, and if so, how much? In other words, the investigator asks what a patient's particular life style is in terms of occupational function, so that therapy can be structured for him to build upon his experiences for improved function.

Method

The first task is identification of sources for such a history. The patient is actually the only witness to all of his own life experience. In addition, there may be observing witnesses such as parents, teachers, employers and possibly some recorded documents offering second party reports of the patient's history. The literature indicates that the patient's self-report of his social life experience is the historian's best and most useful resource. Such a report should be elicited with some assurance that the reporter (the patient) is not giving false or incomplete data.

The second task then for the history-taker is structuring reliability into the data-gathering procedure. The rules of data-collecting indicate that honest and complete self-reports depend upon several variables. For example, the respondent must be motivated to report his history and he must have confidence that the material will not be misused. He should have memory and communication ability free of disabling dysfunction so that he is able to give data.[9]

Even when these factors are in good order and the respondent is willing and able to report, major hurdles remain before the data meets scientific standards. Historians warn that facts do not speak for themselves but must be carefully selected, organized, analyzed and synthesized into meaningful statements in order to be useful.[10]

Selection of Data

Obviously it would be absurd for the investigator seeking to appraise occupational history to permit his data-source (the patient) to ramble along through hours and hours of self-report hoping that the process would yield some useful data. Consequently, the therapist is forced to implement a system for guiding the self-report into areas where the yield will be greatest and into another system to analyze the gathered data into useful statements.

The system most commonly used for the first situation is the interview. Interviews can be conducted in many ways varying according to question construction and degree of structure they impose on the self-report. The more rigid the interview structure (i.e. fixed response type interviews) the more limited but reliable the data are. The less structured the interview form the more it provides for comprehensive data but also the more open it is to distortions and contamination.[11] Since the scope of experience we wish to sample in the the occupational history is broad and general, the data selection method employed has had to be semi-structured. That is, specific questions are asked but the interviewer is free to probe and rephrase questions for the particular material to be elicited. Consequently, all of data selection cannot be built into the interview instrument (the set of questions) but is dependent upon the skill of the interviewer as well as a knowledge of what to ask, how to ask it and what sorts of life experiences are most important to know about. This and all subsequent steps in the history taking process rely heavily on the preparation of the investigator as the knowledge of the process under investigation guides each step and influences the outcome.

Analysis

Analysis of history data is perhaps the most difficult step in this evaluation process. Some points are obvious as the data accumulates, others more obscure and resistant to appraisal. The total importance and meaning of data appear gradually.

This material is elicited according to a pre-arranged order and commonly lends itself to analysis according to patterns of learning, growth and change in the life course. The four basic foci in analysis of data appear as follows:

1. Learnings and socialization in childhood roles.
2. Exploration and decision process around issue of occupational choice.

3. Patterns of achievement and failure and environmental conditions which appear to influence.

4. Course of movement, and solidification or lack of it, in period of adult occupational roles.

Case material selected to exemplify these first attempts at occupational history-taking follows before a discussion of the results and their application to treatment.

Occupational History Case

This case involves a 22-year old schizophrenic male who was referred for evaluation of his potential as a worker and as a college student. He was living at home with his parents and was receiving regular outpatient psychotherapy. He was unemployed and not in school, a situation that had existed for approximately one year. Investigation of his current level of function revealed that he stayed close to home except for occasional outings, had few household responsibilities and was financially dependent on his family. He had few hobbies and spent the majority of his time alone reading. He was able to maintain good grooming, hygiene, and eating habits but was quite casual about his scheduling of time which was consistant with his loosely structured daily activities. He had a few long-term friendships and dated occasionally. His most frequent contacts were his family with whom he seemed to be getting along fairly well. Even though he was not in school, he identified himself as a sort of student; one who selected his material and read independently in preparation for work in the computor-electronics field. His discription of this preparation process aroused serious questions as to the practicality of such an approach and his history was examined in search of clues to a surer way to help him become occupationally functional.

Summary of History Findings

He had been a bright and promising youngster, active in school and boy scouts, and with other special interests such as hiking and camping. He showed early academic potential, made good grades and found school work easy. He was especially good in math. Because he was an asthmatic child, he did not participate in the more active competitive sports but liked mental competition such as chess. As he progressed through school he broadened the scope of his interests to include music, the school band, and social club member-

ship. He continued to do well in school but was informed that his IQ was extremely high and that he should be in the top 1% of his class. In general, the range of his interests, his free exploration of his environment, his feelings of competency were evidence of his early foundation for achievement.

His high school and college experience suggested that his early promise had been highly dependent upon the close homogeneous culture of his neighborhood schools where he had been surrounded by children like himself. When he entered a large public high school he was at a loss to know how to behave within a broader social class representation. The boys his age were striving to prove themselves through behavior that he did not consider proper or fitting for himself. After some struggle, he began to find his identity as a musician and he dreamed of being a career performer. He was talented and received important support from his peers and teachers. As his occupational choice crystalized his parents raised powerful objections, demanding that he consider only the "professions" (i.e. medicine or law). Their intentions were so firm that he could not overcome them. His grades had fallen to C's so his parents had him transferred to an exclusive private school to prepare for college.

The private school culture supported him as elementary school had and his performance once again improved. He was surrounded by children from upper-class families who had been placed in the school for reasons similar to his and he made friends readily. He learned to play a new instrument and became more than ever involved in academic work. He was even able to enter into successful amateur business ventures in the summers with a classmate.

After graduation he entered another large impersonal educational institution four hundred miles from home. He rapidly became lost, lonely and barely functional as a college student. He never made another occupational choice although he gave some serious thought to a literary career based on his one positive experience in an English literature course. By the end of the first year, he flunked out of school and returned home to work as a busboy all summer. In the fall he left home again and attempted to make up his grades in a junior college. He was unable to manage the transfer back into the first university and essentially abandoned his hopes for finishing school. In the following two years he did not return to school but continued the ritual of working summers in unskilled jobs while living at home and going north in the fall each year, and spending the winter in a futile and bizarre way. One year he took his summer earnings, bought fishing and camping equipment, and started out for Alaska hoping to live as a fisherman.

There was one time in those years when he said he was happy and productive. It was a period of two months when he had signed on with a sideshow troop performing and serving as roustabout. The elements of the job that were so important to him were: (1) his boss, a stern, honest, compassionate man made life bright and was fatherly to the patient; (2) the fact that he was a member of a closeworking group and probably the fact that (3) in a small way he was realizing part of his career dream of being an entertainer.

Finally, one year before he was seen, he received an ultimatum from his parents that either he return to school, get a permanent job, or seek psychiatric help. He tried once again to replay the role of student, was again unsuccessful and at the end of six weeks living away from home, he was overtly psychotic and had to accept the only remaining alternative: to live at home in the role of dependent child and to engage in psychotherapy.

Summary of Findings and Recommendations

Some of the conclusions reached after analysis of his history were as follows:

1. The respondent was seen as functioning at a deficit level in comparison with earlier history. He had arrived at that level after a series of disabling occupational role failures and was considered ill-prepared for rapid movement back into either the worker or the student role.

2. He was capable of a higher level of function when provided with support for taking gradual small steps outward, renewing his contacts in the community from his home base, and proceeding again with occupational choice exploration.

3. His potential for the worker role was greater than his potential for the student role at the time he was seen, but any movement into employment would have to be accompanied by clarification of objectives, and assistance in job-seeking. It was crucial that he find a position meeting his particular needs for task, supervision, structure, and status while offering an opportunity for use of his rather exceptional mental and creative skills.

Discussion

Probably the most significant information gained through occupational history-taking with this patient concerned his limited capacity for role flexibility. In instance after instance he had been unable to sustain achievement in environments that failed to provide: (1) regular support and feedback from a peer group fairly homogeneous with himself; (2) regular recognition and feedback from supportive role models and authority figures; and (3) a living arrangement which duplicated a family-like structure. He was bright, attractive, had numerous skills and interests but had suffered enough failures to make risking new attempts at occupational function a highly threatening prospect for him. He had approached occupational assessment with some trepidation but was anxious to revise his failure pattern and willing to approach the situation fairly realistically.

In this case the history findings were submitted to his psychiatrist in the form of a consultation and reported directly to the patient in a counseling session where plans were formulated for his next moves.

Since he had been an active participant in the history-taking process it was possible to discuss openly with him findings and suggestions, and to help him build an awareness of his own requirements for role function. He was advised to increase gradually his involvement with task-oriented roles on a non-pay basis in areas such as a drama workshop, or volunteer service, keeping his homebase intact as a stabilizing factor and moving out cautiously. His history indicated that his capacity for living away from home while establishing new student or worker roles was extremely low. In addition, the issue of job choice was discussed in anticipation of future employment. He was able to incorporate the new information he had about himself and his environmental needs and begin to translate this into more appropriate and feasible goals in terms of occupation.

The case presentation above has been recounted at some length in order to illustrate the particular usefulness of historical data to an occupational therapist. The course taken following assessment was unusual in that it involved counseling rather than clinical treatment of the patient.

Additional uses of the history data are: (a) contracting with patients about treatment goals during hospitalization; (b) structuring the clinic experience to nurture the development of occupational skills; and (c) as an explanation for current deficits and strengths discovered in total case assessment.

Conclusion

We are only at the first phase of knowledge in this form of clinical assessment. At the present time we have identified some areas of history that appear to have a high potential for yielding data useful in understanding the occupational deficits found in patients. We have found that data is accessible in most cases if appropriate methods are used to obtain it. We are beginning to see the need for the occupational therapist to conduct his own history-gathering because he requires specific knowledge of the patient to form the basis for application of his valuable and unique service as a treatment agent.

BIBLIOGRAPHY

1. Caplow, Theodore. *The Sociology of Work.* New York: McGraw-Hill, 1954.
2. Nosow, Sigmund and Form, William. *Man Work and Society.* New York: Basic Books, Inc., 1962.
3. Simmons, Ozzie S. *Work and Mental Illness.* New York: John Wiley & Sons, 1965.
4. Toby, Jackson. "Some Variables in Role Conflict Analysis." In *Problems in Social Psychology,* edited by Backman, Carl W. & Paul F. Secord. New York: McGraw-Hill, 1966.
5. Vinenberg, Shalom. "Rehabilitation: A Means to What End?" In *Current and Future Trends in Rehabilitation as They Affect Occupational Therapy in Rehabilitation Facilities.* Arkansas: Arkansas Rehab. and Teaching Center, 1967.
6. Super, Donald E. et al. *Career Development: Self Concept Theory.* New York: College Entrance Exam Board, 1963.
7. Ginzberg, Eli. *The Development of Human Resources.* New York: McGraw-Hill, 1966.
8. Tiedeman, David and O'Hara, Robert P. *Career Development: Choice and Adjustment.* New York: College Entrance Exam Board, 1963.
9. Richardson, Stephen A., Dohrenwend, Barbara S., & Klein, David. *Interviewing: Its Forms and Functions.* New York: Basic Books, Inc., 1965.
10. Barzun, Jacques & Graff, Henry E. *The Modern Researcher.* New York: Harcourt, Brace & World, 1957.
11. Selltiz, Claire & Jahoda, M., Deutsch, M., Cook, S. W. *Research Methods in Social Relations.* New York: Holt, Rinehart and Winston, 1965.

Temporal Adaptation: Application with Short-term Psychiatric Patients

(psychiatry, time, adaptation)

Ann Neville

This paper begins with a literature review to investigate temporal dysfunction and its relationship to psychopathology and to adaptation. A specific program begun in a short-term hospital with psychiatric patients is then described. This program uses temporal adaptation as a framework for assessing patients' use of time and for developing methods to increase productive use of time.

Activity histories provide the occupational therapist with important information about patients—their work, their interests, their education, and their use of time. In assessments of psychiatric patients in a short-term hospital, the patients' use of time attracted this author's attention.

Kielhofner, in his article on temporal adaptation (1), provides a conceptual framework for looking at time. Learning, culture, homeostasis, social roles, and habits are discussed by Kielhofner as important in how patterns of activity and time

Ann Neville, M.S., OTR, is an Occupational Therapist on the inpatient psychiatric service of the Department of Medicine, Lenox Hill Hospital, New York, New York.

May 1980, Volume 34, No. 5

are integrated for successful adaptation. This framework provides a useful basis upon which to devise an evaluation and treatment program for patients.

This paper begins with a literature review to further investigate temporal dysfunction and its relationship to psychopathology and to adaptation. A specific program started in a short-term psychiatric hospital using temporal adaptation as a framework for assessing patients' use of time and developing methods to increase their productive use of time is described.

Two types of problems presented by psychiatric patients appear in the review of the literature. One relates directly to their psychopathology, which may be organic in origin, and the second relates to problems in development that result in poor socialization and an inability

to solve problems, set goals, and implement these goals. It is important for the occupational therapist to recognize the difference between these two types of problems. The former will diminish as psychopathology is reduced, whereas the latter problems are areas in which occupational therapy can provide assistance (Kielhofner, G, personal communication).

Psychopathology and Time Distortions

Distortions in the experience of time occur in many types of psychiatric disorders. Some distortions clearly have an organic basis such as memory difficulties related to ECT (electric shock therapy), and alcohol and drug reactions. These disorders may show marked impairment on the mental status examination (a test of cognitive functions—attention, ability to abstract, and comprehension) in orientation to time, place, and person.

Other distortions may be experienced more subjectively; stress and anxiety may contribute to this type of distortion. A striking account of a distorted time experience is reported by a patient in her diary:

Julia lives in a strange time world. Everyday is a thousand years, yet the days behind me all collapse into nothing, like a pack of cards. Every-day is so long that a normal human being can't imagine it. Every moment is the same way—long. Nothing within this time world has any meaning for me, which is why the time is so long .... (2)

Time perception shows no direct sensory basis (3). However, the perception of time is connected with exteroceptive sensory organs (sight) as well as proprioceptive organs (sensitivity to alternating rhythms of expectation) (4). Lesions in the brain, primarily in the temporal and occipital region, produce disturbances in perceptual skills that interfere with experiencing time. Sequencing, visual and spatial relations, position in space, and movement in space are perceptual skills relevant to time (5).

Many studies of time perception in schizophrenic patients have been reported (6-8). The results are inconsistent because of problems in terminology, a lack of uniform definitions for terms such as time sense, time orientation, and time perception, and because of differences in experimental methods.

A recent study (9) excluded schizophrenic patients with organic signs. The results showed little or no difference between the schizophrenic population and the normal population in time estimation. Thus, time distortions may have an organic component.

Time distortions and their relation to perceptual motor skills is an area for further study. Sensory integration evaluation and treatment may be a beneficial first step in treatment of time dysfunction. Lorna Jean King, in her recent symposium on "Sensory Integration as a Broad Spectrum Treatment Approach," (10) does not see sensory integration in conflict with other frames of reference but as

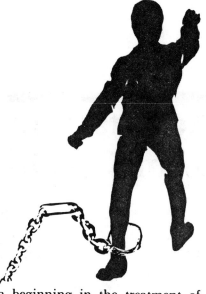

a beginning in the treatment of schizophrenia. This, however, is only a hypothesis that needs testing and verification.

Future Time Perspective and Adaptation

The studies above that emphasize the microstructure of time (time estimation and time duration) have inconclusive results. They are related directly to the symptoms of the psychopathology. In addition, they fail to emphasize the meaningful events that define a person's past, present, and future. These events, called *macro-events* (1), provide persons with a sense of continuity when viewing their past, present, and future. A distortion in this time sense of macro-events can significantly affect ways of coping and adapting to the environment. The importance of these macro-events has been overlooked by the psychiatrist who traditionally has confined the evaluation of time to the mental status examination.

The ability to project into the future is the temporal mode most deficient within a number of different categories of psychiatric diagnoses (12). Several studies have related future time perspective to schizophrenia, depressive states, suicidal potential, and degree of thought disturbance: for instance, in one study of schizophrenia (13), future time perspective is defined and rated

on concepts of "coherence" and "extension." Coherence is the degree to which subjects are able to organize events in the future. Extension is the length of time subjects are able to project themselves into the future. The authors reported significant differences in coherence and extension between schizophrenic and normal people (13).

These methods were also used in a study to measure future time perspective in depressed as well as in schizophrenic persons (14). In addition to supporting the previous findings of differences between schizophrenic and normal persons, on measures of extension the authors found depressed persons were less able to project themselves into the future than schizophrenic persons. Schizophrenic persons, on the other hand, showed more difficulty in coherence—organizing their life events logically. However, those with psychotic depressions showed more disturbance in this area than neurotic depressions. From these studies schizophrenic and depressed persons appear less oriented toward the future than normal persons.

Suicidal potential and its relationship to future time perspective has also been investigated (15). Yufit and others found that persons with serious suicidal intent were less able to establish plans and have hope for the future and were extremely limited in their future time perspective.

Fink's study (16) shows a relationship between future time perspective and activity in elderly subjects. Half of the subjects were institutionalized, and half were residents in the community. Activity was measured by the hours subjects spent working (occupation), engaging in a hobby, or participating in an activity related to the organization of the institution. A positive correlation was found between the number of hours devoted to work (for financial gain) and hobbies, and future emphasis as measured on a time perspective scale. Significant negative correlations were found between these variables and past emphasis. No significant correlations were obtained between organizational activity within the institution and past or future emphasis. The authors concluded that not only activity, but also interest and motivation were correlated to future emphasis. They proposed that an activity program geared toward productive work involving monetary return be developed within the institution.

The above studies add to the understanding of temporal adaptation, with future time perspective a critical dimension to adaptation, linking the future to the present. Future time perspective is important to consider when asssessing patients' use of time, their ability to set and organize goals, and their ability to implement them into purposeful activity.

Future time perspective has been used primarily in the above studies for its diagnostic implications only. This author proposes using future time perspective as an indicator of a person's ability to adapt to his or her environment.

Implementation

A short-term inpatient unit at Payne Whitney Psychiatric Clinic provided the setting for the implementation of the time management program. The need to further assess patients' use of time became apparent after reading their comments on the activity history, a part of the initial evaluation given in occupational therapy. Patients frequently left blank, crossed out, or responded "no way, too personal," or "this is my problem," to the section where

they were asked to complete a schedule of a typical weekday and weekend day before being hospitalized.

A group was organized with a focus on leisure time skills as a first attempt to respond to the need for productive use of time. Patients participated in a planned activity that was followed by a discussion. Although active participation ensued, the group did not help individuals with their personal time management problems. A more thorough evaluation of this area of the patient's life seemed necessary together with restructuring the occupational therapy program to emphasize the temporal dimension.

The time management group was organized for patients who, according to the occupational therapy intake information, had problems managing their leisure and work time outside the hospital. It met for 1 hour once a week until the author left the setting, a period of about 8 months. It was based upon a two-part time-oriented evaluation and implementation.

The group's goals (terminal behaviors) were for the patient to be able to: 1. indicate how time was spent outside the hospital; 2. classify activities in relation to work, play, and self-care (patients have a difficult time identifying what is work, play, or self-care); 3. identify a need for change; 4. formulate goals for one's self; 5. organize these goals into priorities; 6. formulate specific activities to accomplish these goals; and 7. begin working on these activities.

Group Format. At the beginning session, the patients were told about the group's purposes—to look at how they spend their time outside the hospital and to identify what they would like to change, and how they would implement these changes. Responsibility for identifying

problems with time management was placed upon the patient. Motivation is also important if change is to occur. Patients who were in the group the first week were requested to instruct new members about the group. Continual restatement of the goals was helpful, not only for the old members to refocus their goals, but also for the new members by providing a rationale for the process of examining their use of time.

After the introduction to the group patients were given a folder with a series of activities to complete. The "pie of life" (17) activity consists of a circle divided into 24 equal sections corresponding to 24 hours. The patients were instructed to fill in each section with how they spent their time before they were hospitalized; to color each area with a coded color; to count and record the number of hours spent in each activity; and, after having a look at their previous use of time, they were asked if they were satisfied with how they are spending their time and what they would like to see changed. This activity is graphically useful in revealing the areas of dysfunction.

The second activity emphasizes goal setting and is a simplification of Alan Lakein's steps to time management (18).

Further assessment of time use is individualized and is based on the patient's awareness of problems and need for change. For example, some patients have worked on vocational tests, work evaluations, and activities related to leisure interests. Some have explored various community agencies or programs to achieve a goal.

Outcome or Results. Initially, some patients responded negatively to the group and walked out of the room. It was apparently threatening for them to examine their use of time publicly. For those who stayed and followed the time-management evaluation, problems were identified faster and intervention could occur more quickly. The first step in making a change is being aware of the problem. Because it is difficult to deny a problem with time management when it is so clearly defined by the time schedule of the patient, the evaluation format revealed temporal adaptation problems in one session. For example, a young patient who spent his day at home watching TV revealed his low self-image was caused by his weight problem; the patient would not go out because of his appearance. In the group discussion (which occurred in each session) another patient suggested he contact Over-Eaters Anonymous to help him achieve his goal of losing weight. The patient looked up the telephone number of this organization in the phone book but became resistant when it was time to make the call because he had never used the telephone. The patient role-played the situation and was able to follow through on the call. Through identifying a problem with use of time, other problems were identified—a weight problem, poor self-image, and lack of communication skills via the telephone. As Kielhofner states (1), the temporal adaptation frame of reference focuses on an important dimension of one's life, a dimension that encompasses all areas of occupational therapy.

However, a time management program cannot be handled effectively in just a one-hour weekly session, for it must encompass all areas of a person's life. Patients should make some decisions and have responsibility for using their time more productively. Time management could become the central theme around which to structure the entire occupational therapy program.

Plans are to use this time evaluation with all patients as part of the initial occupational therapy evaluation upon admission. In addition, many of the methods used in the future time perspective studies such as time questionnaires, story completions, and future autobiographies could be incorporated into the program. The remainder of the program could be divided into work, leisure, and self-care modules with patients attending one, two, or all three areas. These areas would be divided into activities such as recreational therapy, dance therapy, and crafts, with referrals based on individualized needs, rather than on the traditional group approach. It appears that an individualized program, not group-oriented activities, may be more appropriate for patients in a short-term hospital setting.

Summary

Future time perspective, defined as an ability to project into the future and to logically organize future events, is deficient in a number of people. Understanding the future time perspective of patients may help improve their ability to engage in purposeful activity in their every day schedules. Development of programs emphasizing work, play, and self-care in relation to future orientation seems indicated, especially where length of hospital stay is short.

Acknowledgments

The author wishes to acknowledge Sharon Coleman, Ph.D., for her editorial assistance, and Susan B. Fine, M.A., OTR, FAOTA, and Gary Kielhofner, M.A., OTR, for their support and encouragement.

This article is based on a presentation given at the AOTA 58th Annual Conference, San Diego, California.

REFERENCES

1. Kielhofner G: Temporal adaptation: a conceptual framework for occupational therapy. *Am J Occup Ther* 31: 235-242, 1977
2. Hartocollis P: Time and affect in psychopathology. *J Am Psychoanal Ass* 23: 383-395, 1975
3. Dobson W: An investigation of various factors involved in time perception as manifested by different nosological groups. *J Gen Psychiatr* 50: 277-298, 1954
4. Edelstein E: Changing time perception with anti-depressant drug therapy. *Psychiatr Clin* 7: 375-388, 1974
5. Schecter DE, et al: Development of the concept of time in children. *J Nerv Mental Dis* 121: 301-310, 1955
6. Densen M: Time, perception, and schizophrenia. *Percept Mot Skills* 44: 436-438, 1977
7. Goldfarb S, et al: Time perception of alcoholics and other psychiatric patients. *J Genet Psychol* 125: 315-318, 1974
8. Johnson JE, Petzel T: Temporal orientation and time estimation in chronic schizophrenics. *J Clin Psychol* 27: 194-196, 1971
9. Crain P, et al: Temporal information processing and psychopathology. *Percept Mot Skills* 41: 219-224, 1975
10. King LJ: Symposium: Sensory integration as a broad-spectrum treatment approach. King of Prussia, PA: Continuing Education Programs of America, 1978
11. Wallace M, Rabin A: Temporal experience. *Psychol Bull* 57: 213-236, 1960
12. Braley LS, Freed N: Modes of temporal orientation and psychopathology. *J Consult Clin Psychol* 36: 33-39, 1971
13. Wallace M: Future time perspective in schizophrenia. *J Abnorm Social Psychol* 52: 240-245, 1956
14. Dilling CA, Rabin AI: Temporal experiences in depressive states and schizophrenia. *J Consult Psychol* 31: 604-608, 1967
15. Yufit RI, et al: Suicide potential and time perspective. *Arch Gen Psychiatry* 23: 158-163, 1970
16. Fink H: The relationship of time perspective to age, institutionalization, and activity. *J Gerontol* 12: 414-417, 1957
17. McDowell CF: *Leisure Counseling: Selected Lifestyle Processes*, University of Oregon, Portland, OR: Center of Leisure Studies, 1976, p 83
18. Lakein A: *How to Get Control of Your Time and Your Life*, New York: Alan Lakein & Co., 1973

The American Journal of Occupational Therapy

A WORK ACTIVITY PROGRAM FOR FORMER MENTAL PATIENTS

Arlene Price, O.T.R.
Connie Rance, O.T.R.
Joel Pribnow, M.A.

■In February 1972 the multidisciplinary aftercare team of the inpatient psychiatry service at Hennepin County Medical Center in Minneapolis designed and implemented a work activity program for former psychiatric patients with poor employment histories. The program was to provide a supportive atmosphere in which clients could learn and develop socialization and work skills in a simulated work setting.

The program is located in a social rehabilitation center in the inner city. It is set up like a small manufacturing company, with clients working on an assembly line to produce handcrafted goods, primarily patchwork quilts and placemats. There is also some contract work with local industry. Currently clients do collating for a real estate firm and disassemble light meter boxes so that the parts can be sold as scrap metal.

Staff of the program include a director with a master's degree in vocational rehabilitation and a master's-level registered occupational therapist who work full time. Work study students from local universities, volunteers from the community, and the aftercare nurse from the inpatient psychiatry service at the center work part time. There is also one CETA position, currently filled by a mental health worker. The aftercare team continues to serve as consultants to the staff.

The program operates four days a week, from 9 to 11 a.m. Twenty-five clients currently participate; they keep track of their hours on a time clock and receive a small wage, 60 cents an hour, paid every two weeks. Those who have perfect attendance and are punctual for two consecutive weeks receive a bonus, equivalent to one day's wages. Although the salary is small, it has helped improve the self-esteem of many of the workers; they are gratified to hold a paid job.

The clients are referred from the mental health services at the center, the division of vocational rehabilitation, board-and-care facilities, and the county welfare system. All clients have a history of previous hospitalizations, are unemployed and have been unable to hold a job, and have been unsuccessful in other vocational programs. Their chronic adjustment problems have made integration into the community difficult.

A total of 75 clients have participated in the program. They range in age from 18 to 70 years; the majority are between 30 and 55. Most are white and live in efficiency apartments or in board-and-care homes. Sixty per cent are men, and approximately 95 per cent receive some form of public assistance. Most have chronic to severe psychiatric disturbance, primarily schizophrenia, and approximately 95 per cent are receiving psychotropic medication.

After a client is referred to the program, he completes an application and an interview and works for one week in a variety of tasks. At the end of the evaluation period staff assign him to an appropriate activity. The staff make daily notes on each client's performance and give him feedback on his progress. After three months in the program the clients are re-evaluated on the basis of their attendance, personal appearance, social skills, quality of work, attitude, and stability.

The production tasks range from the simple and repetitive, such as cutting patchwork squares, to the more complex operation of running a sewing machine. Clients begin work at the level of their ability and move to more complex tasks as their skills improve. There are no specific time limits on patients to progress through the levels of activity.

A unique feature of the program is home visiting. Within two weeks after the client is accepted in the program, a staff member visits the client's residence in order to better understand his life style. The visits also provide support for the client living in a new setting and help staff evaluate future placements.

Marketing the craft products, which involves developing and maintaining outlets in the business community for their sale, creates incentives for work, instills pride in clients, and promotes good relations with the community. Currently quilts and placemats are sold directly to two shops, are sent to two others on a consignment basis, and are sold periodically at special sales in shopping centers. Approximately 10 per cent of the program's funding comes from the sale of products. The division of vocational rehabilitation provides 35 per cent of the program's funds and Hennepin County provides the rest.

The ultimate goal of the program is to place the clients in sheltered workshops, vocational training programs, or competitive employment. Seven clients have graduated from the program and moved into competitive employment, six into sheltered workshops, and three into training programs. Although the figures are modest, one must remember that these are individuals who had not succeeded in or qualified for traditional rehabilitative programs. Ten clients dropped out of the program and five have been placed in the transitional program for work activity clients who can assume a higher level of responsibility and are awaiting placement in community programs or employment.

The clients' enthusiastic attendance at the program and increased socialization indicate that it is successful. Part of the success can be attributed to the individual support offered by staff and the flexibility of the organizational structure. When clients are placed in another workshop or job, the work activity program staff help the client and his new employer solve any adjustment problems that occur. If a client is unsuccessful in his new placement, he can return to the program and work

Mrs. Price and Ms. Rance are consultants to the work activity program and are staff members of the inpatient psychiatry service at Hennepin County Medical Center, 701 Park Avenue South, Minneapolis, Minnesota 55415. Mr. Pribnow is the director of the work activity program.

toward another placement. To date seven clients have returned to the program.

Future plans include expanding the program to five mornings a week for the better-functioning clients and offering an afternoon shift for those who are functioning at a lower level. The afternoon session may become a maintenance program for the long-term client who cannot advance from a work activity status to transitional or competitive employment. The clients in the morning session could work as leaders during the afternoon session and thus develop supervisory skills and increase self-confidence.

As state hospitals close and community treatment develops, program planners must include work activity programs as part of the community plan. Staff, clients, and businessmen involved in this project are convinced that work activity programs can meet the basic human needs of self-esteem and personal acceptance for a population of minimally functioning former psychiatric patients who have not benefited from traditional vocational rehabilitation programs.

E. PAUL TORRANCE

Reprinted with permission from the author and *The Journal of Creative Behavior*

Sociodrama as a Creative Problem-Solving Approach to Studying the Future

The term "futuring" is being heard more often as people recognize the importance of studying the future and as we develop skills for doing so. A new profession of futurists — people working in such fields as forecasting, policy research, futuristics, etc. — has been developing. Futurists stress future alternatives, opening up possibilities, imagining "unimaginable worlds," and fitting us all into them. They do not wish to ignore the past or to manipulate the future, but try to keep us from letting the future take us too much by surprise and show us that choices being made today influence what will happen tomorrow.

The idea of futures studies in schools was advocated in the 1930's and 1940's but the idea failed to catch on then. Now the need for futures studies is more obvious and we also know more about the abilities, skills, and methods required in such studies. Almost all of the programs that have been developed for teaching creative thinking and creative problem-solving have emphasized these abilities and skills. A variety of ways for teaching children to study the future have been suggested; however, fundamental to all of these methods is the ability to solve problems creatively. Children who have learned and can practice creative problem-solving skills will be able to solve future problems. They will be better prepared to cope with situations where basic information has changed, as it were, overnight.

FUTURISM IN CHILDREN'S SOCIODRAMATIC PLAY

Young preschool children are studying the future when they engage in spontaneous sociodramatic play or role playing. Two- and three-year-olds derive a great deal of satisfaction

Volume 9   Number 3   Third Quarter

from playing mother and father and other adult family roles. However, two or three years later these same children seem to take these roles for granted and, though they still make use of them, it is not with the same excitement. The child's social world is expanding and so is his concept of the future.

Since sociodramatic play is such a natural way of exploring and studying the future, the procedures suggested here seem very natural. The child entering kindergarten or first grade already has the intellectual skills for engaging in this kind of study. By adding to it the discipline of creative problem-solving, it should become increasingly productive as the child develops and matures. It should also be a useful technique with adults.

SOCIODRAMA AS A CREATIVE PROBLEM-SOLVING PROCESS

In *Creative Learning and Teaching* (Torrance & Myers, 1970) I described sociodrama as a creative problem-solving process. Sociodrama at its best is a group creative problem-solving process, and the problem-solving process in sociodrama can be as deliberate and as disciplined as any other creative problem-solving approach. The general principles of sociodrama have been formulated by Moreno (1946) and have been refined by Moreno himself (1952), Moreno and Moreno (1969), Haas (1948), Hansen (1948), Klein (1956), and others.

Sociodrama can be conducted in the ordinary classroom or in practically any other physical setting, if the director or teacher can create the proper atmosphere. Some children and adults find it easier to identify with a role if they are furnished with a single, simple stage prop, such as a cap, helmet, shoe, coat, or even superman gear. The director must be imaginative in transforming an ordinary desk and chair into a ship or a jet aircraft or whatever the occasion calls for.

The objective of sociodrama is to examine a group or social problem by dramatic methods. In the case of futuristic sociodrama, the problem focus is a problem or conflict which is expected to arise out of some trend or predicted future development. Multiple solutions may be proposed, tested, and evaluated sociodramatically. As new insights or breakthrough in thinking occur, these too can be practiced and evaluated. The planning, selling, and implementing stages of problem-solving can also be practiced and tested. The production techniques and their power to induce different states of consciousness facilitate creative breakthroughs and increase the chances that creative solutions will be produced.

A number of things can be done to produce readiness for sociodrama. Perhaps the most important thing is to set aside one or more periods prior to the sociodrama for a free and open discussion of the problem to be studied. Efforts should be made to generate as much spontaneity as possible in these discussions. This is a part of the process of becoming aware of puzzling situations, gaps in information, conflicts, dilemmas, and the like. The problem selected for sociodramatic solution should be one that the group members have identified as important to all or most of them.

Although not necessary, the use of music, lights, and decorations can do much to set the right mood for a sociodrama.

The steps in the problem-solving process in sociodrama are quite similar to those formulated by Osborn (1963) and Parnes (1967) for creative problem-solving.

Step 1. *Defining the Problem.* The director, leader, or teacher should explain to the group that they are going to participate in an unrehearsed skit to try to find some ways of solving some problem of concern to all of them. It is a good idea to begin by asking a series of questions to help define the problem and establish the conflict situation. At this point, the director accepts all responses to get facts, to broaden understanding of the problem, and to word the problem more effectively, and asks other questions to stimulate or provoke further thinking about the real problem or conflict. This produces what Parnes (1967) refers to as "the fuzzy problem" or "the mess" and leads to the establishment of the conflict situation (statement of the problem).

Step 2. *Establishing a Situation (Conflict).* Culling from the responses, the teacher or director describes a conflict situation in objective and understandable terms. No indication is given as to the direction that the resolution should take. As in creative problem-solving, judgment is deferred. The conflict situation is analogous to problem definition in the creative problem-solving model.

Step 3. *Casting Characters (Protagonists).* Participation in roles should be voluntary. The director, however, must be alert in observing the audience for the emergence of new roles and giving encouragement to the timid person who really wants to participate and is saying so by means of body language. Rarely should roles be assigned in advance. Several members of the group may play a particular role, each trying a different approach.

Step 4. *Briefing and Warming Up of Actors and Observers.* It is usually a good idea to give the actors a few minutes to plan the setting and to agree upon a direction. While the actors are out of the room, the director should warm up the observers to the possible alternatives. Members of the audience may be asked to try to identify with one or the other of the protagonists or to observe them from a particular point of view. When the actors return to the room, they can be asked to describe the setting and establish more fully their role identities. A brief but relaxed procedure, it warms up both the audience and the actors.

Step 5.
Acting Out the Situation. Acting out the situation may be a matter of seconds or it may last for 10 or 20 minutes. As a teacher or leader gains experience as a sociodrama director, he will be able to use a variety of production techniques for digging deeper into the problem, increasing the number and originality of the alternatives, getting thinking out of a "rut," and getting group members to make bigger mental leaps in finding better solutions. The director should watch for areas of conflict among group members, but not giving clues or hints concerning the desired outcome. If the acting breaks down because a participant becomes speechless, the director may encourage the actor by saying, "Now, what would he do?" or turning to another actor and saying, "What happens now?" If this does not work, it may be necessary or desirable to "cut" the action. The use of the double technique may also be used to cope with such a crisis.

Efforts should be made to maintain a psychologically safe atmosphere and to give freedom to experiment with new ideas, new behavior, new ways of solving problems. It is in this way that participants come to "see and feel" other ways of "behaving" and get away from "more and better of the same" inadequate behavior.

Step 6.
Cutting the Action. The action should be stopped or "cut" whenever the actors fall hopelessly out of role, or block seriously and are unable to continue; whenever the episode comes to a conclusion; or whenever the director sees the opportunity to stimulate thinking to a higher level of creativity by using a different episode. A description of some of these production techniques will be given later.

Step 7.
Discussing and Analyzing the Situation, the Behavior and the Ideas Produced. There are many approaches for discussing and analyzing what happens in a sociodrama. Applying the creative problem-solving model, it would seem desirable to formulate some criteria to use in discussing and evaluating alternatives produced by the actors and audience. In any case, this should be a rather controlled or guided type of

discussion wherein the director tries to help the group rede-fine the problem and/or see the various possible solutions indicated by the action.

Step 8. *Making Plans for Further Testing and/or Implementing Ideas for New Behavior.* There are a variety of practices concerning planning for further testing and/or implementa-tion of ideas generated for new and improved behavior resulting from the sociodrama. If there is time or if there are to be subsequent sessions, the new ideas can be tested in a new sociodrama. Or, plans may be related to applications outside of the sociodrama sessions. This step is analogous to the selling, planning, and implementing stage in creative problem-solving. For some time, role playing has been a widely used technique for preparing people to sell and/or implement new solutions. What happens in Step 8 of socio-drama is quite similar to what has happened through this particular use of role playing.

As Stein (1974) indicates, most discussions about role playing, psychodrama, and sociodrama as techniques for stim-ulating creativity discuss potential usefulness for hypothesis formation. Usefulness at the hypothesis making (solution finding) stage is obvious, because playing a role permits a person to go beyond himself and shed some of the inhibi-tions that stifle the production of alternative solutions. Playing a role gives a person a kind of license to think, say, and do things he would not otherwise do. In my experi-ence I have found that the sociodramatic format can facilitate all other stages of the creative problem-solving process as well. Children who have internalized and practiced the crea-tive problem-solving process move spontaneously into such stages as developing criteria, evaluation of alternatives, and implementing solutions when engaged in sociodrama.

DIFFERENT
STATES OF
CONSCIOUSNESS
There is considerable evidence to indicate that the produc-tion of breakthrough ideas usually occurs during states of consciousness other than the ordinary, fully rational state. Gordon (1961), for example, has maintained that "in the creative process the emotional component is more important than the intellectual, the irrational more important than the rational."

He states further that these emotional, irrational elements can and must be understood in order to increase the proba-bility of success in a problem-solving situation. He explains that these ideas must be subjected to logical, rational tests once they have been produced but that this is not the way breakthrough ideas occur.

The term "arational" rather than "irrational" would probably be more appropriate. Some psychologists would attribute the phenomena to a difference in the way the brain processes information. Ornstein (1972) and others explain much of what happens in terms of the differential functions of the right and left hemispheres of the brain. The left hemisphere processes information by means of the ordinary mode of consciousness — the analytical, logical, sequential way of thinking that most of us have learned to take for granted. The right hemisphere of the brain, it appears, operates in a very different way — another way of perceiving reality, of processing information. Rather than processing information linearly and sequentially, it processes information globally, non-linearly. It does not deal very much with words but rather with spatial form, movement, and experience. It processes information more diffusedly and its responsibilities demand a ready integration of many inputs simultaneously. Its functioning is more holistic and relational. There are some indications that this functioning can be facilitated through states of consciousness other than ordinary awareness. Such states of consciousness as heightened awareness, rapture, regression, meditation, reverie, and expanded awareness would appear to be especially facilitative.

It is my hypothesis that sociodrama can facilitate the induction of these states of consciousness, if the sociodramatic director employs those production techniques that encourage the above states of consciousness. In the section that follows, I shall identify and describe briefly some of the production techniques that would seem best to facilitate the induction of these states of consciousness and thus the production of breakthrough ideas that could not be produced by logical reasoning.

SOCIODRAMATIC PRODUCTION TECHNIQUES

A variety of production techniques have been developed by Moreno (1946, 1969) and his associates. Some of them seem much better than others for engendering different states of consciousness and facilitating the production of creative ideas. I shall identify and describe briefly some of these along with a few that my students and I have invented.

Direct Presentation Technique

Direct Presentation Technique (Moreno & Moreno, 1969). Group members are asked to act out some problem situation, new situation, conflict situation, or the like related to the statement of and/or solution of the problem under study. In using sociodrama to study the future, problem situations will usually be anticipated future problems of concern to group members.

The following are good sources of such problems:

The Futurist and many other materials published by World Future Society, 4916 St. Elmo Avenue (Bethesda), Washington, D.C. 20014.

Footnotes to the Future published by Futuremics, Inc., 2850 Connecticut Avenue, N.W., Washington, D.C. 20008.

Futureport published by Future Forum, 12 Shattuck Street, P. O. Box 1169, Nashua, N.H. 03060.

Futuribles (cards containing 288 possible futures) published by Cokesbury Press, P. O. Box 840, Nashville, Tenn. 37202.

Future Planning Games Series published by Greenhaven Press, Box 831, Anoka, Minn. 55303.

While the direct presentation production technique can usually be counted upon to produce increased alertness and even expanded awareness at times, it is not as likely to induce other states of consciousness as some of the other production techniques. At times, however, actors become so caught up in the sociodrama that they seem to lose ordinary awareness, at least for a time, and new insights burst forth.

Soliloquy Technique   *Soliloquy Technique.* In the soliloquy, the actors share with the audience their normally hidden and suppressed feelings and thoughts. The actor (protagonist) turns to one side and expresses his feelings in a voice different from that used in the dialogue. One type of soliloquy may take place immediately after the enactment of a conflict situation. The protagonist may be walking home, driving, riding a bus, trying to study, or just engaging in reverie. On the three-level stage, the actor performs on the lower, larger level. In another type of soliloquy, the portrayal of hidden, unverbalized feelings and thoughts are portrayed by side dialogues parallel with other thoughts and actions. It permits the actors to share experiences which they feared to bring to expression or failed to perceive in the direct presentation.

This production technique frequently evokes original ideas which later stand the test of logic. The states of consciousness most likely to be induced are reverie, internal scanning, fragmentation, and regression. In the terminology of creative problem-solving, incubation is likely to occur both among the actors and the audience. The time out for soliloquy, though brief, gives a chance for the incubation process to operate and new ideas may burst forth and then be applied immediately in the ongoing dramatization.

Double Technique

Double Technique (Toeman, 1948; Moreno & Moreno, 1969). In this production technique, one of the actors in a conflict situation is supplied with a double who is placed side by side with the actor and interacts with the actor as "himself." The double tries to develop an identity with the actor in conflict. By bringing out the actor's "other self," the double helps the actor achieve a new and higher level of creative functioning. The Actor-Double situation is usually set up following the use of a Direct Presentation after the actor has withdrawn from the conflict. He imagines himself alone in the woods, walking along the street or in a park, or sitting at home. This production technique may also be used following the Soliloquy technique to speed up or facilitate the production of alternative solutions.

The whole idea of Double Technique (Toeman, 1948) is rooted in ideas concerning creativity in altered states of consciousness. The idea appears in the mythology of many different cultures. Many highly creative people have reported having doubles. The famous French author, de Maupassant, reported that his double would come into his room and dictate his work to him. In executing the Double Technique, the protagonist and the double are on the stage together and the double acts as the protagonist's invisible "I," the alter ego with whom he talks at times but who exists only within himself. This invisible double in sociodrama is projected into space, embodied by a real person and experienced as outside of the protagonist. The double may try to stir the protagonist to reach deeper levels of expanded consciousness. He reaches for those images which a person would reveal when talking to himself in privacy. It is a shared task. In one sense, it is dyadic brainstorming at a very intense level. The protagonist may experience many kinds of resistance. The double makes use of this resistance to suggest even more diverse ideas or solutions and to work through to deeper and more expanded states of consciousness.

Any one of several states of consciousness may emerge. The most likely include: expanded consciousness, internal scanning, stored memories, reverie, suggestibility, regression, and rapture.

In using sociodrama as a deliberate method of solving problems creatively, the sociodramatic director may instruct the double and the protagonist to engage in dyadic brainstorming for alternative solutions. At times, it may even be useful to have someone record the alternatives produced. At the end of the dyadic brainstorming, the audience can be given an opportunity to add alternatives that did not occur on the stage.

Multiple Double Technique

Multiple Double Technique (Moreno & Moreno, 1969). This is a variation of the "standard" double technique and is especially useful for bringing different points of view to bear on a conflict situation and provides a good vehicle for group brainstorming. The actor in the conflict situation is on stage with two or more doubles of himself. Each portrays another part of the actor (different moods, different psychological perspectives, etc.).

This production technique is especially effective when turned into a group brainstorming session, involving from three to six people. The traditional rules of brainstorming may be applied or they may be relaxed. If brainstorming rules (Osborn, 1963) are relaxed and negative criticism occurs, one of the doubles can talk back in a way that is not possible in ordinary brainstorming. This may heighten the conflict and lead to a kind of arousal which will produce breakthrough ideas. After such a brainstorming session, additional ideas may be obtained from members of the audience who were identifying with one of the actors.

Identifying Double and Contrary Double Technique

Identifying Double and Contrary Double Technique (Pankratz & Buchan, 1965). This technique is a variation of the Multiple Double Technique. The protagonist is given an identifying double and a contrary double to represent the "good" and "bad" parts of his thoughts. These two doubles are encouraged by the director to influence the protagonist. The doubles may be quite forceful with their lies, promises, and distortions. The protagonist is encouraged to evaluate carefully both sides of the issue or conflict.

Mirror Technique

Mirror Technique (Moreno & Moreno, 1969). In this production technique, another actor represents the original actor in the conflict situation, copying his behavior patterns and showing him "as in a mirror" how other people experience him. This technique may help the audience and actors become aware of emotional blocks to conflict resolution.

In sociodrama, I have found the Mirror Technique less frequently useful than in psychodrama. However, I have found that an effective variation of the Mirror Technique can be produced in sociodrama when the protagonist leaves a conflict situation involving two or more alter egos. The alter egos can then mimic, as frequently occurs in real life, the behavior of the protagonist. This variation of the Mirror

Technique makes it clear to the group that more of the same kind of behavior will only make matters worse and that the problem situation should be restructured and the problem redefined. Once this happens, the group is ready to produce and test solutions quite different from the ones being used.

The Mirror Technique may be used in sociodrama when the protagonist cannot represent his role. The mirror may be exaggerated, employing techniques of deliberate distortion in order to arouse the protagonist or a member of the audience to correct what he feels is not the accurate enactment and interpretation of the role. In sociodrama, the audience may become the protagonist and react to two or more mirror presentations of some human drama relevant to the central conflict.

Role Reversal Technique

Role Reversal Technique (Moreno & Moreno, 1969). In this particular technique, two actors in the conflict situations exchange roles — a mother becomes the child and the child becomes the mother; a teacher becomes a pupil and a pupil becomes a teacher, etc. Distortion of the "other" may be brought to the surface, explored, and corrected in action, and new solutions may emerge. In sociodrama, representatives of different social roles should reverse roles. For example, a black person should play a white person's role and vice verse.

Moreno and Moreno (1969) considered role reversal the direct route to the co-conscious and the co-unconscious. Many workers have reported that through role reversal they can get to preconscious thinking within a single one-hour session. By reversing roles one actor tries to identify with another. Experience has shown that persons who are intimately acquainted reverse roles more easily than those who are separated by a wide psychological, ethnic, or cultural distance. In sociodrama, however, there are values to be derived from errors in identification due to this distance and misunderstandings can at times be reduced.

Future Projection Technique

Future Projection Technique (Yablonsky, 1974). In using sociodrama to study the future, this production technique is of course, quite basic. In it, the actors show how they think the conflict will "shape up" in the future. An intense, effective warm-up is highly essential and the known particulars and specifics of the situation should be given. Generally this will involve dyadic brainstorming between the director and the protagonist. However, the audience may also help construct the future situation, pooling their already acquired information about the future. Daydreaming, expanded awareness, internal scanning, and stored memories are the major states of consciousness likely to be tapped by this production technique.

Auxiliary World Technique. The entire future world of the protagonist is structured through a series of acts or episodes as he envisions them. Each of these acts should portray some part of the protagonist's future world that is likely to influence the behavior of members of the group and have consequences for the resolution of the conflict situation. Basically, this production technique facilitates daydreaming, internal scanning, and expanded awareness.

Magic Shop Technique (Moreno, 1946). The Magic Shop Technique is useful in providing groups with insights into their real goals and desires in life. In studying the future, it provides a natural vehicle for testing out and evaluating new alternative life styles. The group or a representative of the group is confronted by the proprietor of the Magic Shop, who may be either an auxiliary ego or the director. In this confrontation, the proprietor offers the group anything that they may want in the future, such as an end of racial discrimination, elimination of pollution, increased intelligence or creativity, a particular style of life, and the like. The proprietor demands as payment something that the group may also value, such as leisure, a high standard of living, etc. This places the group in a dilemma and usually brings about immediate introspection or internal scanning. The result of this confrontation is an acceptance or rejection of the "bargain" or, as occurs in many cases, the inability of the customer to make a decision. To push thinking further, such techniques as Soliloquy, Double, Multiple Double, etc. may be used to facilitate meditation, daydreaming, and expanded awareness.

High Chair and Empty Chair Techniques (Lippitt, 1958). These production techniques are especially useful with groups lacking in self confidence about their futures. In the Empty Chair Technique, the protagonist acts out problems by imagining his enemy seated in an empty chair on the stage, and he interacts with the "phantom" being (common enemy), even to the extent of reversing roles and, in the phantom role, interacts with the imaginary other person in the role of the one who is absent.

In the High Chair Technique, either an ordinary chair is placed on a box so that when the protagonist sits on it he is higher than anyone else seated, or he stands on a chair so that he stands higher than anyone else on the stage.

Auxiliary World Technique

Magic Shop Technique

High Chair and Empty Chair Techniques

This is a useful technique for helping a protagonist acquire a feeling of power needed to deal effectively with enemies or strange future situations. The group can then brainstorm analogues to the high chair which will give equivalent advantages.

Dream/Fantasy Technique

Dream/Fantasy Technique (Z. T. Moreno, 1959). This production technique allows a group to enact its dreams and hopes and test and change them. Or it may put its delusions and fantasies about the future to a test. This technique is good for encouraging "freewheeling" and "wild ideas" which, once they are produced, can be tamed or modified.

Therapeutic Community Technique

Therapeutic Community Technique (Moreno & Moreno, 1969). This production technique projects a community in which disputes, conflicts, etc. between individuals and groups are settled under the rules of therapy instead of the rules of the law. In a difficult, depressing situation when few constructive solutions have been produced, the use of this technique is useful for ending the session on a "high, hopeful note."

Sociodramatic Dance Technique

Sociodramatic Dance Technique (Fine, Daly, & Fine, 1962). In this production technique participants sit in a circle and listen to music. They become warmed up at their own pace. It can be combined with other production techniques such as double ego, multiple role playing, etc. It is a non-verbal approach that is useful for emotional expression, or learning new behavior. It is facilitative of a variety of states of consciousness (expanded awareness, reverie, regression, etc.).

"Silent" Auxiliary Ego Technique

"Silent" Auxiliary Ego Technique (Smith, 1950). In this production technique, the actors communicate by gesture rather than speech and activities are suggested in the same manner. States of consciousness such as heightened alertness and expanded awareness should be encouraged.

Magic Net Technique

Magic Net Technique (Torrance, 1970; Torrance & Myers, 1970). This is especially useful for warm-up purposes in heightening anticipation and expectations. About five volunteers are given the "Magic Net" (pieces of nylon net in various colors). Having created an atmosphere of "magic," these volunteers imagine that they have been transported into some future and are asked to name their future roles. The director then gives the group a future problem and the audience is asked to make up a story to solve the problem, using the characters that have been transformed by the magic net. The storyteller (problem-solver) is also supplied with a magic net, distinctly different from those of the role players. As the storyteller relates the story, the actors mime the action. This technique is especially useful with disadvantaged children, some emotionally disturbed children, and mentally retarded children.

REALITY LEVEL SOCIODRAMA An entire classroom, school, or, other learning situation may be turned into a sociodrama stage through Reality Level Sociodrama. Perhaps the most commonly practiced Reality Level Sociodrama has been the application of the Role Reversal technique to real life situations. In the home, the father and the mother may reverse roles or one of the children may exchange roles with one of the parents. In the school, the teacher may take the role of a student and the student may take the role of the teacher. Reality Level Sociodrama may be more inclusive, however, and involve an entire class in establishing a community or some other social group faced with a future problem. A very powerful description of Reality Level Sociodrama is found in *A Class Divided* by Peters (1971). For one week the teacher treated as inferior all children with brown eyes and as superior children with blue eyes. Later, the direction of the prejudice was reversed and the brown eyed children became the favored group and the blue eyed ones became the disfavored group. Such real-life experiments could be made more powerful by injecting the creative problem-solving process to understand the problems involved, define them, search for solutions, evaluate alternatives, and to test the best alternatives.

REFERENCES BLATNER, H. A. *Acting-in: practical applications in psychodramatic methods.* NYC: Springer, 1973.

FEINBERG, H. The ego building technique. *Group Psychotherapy*, 1959, *12*, 230-235.

FINE, R., DALY, D. & FINE, L. Psychodance, an experiment in psychotherapy and training. *Group Psychotherapy*, 1962, *15*, 2-3-223.

FRIELDS, G. *Sociodramatic play: a framework for a developmental preschool program.* Dubuque, IA: Kendall/Hunt, 1974.

GORDON, W. J. J. *Synectics.* NYC: Harper & Row, 1961.

GREENBERG, I. A. (ed.) *Psychodrama: theory and therapy.* NYC: Behavioral Publications, 1974.

HAAS, R. B. The school sociatrist. *Sociatry*, 1948, *2*, 283-321.

HANSEN, B. Sociodrama: A methodology for democratic action. *Sociatry*, 1948, *2*, 347-363.

KLEIN, A. F. *Role playing in leadership training and group problem solving.* NYC: Association Press, 1956.

LIPPITT, ROSEMARY. The auxiliary chair technique. *Group Psychotherapy*, 1958, *11*, 8-23.

MAIER, N. R. F., SOLEM, A. R. & MAIER, A. A. *Supervision and executive development: a manual for role playing.* NYC: John Wiley, 1956.

MORENO, J. L. *Psychodrama. First Volume.* Beacon, NY: Beacon House, 1946.

MORENO, J. L. Psychodramatic production techniques. *Group Psychotherapy*, 1952, *4*, 243-273.

MORENO, J. L. & MORENO, Z. T. *Psychodrama. Third Volume.* NYC: Beacon House, 1969.

MORENO, Z. T. A survey of psychodramatic techniques. *Group Psychotherapy*, 1959, *12*, 5-14.

ORNSTEIN, R. E. *The psychology of consciousness.* San Francisco: W. H. Freeman, 1972.

OSBORN, A.F. *Applied imagination.* (3rd. ed.) NYC: Charles Scribner's. 1963.

PANKRATZ, L. D. & BUCHAN, G. Exploring psychodramatic techniques with defective delinquents. *Group Psychotherapy*, 1965, *18*, 136-141.

PARNES, S. J. *Creative behavior guidebook.* NYC: Charles Scribner's, 1967.

PARRISH, M. M. Psychodrama: Description of application and review of techniques. *Group Psychotherapy*, 1953, *6*, 63-89.

PETERS, M. R. *A class divided.* Garden City, NY: Doubleday, 1971.

SHAFTEL, F. R. & SHAFTEL, G. *Role playing for special values.* Englewood Cliffs, NJ: Prentice-Hall, 1967.

SMITH, M. R. The "silent" auxiliary-ego technique in rehabilitating deteriorated mental patients. *Group Psychotherapy*, 1950, *3*, 92-100.

STEIN, M. I. *Stimulating creativity.* Volume 1. NYC: Academic Press, 1974.

TOEMAN, Z. The "double situation" in psychodrama, *Sociatry*, 1948, *1*, 436-446.

TORRANCE, E. P. *Encouraging creativity in the classroom.* Dubuque, IA: Wm C. Brown, 1970.

TORRANCE, E. P. & MYERS, R. E. *Creative learning and teaching.* NYC: Dodd, Mead, 1970.

YABLONSKY, L. Future-projection technique. In GREENBERG, I. A. (ed.), *Psychodrama: theory and therapy.* NYC: Behavioral Publications, 1974.

YABLONSKY, L. Psychodrama lives! *Human Behavior*, 1975, *4*(2), 25-29.

Dr. E. Paul Torrance, Dept. of Educational Psychology.
Address: The University of Georgia, Athens, Georgia 30602.

Reprinted with permission from the Journal of Creative Behavior, 1975, 9(3), published by the Creative Education Foundation, Buffalo, New York.

Modification of the Employment Handicaps of Psychiatric Patients by

BEHAVIORAL METHODS

Fraser N. Watts

Vocation rehabilitation needs to be more concerned with identifying and correcting specific employment handicaps. The principles of behavior modification are likely to be of value and a review of the literature indicates a number of promising applications. Methods of behavioral training can be used to improve inadequate social behavior or poor concentration. Incentives can be used to improve work effort. Graded exposure can reduce anxiety about work. Finally, methods such as behavioral counseling can help patients to find a job. The wider use of behavioral methods to improve specific work handicaps should be encouraged.

Although the use of industrial therapy units in mental hospitals has been increasing (1), there is very little evidence that this, or indeed any other measure, has much effect on the numbers of patients who return to employment (2, 3). There is thus an urgent need to consider how more effective methods of preparing such patients for re-employment can be developed.

If industrial therapy units revised their approach to prepare people for employment more explicitly, their effectiveness could be increased. There are two main components in such an approach:

1. Identifying the areas of poor functioning that will prevent the patient from achieving or sustaining employment.
2. Taking whatever remedial measures are

Fraser N. Watts, Ph.D., is Principal Psychologist at King's College Hospital, Denmark Hill, London, SE5, England.

necessary to help the patient overcome these deficits. An active remedial approach to employment handicaps could lead to more individually centered rehabilitation programs than those usually adopted at present. Different programs could be set up for patients with different problems.

In order to identify a client's problem areas, two sources of data can be used. First, by interview with the client, obtain an account of the difficulties the client has experienced with jobs over the course of his work history, paying particular attention to the reasons he left the jobs. Second, observe the patient's job functioning difficulties in a simulated work environment. Such an environment would need to be as realistic as possible, in both terms of general organization and kind of work, if the assessments were to be of value. Rating scales for codifying observations of job functioning that have acceptable reliability and validity already exist (4, see also *Related Reading*).

The information from these data sources would then need to be interpreted against the background of a general theory of employability that would indicate how seriously particular deficits affect a patient's chances of obtaining employment. The evidence indicates that enthusiasm, social relationships, and response to supervision are more important than task performance (3). As understanding of employability improves, it will become possible to select the targets of remedial programs for individual patients more rationally. It is probably possible to achieve only relatively small and specific improvements in vocational functioning, and those will need to be carefully chosen to have the maximum effect on the patient's chances of employment.

In developing remedial programs for such deficits, the general principles of behavior modification (5) are likely to be of value. These have shown sufficient promise in the modification of other handicaps to justify their application to deficits in employability. The remainder of this paper will be devoted to illustrating the application of these principles to five common problem areas: social behavior, concentration, work effort, anxiety, and job finding.

Social Behavior

Assertive behavior has been the most common target of social training. Significant improvements in assertiveness can be obtained by using coaching and rehearsal methods (6). Modeling and video-tape feedback may be useful additional ingredients in assertive training, although their value has not been well demonstrated. Importantly, it has been shown (6) that training in assertive behavior can have effects that extend to real life situations. This is obviously less easy to obtain than a change in behavior during the training sessions. There is good reason to hope that similar training methods will be able to modify vocationally relevant social behavior.

Some patients' employability is reduced by grossly inappropriate social interactions with their supervisors, ranging from being unable to speak to the supervisors about anything at all, to being unable to refrain from saying something, however unnecessary, whenever they see the supervisor. Inappropriate social interactions with co-workers also can prevent a person from fitting into a job. Social training is most effective when clients are asked to modify their behavior in quite limited and specific ways in order to be more appropriate. It is unrealistic to expect a complete change of social style. Fortunately, a few limited changes are sometimes sufficient to bring people's social behavior within acceptable limits.

A specific aspect of social behavior that is often poor in clients who have been out of work for some time is behavior at job interviews. Many of the people who have this difficulty display good social behavior in other situations, and are therefore relatively easy to help. The client problems vary from giving monosyllabic answers to questions, to talking too much about inappropriate material such as their medical symptoms. Because this is a common area of difficulty, it is feasible to provide coaching and rehearsal on a group basis.

Concentration

Inadequate task performance often can be traced to poor concentration on some part of the task. For example, difficulty with concentrating on instructions for a new job or with noticing errors in performance are common. A similar strategy of coaching and structured practice can result in improvements in these problems too.

The first stage is to make certain the patient is quite clear about what aspect of his or her performance needs to be improved. Then a strategy could be suggested that might help the patient to overcome the problem in concentration. People who find it hard to concentrate on instructions for new jobs might be advised to rehearse them, either aloud or to themselves, immediately after being instructed. Patients who failed to notice errors in their work could be advised exactly how to check their work.

It is helpful to follow this with closely supervised work practice that has the sole aim of improving the particular problem concerned. Immediate feedback can then be given on how successful the patient is in improving his performance in the way suggested. This is more likely to be effective than general advice given in the course of the normal work routine. It is also helpful for the work practice to be centered on problems of graded difficulty. If the problem was one of concentrating on instructions, the instructions could be graded by length and complexity, starting with the simple ones. A "graded training" approach helps to ensure that the patient learns to perform successfully.

A similar graded training approach can be used for the related problem of sustaining concentration for an adequate span of time. Rather than simply encouraging the patient to concentrate for longer periods of time, a specific length of time would be set for concentrating. This would initially be something that could easily be managed, and would be gradually extended as concentration improved. If necessary, some other help would be given, such as training in switching attention away from distracting thoughts, using the thought-stopping technique developed by Wolpe (7). While it is unlikely that all concentration problems in psychiatric patients would respond to this kind of approach, there are cases where it could result in considerable improvement.

Work Effort

Improving productivity is the best developed area of remedial work in rehabilitation. Productivity is poor for various reasons. Of the two obvious reasons, working slowly and not working continuously, the latter is more likely to make a person unemployable (8). However, the total amount of work done is a relatively simple variable to measure and has been the most common target variable in programs designed to improve work effort.

A number of published reports have illustrated the use of incentives to increase productivity. To be successful, an incentive needs to be found that is powerful enough to affect the patient's behavior and that the therapist can regulate. This is less easily achieved in a rehabilitation unit situated outside residential institutions. However, staff attention is an incentive that is an exception—it is something that the staff can control and is usually valued by the patients.

The method of giving social attention reported by Taylor and Parsons (9) for "Patient 1" is simple and effective. A chart was placed on the wall that showed a record of the amount of time spent working each day. The entire staff was instructed to comment on this and engage in social interaction as long as the amount of time was being maintained or increased, but to withhold attention if it fell from the previous day's level. Similarly, Wing and Freudenberg (10) report positive effects on productivity for a "social stimulation" procedure. This was a general package involving a number of ingredients, one of which was encouragement from the supervisor for good performance. This study also illustrates one of the problems of incentive schemes. When the social stimulation was withdrawn, productivity fell to its previous level. This is the fate of many incentive (or "reinforcement") programs unless they can be provided on a permanent basis as a "prosthetic environment" (11). One way to avoid this problem is to fade out the incentives gradually and to train the patient to "reinforce" himself after external incentives have been withdrawn.

Although tangible incentives have often failed to produce significant results (12), there are circumstances in which they have a powerful effect. Zimmerman and others (13) obtained good results using a token economy in a sheltered workshop for retardates. It is noteworthy that this study was conducted in a community, rather than in an institutional setting, where the relatively free availability of most tangible rewards would tend to lessen the effects of the token economy. In addition, the study included a control condition in which feedback on performance was given by telling patients how many tokens they would earn for their performance. They were able to show that this feedback had significantly less effect than actually giving the tokens.

Anxiety Reduction

A number of patients experience substantial amounts of anxiety about work. Specific anxiety reduction measures can be helpful in cases where the anxiety does not reduce spontaneously as patients get accustomed to working again. Reduction measures are most appropriate when the anxiety is related to some specific aspect of the job, and when the patient recognizes the anxiety as inappropriate.

Of the various available methods of anxiety reduction, graded exposure to the anxiety-evoking cues (that is, "in vivo" desensitization) is the most readily applicable. This method was used, for example, with a patient whose motivation for work was affected by excessive anxiety about making mistakes, switching from one task to another, and working under pressure of time. He worked through a graded series of tasks during a number of sessions, carrying an increasing risk of making mistakes. This brought about a reduction in his work anxiety, and enabled him to progress to a further stage of the rehabilitation program that he had previously considered too stressful. In this way, anxiety reduction can have an important effect on the patient's motivation to work.

Another approach to anxieties about work that has proved helpful is to use the method of modifying self-talk developed by Meichenbaum (14). He has drawn attention to the fact that anxious people tend to undermine their performance by "negative" self-talk, and has provided some encouraging evidence regarding the effects of giving patients constructive self-talk to use. Some patients seem to find it helpful to keep one or two phrases of positive self-talk on their desk or workbench. For example, a client who regularly observed to himself that he could not cope with his work was taught to remind himself instead "I know I can manage this if I don't get flustered."

Techniques of anxiety reduction may be applicable to a wider range of negative emotional reactions. There is now evidence (15) that imaginal desensitization is effective in reducing anger associated with specific social cues. The desensitization hierarchies in this experiment included a number of job-related anger-cues, such as having to take orders and being criticized. If desensitization could effectively reduce the anger or resentment aroused in many rehabilitees, it could be an important factor in increasing their employability. There is little doubt that excessive resentment of criticism and authority is a common employment handicap.

Finding a Job

Even if patients are ready for employment, the task of finding an appropriate job remains. Jones and Azrin(16) reported evidence that the majority of jobs are found through personal contacts and that jobs identified in this way are more likely to lead to actual placements. From this they hypothesize that one of the reasons people have difficulty in returning to work is that they are out of touch with the normal network of job contacts. To overcome this problem, advertisements were placed in local newspapers offering a financial reward to people who were able to supply information leading to a successful placement. This produced significantly more job placements than control advertisements not offering the reward.

This may not be a practical method to operate as a routine service, but it emphasizes the need for rehabilitees to involve people in helping them to find a job. Another way of doing this is reported by Fairweather (17). The patients in the study elected four of their members to serve on an "employment committee." This committee assessed what kind of job each patient needed and then sought out suitable openings through newspapers and by visiting local employers. Although this was an uncontrolled study and no definite conclusions can be drawn, it seems likely that the activities of this committee were partly responsible for the substantial number of patients returning to work. In a community setting, similar results could probably be achieved by involving the patient's family in finding a job.

Besides identifying a suitable job, the activities of the employment committee probably had an important motivational effect. It is not difficult to see that there would be considerable pressure to make use of the job opportunities the committee had discovered. Similar effects were achieved in the token economy reported by Kelley and Henderson (18) by providing tokens for attending job interviews. Social reinforcement for job hunting has been used much less than for improving work effort in rehabilitation units, but it may well have more effect on the rate of re-employment.

More recently, Azrin and others (19) developed a comprehensive program of group behavioral counseling for patients trying to find a job. The program involved attending the group each day until a job had been found. Patients took an average of 14 days to find a job, compared to an average of 53 days for comparable patients not in the program.

Conclusion

These examples do not exhaust the potential application of behavior modification methods to employment handicaps, but it is hoped that they are sufficient to establish the feasibility of applying this approach to specific rehabilitation problems. The success of these methods

in other areas gives reason to hope that they will also be capable of improving patients' vocational functioning. However, this is a question that will need to be settled by empirical investigation. Not all employment handicaps can be modified in this way, but, even if only limited improvements can be achieved, they may be enough to significantly affect whether or not a patient is able to return to work. The behavioral approaches described here deserve wider use. •

REFERENCES

1. Black BJ: *Principles of Industrial Therapy for the Mentally Ill*, New York, Grune and Stratton, 1970
2. Anthony WA, Buell GJ, Sharratt S, Althoff ME: Efficacy of psychiatric rehabilitation. *Psychol Bull* 78: 447-456, 1972
3. Watts FN: Social treatments. In *A Textbook of Human Psychology*, HJ Eysenck and GD Wilson, Editors, Lancaster, Medical and Technical Publishing Company, 1976, chap. 21
4. Griffiths RDP: A standardised assessment of the work behaviour of psychiatric patients. *Brit J Psychiatry* 123: 403-408, 1973
5. Kanfer FH, Phillips JS: *Learning Foundations of Behavior Therapy*, New York, Wiley, 1970
6. McFall RM, Twentyman CT: Four experiments on the relative contributions of rehearsal, modeling, and coaching to assertive training. *J Abnorm Psychol* 81: 199-218, 1973
7. Wolpe J: *Psychotherapy by Reciprocal Inhibition*, Stanford, Stanford University Press, 1958
8. Cheadle AJ, Morgan R: The measurement of work performance of psychiatric patients: A re-appraisal.- *Brit J Psychiatry* 120: 437-441, 1972
9. Taylor GP, Persons RW: Behaviour modification techniques in a physical medicine and rehabilitation centre. *J Psychol* 74: 117-124, 1970
10. Wing JH, Freudenberg RK: The response of severely ill chronic schizophrenic patients to social stimulation. *Am J Psychiatry* 118: 311-322, 1961
11. Kazdin AE, Bootzin RR: The token economy: An evaluative review. *J Appl Behav Anal* 5: 343-372, 1972
12. Goldberg D: Rehabilitation of the chronically mentally ill in England. *Social Psychiatry* 2: 1-13, 1967
13. Zimmerman J, Stuckey TE, Garlick BJ, Miller M: Effects of token reinforcement on productivity in multiply handicapped clients in a sheltered workshop. *Rehabil Lit* 30: 34-41, 1969
14. Meichenbaum DH: Cognitive factors in behavior modification: Modifying what clients say to themselves. In *Advances in Behavior Therapy*, Rubin et al, Editors, New York, Academic Press, 1973
15. Evans DR, Hearn MT: Anger and systematic desensitization: A follow-up. *Psychol Rep* 32: 569-570, 1973
16. Jones RJ, Azrin NH: An experimental application of a social re-inforcement approach to the problem of job finding. *J Appl Behav Anal* 6:345-353, 1973
17. Fairweather GW: *Social Psychology in Treating Mental Illness: An experimental approach*, New York, Wiley, 1964
18. Kelley KM, Henderson JD: A community-based operant learning environment, II: Systems and procedures. In *Advances in Behavior Therapy*, Rubin et al, Editors, New York, Academic Press, 1971
19. Azrin NH, Flores T, Kaplan SJ: Job finding club: A group assisted program for obtaining employment. *Behav Res Ther* 13: 17-27, 1975

RELATED READING
Van Allen R, Loeber R: Work assessment of psychiatric patients: A critical review of published scales. *Can J Behav Sci* 4: 101-117, 1972

R30803

"The recognition that no knowledge can be
complete, no metaphor entire, is itself
humanizing. It grants even to adversaries
the possibility of partial truth, and to
oneself the possibility of error. This
possibility is especially present in large-
scale synthesis. Yet, as the critic George
Steiner has written, 'To ask larger questions
is to risk getting things wrong. Not to
ask them at all is to constrain the life of
understanding.' "

Alvin Toffler. *The Third Wave.*